P9-DZZ-944

ATTENTION DEFICIT DISORDER

Practical Coping Methods

ATTENTION DEFICIT DISORDER

Practical Coping Methods

Barbara C. Fisher
Ross A. Beckley

CRC Press
Boca Raton London New York Washington, D.C.

womens

Acquiring Editor:	N. Frabotta
Project Editor:	Sylvia Wood
Marketing Manager:	Becky McEldowney
Cover design:	Dawn Boyd

Library of Congress Cataloging-in-Publication Data

Fisher, Barbara C.
    Attention deficit disorder: practical coping methods / Barbara C. Fisher and Ross A. Beckley.
        p.   cm.
    Includes bibliographical references and index.
    ISBN 0-8493-1899-0
    1.Attention-deficit hyperactivity disorder. 2. Adjustment
(Psychology) 3. Biological psychiatry. Neuropsychology.
Beckley, Ross A. II. Title.
[DNLM: 1. Attention Deficit Disorder with Hyperactivity.
2. Biological Psychiatry. Neuropsychology. WS 350.8.A8 F533ab
1998]
    RC394.A85F57 1998
    616. 85' 89—dc21
DNLM/DLC   98-7960
for Library of Congress   CIP

Cover illustration: Matthew T. Rivard
© 1999 by CRC Press LLC

No claim to original U.S. Government works
International Standard Book Number 0-8493-1899-8
Library of Congress Card Number 98-7960
Printed in the United States of America 2 3 4 5 6 7 8 9 0
Printed on acid-free paper

3|14|00

Preface

This book has been rewritten no fewer than five times in an effort to keep abreast of current information. It is a compilation of personal/professional experiences, notes, anecdotes, research and hopes that have been stored and shared over the past decade. New research is occurring constantly and this disorder, which has been historically looked upon as a disorder of childhood, is now being widely accepted as one that spans the lifetime. It is a disorder that one is born with, and it does not end with childhood, instead, symptoms develop and change commensurate with the developmental cycles of adolescence, adulthood, middle age and advanced age. This book is meant for parents, children, teachers and ADD adults who are tired of searching and are ready for answers to their many questions about this very diverse and complicated disorder.

Our goal is to demystify the vast amount of information that has been generated and to present this rather confusing disorder in a manner that is both understandable and applicable by providing what we have learned that is helpful in addressing this disorder in the individual's everyday life. This books addresses the questions of why Ritalin does and doesn't work, why ADD is not just a childhood disorder, why ADHD is being over-diagnosed and why so often the person diagnosed and treated with medication is not cured and the story is far from over.

The presence of ADD has broken up marriages, prevented many from attending college, fulfilling their potential, or following the career path that they truly desire. It has made people feel stupid and incompetent. With new perspectives, changes can occur, and people can create the life they want and deserve; they can fulfill their dreams. ADD is a disorder with far-reaching consequences, however, it is also a disorder that can be treated and specific symptoms can be managed. We prefer to think of ADD as a challenge that can be met with good physical health, nutrition, specific coping mechanisms, medication, and, most of all, education and understanding. A good diagnosis identifying all of the various disorders that can complicate the situation is absolutely imperative.

What we provide to the reader in this book in the way of knowledge about ADD has been field-tested in a variety of settings—households, schools, clinics, businesses, colleges, hospitals, and classrooms.

Authors

Barbara C. Fisher, Ph.D, is a fully licensed psychologist who has specialized in neuropsychology for the past 19 years. She approaches Attention Deficit Disorder from a brain-behavior viewpoint and utilizes her knowledge of the brain and neuroanatomy to understand, diagnose, and explain specific symptoms of this disorder.

Dr. Fisher is the author of *Reasons for Misdiagnosis, Approaching ADD from a Brain-Behavior Neuropsychological Perspective for Assessment and Treatment,* and co-author of *We Are Not Getting Older, We Are Just Coming of Age..* She also specializes in the diagnosis of head trauma, as well as Alzheimer's Disorder and Dementia.

A well-known speaker, Dr. Fisher has presented at various workshops with her husband, Ross Beckley, including radio and television, on such varied topics as ADD, Depression and Anxiety, and Comorbid Disorders. She conducts custody evaluations; neuropsychological evaluations; alcohol assessments; and psychological, education, and achievement evaluations. Trained in hypnosis, she is a member of the American Society of Clinical Hypnosis.

Ross Beckley, Ph.D, is a former school teacher, special-education teacher, and teacher consultant for the learning disabled, the emotionally impaired, and educable mentally impaired. Dr. Beckley holds a Ph.D. in Clinical Psychology, a degree in Elementary Education, Master's degrees in Reading and Learning Disabilities, and Marriage and Family Therapy. He also has a specialist degree in Administrative and Organizational Studies. More importantly, Ross is stepdad to an ADD child.

Both Fisher and Beckley are members of the National Physicians Consortium for Attention Deficit Disorder, American Psychological Association, Association of Family and Conciliation Courts, and various support groups for Attention Deficit Disorder. They have been speaking for the past several years on ADD and currently run a successful parent-training program. Together, they operate United Psychological Services and the Attentional Deficit Disorder Clinic in Clinton Township, with a satellite office in Lansing, Michigan.

Acknowledgments

In the completion of this project, we would like to recognize the following individuals for their direct or indirect contribution to this project.

Special recognition is due to:
God, the source

Mr. Phillip Fisher: accountant/bean-counter extraordinaire, father, father-in-law

Mr. Donald Beckley: organizer, critic, cheerleader

Blythe VanderBeek: partner, editor, and friend

Dr. Edna Copeland: expert in ADD and renowned author who first said, "Why don't you two write a book?"

Greer Huntley: typist, proofreader, who always believed in this project

Janine Thomas: M.S.W., colleague, idea person, truth teller

Don Santilli, Chuck O'Connor, Utica Community Schools

Nick Simkins, attorney specializing in head injury

Dr. Akemi Takekoshi: neurologist

Dr. David Villanueva: psychiatrist

Drs. Georgiou and Merschaert: internists and specialists

The many pediatricians and neurologists for their insightful knowledge of clinical aspects of this disorder

Dr. Douglas Davidson: The Union Institute, Western Michigan University

And, last but never least, Laura and Jeff, relentless partners in questions, answers, worries/fears, love, honor, and stars

Contents

1

What is Attention Deficit Disorder?

1.1 What Attention Deficit Disorder (ADD) Was Once Thought to Be

Historically, when Attention Deficit Disorder (ADD) was discussed, we were referring to Attention Deficit Disorder with Hyperactivity (ADHD). At that time there was no awareness of ADD *without* hyperactivity. It was thought that ADD was a psychological or behavioral problem viewed as a disorder of childhood. The symptoms were hyperactivity, overactiveness, and attention deficiency, hence the term ADD.

The theory was that the disorder was the consequence of a system in the brain not being mature — perhaps due to early birth or damage to the brain. That underdeveloped system in the brain was thought to be the Reticular Activating System (RAS), which is involved in general arousal and alertness. In that underdeveloped or immature state, the result was overactive or hyperactive behavior on the part of the child. As this system developed, the symptoms of ADHD and its hyperactive or overactive component would disappear. It was believed that because the system was immature it produced the overactivate and inappropriate behavior characteristic of hyperactivity, a motor-driven activity.

Therefore, ADD was *not* understood as a disorder involving the thought processes but as a disorder linked to behavior with symptoms such as a child who "ran but did not walk" and was continually distracted, not focused, or could not attend to task. These children were seen as behavioral problems as they did not respond to directions, but did as they pleased without obeying the rules and regulations of the family household. The attention disorder was viewed as ADHD; a rather disruptive behavioral problem that was expected to go away once the child reached the later stages of adolescence and the RAS matured and began to function as it should, and no longer produced overactive behavior.

The problem was that ADD and the systems seen did not make sense. Sometimes the behavior would be there and sometimes it would not. There seemed to be no rhyme or reason. It was difficult to diagnose unless the disorder was severe and there were clear symptoms for the doctor or psychologist to observe. Parents did not see symptoms of the disorder but teachers did. Children who should have been able to function better and lead productive lives after adolescence still had problems. ADD children, once they became adults, still had problems and were not like their peers.

1.2   If the Disorder was Over, Why Wasn't It Over?

What was not understood was that ADD was a thinking disorder involving the higher-level portions of the brain, or higher-level functioning of the brain. Further, on reaching adolescence and adulthood this disorder does *not* go away. Rather, it persists throughout the life span and through the aging process. In fact, we have tested individuals in the age range of 70 to 80 years and found clear symptoms of an attentional disorder that had been impacting their lives.

Now we realize that, first, *ADD does not go away* and, also, *there is another disorder with the absence of hyperactivity* (or motor overactivity) entitled Attention Deficit Disorder without Hyperactivity.

1.3   How is this New View or Theory of ADD Known?

Recent research was conducted in which researchers found evidence of *hypofrontality* — a lack of activity in the frontal area of the brain when it should have been activated. Using a computerized technique called the PET scan, researchers were able to measure the brain's use of energy. The PET scan allows the activity of the brain to be measured in response to some sort of task performance. Testing diagnosed ADHD individuals who performed tasks that necessarily require the frontal area of the brain. Hypofrontality was displayed because frontal regions of the brain were not aroused as they should have been for the task performance. This can also be seen on SPECT scans, which measure how the brain is utilizing its energy.

Hypofrontality was then linked to the deficiency of *dopamine* and *norepinephrine*, two neurotransmitters or brain messengers.

1.4   Defining Neurotransmitters or Brain Messengers

The brain contains structures geared to performing specific jobs. All of these structures must be able to communicate with one another to allow thinking and acting to be a smooth operation. It is like a giant communication system, e.g., the Internet or the information highway. The brain transmits messages to itself — it talks to itself; therefore, the brain structures can work only if its communication system is in order.

EXAMPLE

For a car to run, you need fuel and spark. You can have a perfectly fine automobile, but it will not go anywhere unless it has a full tank of gas and a charged battery. The same is true of the brain. The brain can be fine and intact, however, it will not work unless it has fuel and a spark.

The brain talks to itself using two systems, *chemical* and *electrical*. When either of these communication systems breaks down, there is potential for a whole host of problems ranging from emotional disorders to physical disorders to damage to the brain. When people cannot think, or they can't walk or talk or act appropriately or make the right decisions, something has happened to one or both of these systems.

1.5 ADD Has to do with the Way the Brain Talks to Itself Chemically

When the brain talks to itself chemically, it does so through what we call *neurotransmitters* or *brain messengers*. These neurotransmitters allow the communication system or information highway to transmit messages between different brain structures. Each brain structure has a specific job that allows the body to walk, talk, think, learn. The brain structures are connected by neurons. It is the neurotransmitters or brain messengers that allow information to travel from one neuron to another. When defining neurons, see the brain activity as a series of steps:

1. Neurons are composed of a cell body connected to an axon that connects to another cell body that connects to an axon and so on (Figure 1.1).
2. The neurons have projections called dendrites, or branches, whose primary function is to receive information from other cells and pass this information along to the cell body.
3. Electrical changes occur in the nerve membrane that result in information being passed along the axon to the nerve terminal located at the end of the axon.
4. It is the change in membrane permeability at the nerve terminal that triggers the release of the neurotransmitter substance.

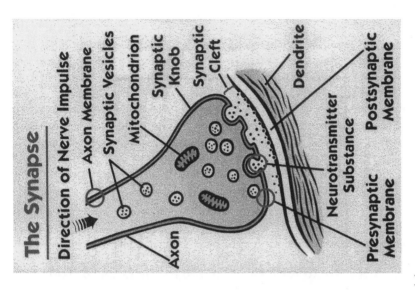

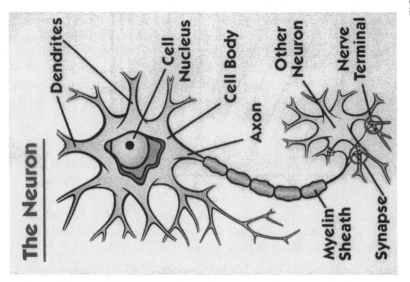

FIGURE 1.1

5. When the transmitter substance is released from a nerve terminal it diffuses across what is called a synaptic cleft to the postsynaptic membrane where it stimulates the receptor site (or receiver of the information).

6. The synaptic cleft is the area between what are called the pre- and postsynaptic membranes. These are terms used to delineate the area sending the message and the area receiving the message.

While this is all very complex, the idea is that neurons respond to input from several sources and, as a result, modulate, impact, or affect the cells to which they project. All of this communication is linked in an intricate network. Neurotransmitters can be released from dendrites, the cell body, as well as the axons. These synapses over which the transfer of information occurs can happen at all of these release sites. This demonstrates the interconnectivity of the brain.

Finally, there are billions and billions of neurons, more than you will ever need in your lifetime, all connecting and interacting and allowing you to operate effectively and efficiently in your environment. That exemplifies the interconnectivity within the brain.

For the brain to work, it needs to be able to send messages across the billions of neurons that make up its thinking areas. If there is a chemical imbalance, the brain is unable to send and receive the messages it needs to work properly.

1.6   Where Does this Fit in With ADD?

In review, the hypofrontality theory refers to the idea that its presence is due to a lack of arousal of the frontal area of the brain that is necessary to perform a task at hand. The frontal area or structure is not aroused due to the failure of a chemical messenger that results in a failed communication system. The failure of this chemical messenger in the system is called a *biochemical imbalance*. This means that a chemical messenger system is not working due to a problem with its delicate balance.

Neurotransmitters are like dominoes, each has a direct effect on its neighbors, and some excite, some inhibit. Some inhibit more excitation. Some excite more inhibition. All are delicately balanced and necessary to maintain the communication system between the neurons to allow the brain to talk to itself.

The chemical messengers, or neurotransmitters, that operate in the frontal area of the brain are predominately dopamine and norepinephrine. These are the neurotransmitters isolated to date that are thought to be involved in ADD. The job of dopamine and norepinephrine is arousal and alertness, and when the substances are not fully available, the brain is not aroused and alert — in essence, it is sleeping.

The definition of ADD is the presence of a genetic biochemical disorder (passed from one generation to another) that does not allow people to work to their potential. Because it is the biochemical system that is affected, this is not a disorder involving any damage to the brain. Rather, the brain is intact, just not able to work to its potential.

ADD is described as an inequality of the chemical balance needed to transmit messages within the intricate structure of neurons within the brain. The brain is not working to its maximum efficiency and strength. Thus, it becomes very important to separate out an attentional disorder from any other neurological process that may be occurring within the brain. We must rule out any other intervening variables or issues to truly rule in an attentional disorder; such as

- Congenital factors of low birth weight
- Fetal alcohol syndrome
- Prenatal difficulties
- Neurological insult
- Toxins
- Environmental agents
- Allergies
- Emotional/familial factors

The challenge is to differentiate an attentional disorder from one that is due to some other source.

Two other points are important regarding the discussion of biochemical imbalance.

1. ADD is defined as a biochemical imbalance but it is not an exact science. Sometimes there is more of the neurotransmitter at the receptor site where the neurons talk to each other and sometimes there is less. As a result, the symptoms of ADD can vary from day to day, hour to hour, minute to minute, and structure to structure.

2. The symptoms of ADD cannot always be seen. If something is externally stimulating and truly exciting it will bypass this system and the symptoms of ADD will not appear. We do not know exactly how this happens in the brain, only that the phenomenon does exist and can clearly be observed.

1.7   When are the Symptoms of ADD Seen?

- When things are peaceful and quiet and boredom sets in
- When tasks are mundane and humdrum

- When routine paperwork must be done
- When studying or homework must be done
- Midway through a project but not in the beginning when things are exciting
- When a business has become established but not when it is first beginning or being planned

This is why kids can sit and not move an inch when in front of a TV set or Nintendo for hours but will move constantly in a class situation. This is also why adults can start things but not finish them or follow through or complete them. It's when things become boring and/or less exciting that symptoms of ADD become obvious.

EXAMPLE
One woman and her ADD son, who was extremely slow moving and slow thinking, were racing across town through traffic to make an appointment. As the car roared up to the curb and stopped, she practically threw the child out of the car to hurry to the appointment. She watched helplessly as he slowly climbed the steps. She thought to herself, "he is going to be even later than he already is." Yet this same child who walked so slowly to his appointment can sit in front of a NINTENDO and move his fingers like lightning.

This is a perfect example of how something can downplay the symptoms of ADD. It explains why this disorder has been so difficult to diagnose based on self-reported symptoms. Another example is an adult with ADD who is starting a new business. Talk to him the first month and he is so excited; charged with energy and ideas. Talk to him a month later and he has a million excuses for why things did not work out. He exhibits little interest in continuing the project.

Often, people will deny their ADD by describing an activity on which they can remain intently focused. However, it is important to note whether the task is interesting to them. Such differences are found between subjects, for instance, reading and math. A person who loves numbers can remain focused on math and yet not be able to pay attention long enough to learn to read. We assume that they do not have ADD because they can sustain attention to task in one subject area. The common misassumption is that a child does not have ADD because he is able to sit in front of the TV set for hours and maintain a healthy level of attention. The TV is stimulating. Topics of interest are stimulating. The disorder will not be seen at these times. This impacts the decision on when to medicate. If the situation is stimulating in and of itself, or, as we say, externally stimulating, then the person would not need medication as the brain is already aroused and working.

As if to complicate things, in addition to dopamine and norepinephrine, a third neurotransmitter, serotonin, has also been found to be involved in this disorder. Serotonin, however, has less impact on the thinking aspects of ADD and more on the behavioral aspects of impulsivity and inappropriate, problematic behavior. These neurotransmitters are also co-related or connected with a number of other emotional disorders, as well as neurological disorders.

The lack of serotonin further disrupts the delicate balance that allows the person to operate on a fairly normal basis by involving not only emotional but behavioral brain messengers. This creates an imbalance that ricochets down the line and creates more imbalance and the presence of other disorders as well as physical symptoms. This is why ADD is not often found by itself. It becomes easy to see why ADD is so complex and tends to be present with other coexisting conditions as well. The idea being that when the system is impacted in some manner, the delicate balance that is there is destroyed. This can then create further disorders associated with the same neurotransmitters. There are many disorders associated with the neurotransmitters dopamine, norepinephrine, and serotonin. This is why we tend to see ADD coexist with such disorders as

- asthma
- allergies
- manic-depression
- schizophrenia
- thyroid disorders
- anxiety and depression

This distinction among the various disorders is a key element in determining how and when to medicate. Medications designed to trigger one neurotransmitter system will not be helpful if it is not the neurotransmitter that is out of balance. For example, administering serotonin will not be helpful for the thinking problems associated with ADD but will be helpful with emotional issues and impulsivity. Knowing which neurotransmitter system is involved helps to determine which medication will work. Medications must impact the correct neurotransmitter systems to create the expected balance and change.

As a side note, there is a considerable amount of research that examines how different emotional disorders impact this messenger system, disrupt balance, and create thinking problems. One example is Post-traumatic Stress Disorder (PTSD) which displays symptoms similar to those of ADD.

With PTSD, a highly stressful event has altered the system's balance and, as a result, the person has difficulty concentrating, sustaining attention and focus to task, and completion of work. Another example is when injury to the brain also affects the delicate chemical balance of the neurotransmitters dopamine, norepinephrine and serotonin, creating symptoms similar to that of ADD.

So with all of this confusion, how is the correct diagnosis determined?

What symptoms are due to ADD and which are due to something else? This is the reason for specific evaluation using testing, not self-report measures, as well as knowledge of the other disorders and what the symptoms look like.

By understanding that there is an imbalance in the system of neurotransmitters (dopamine and norepinephrine) that serve the functions of arousal and alertness in the frontal and parietal areas of the brain, it can be seen how the brain would be sleeping in these higher-level, higher-functioning, thinking areas of the brain. Therefore the theory emerged that ADHD did not disappear with adulthood and the maturity of the RAS system. Rather, the overactivity became more repressed toward normalcy, meaning that the individual did not continue to display those symptoms of running and moving from thing to thing, task to task, and object to object at a fast and furious pace. Although, in adulthood, remnants can be observed in the quickness of task performance, fidgetiness and somewhat constant movement.

The theory then is substantiated that ADD is a medical biochemical disorder, involving the highest-level thinking areas of the brain, and not a behavioral disorder as once thought. True, behavioral symptoms associated with ADD can be experienced with the disorder, but the key issue is that ADD is a thinking disorder and that someone does something not because they want to, or for an emotional reason, but due the incorrect systematic operation and activity of the brain.

That is not the end of the whole story. If the brain messengers dopamine and norepinephrine have an impact on the frontal area of the brain, and the hypofrontality creates the higher-level-thinking disorder of ADD or ADHD, then wouldn't it also affect the other thinking areas of the brain that use these same neurotransmitters? Hypofrontality defines the lack of dopamine and norepinephrine primarily in the frontal area of the brain. However, the effect can also be seen in the parietal area of the brain. This defines the basis for the anatomical differences between the two subtypes of ADD: ADHD and ADD without hyperactivity (ADD). It has been found through both clinical research and studies of medication that ADD without hyperactivity is more closely related to the parietal area of the brain and the neurotransmitter norepinephrine, while ADHD is found to be more related to the frontal area or processes and the neurotransmitter dopamine.

Before this biochemical discussion is ended, note that although the SPECT scan research began this entirely different way of looking at ADD, it has not proven totally reliable under recent research. This is due to a number of issues, but mainly the measurement of brain functioning. We are not always measuring what we think we are measuring. For example, the person is given a task to do and SPECT measures what part of the brain is being used at that point in time. But what if the part of the brain that we would expect to be used to complete the task is not being used? Thus, the theory of hypofrontality emerges — this area of the brain is not being used for a task historically seen as involving frontal functions. However, what if the task can be accomplished just as well using the parietal area? Does this mean that the brain is not functioni g properly or that the task is not predominantly a task of frontal processes? This becomes the dilemma and basis for the controversy in the use of SPECT for ADD. The SPECT exam, however, is wonderful for diagnosing biochemical disorders such as Bipolar Disorder, Schizophrenia, Obsessive Compulsive Disorder and so on. The SPECT scan is known as a leading measure to diagnose the effects of head injury. However, for ADD, things are just not that simple. Thus, the situation becomes even more complex. However, the theory is being backed and substantiated by recent research using many other methods — one of which is the evoked potential studies and (quantitative or computerized electroencephalogram (QEEG) studies, to determine that the theory is, in fact, correct. Such measures, however remain problematic in being able to specifically quantify symptoms, thus the primary role of measurement remains the paper-and-pencil neuropsychological methods, augmented and assisted by the above types of medical testing.

Understanding the biochemical theory of an ADD, the structures involved, and what their job is really provides a clear picture of ADD and what it means for people diagnosed with this disorder with regard to their everyday lives. To understand the structures involved in ADD, it is necessary to know how the brain works in a general fashion. The following section will discuss how the brain works and how it takes in information.

1.8   Basic Information and the Brain

The brain is divided into four lobes or areas that represent the cortical or thinking areas. They are the frontal, parietal, temporal, and occipital lobes.

The frontal lobe is the president or supervisory area of the brain. Its job is to integrate all of the information and make sense out of it so it can be of use. The frontal area pulls together all of the information from the other areas of the brain, somewhat like taking all of the ingredients to make a cake, putting it together, and then baking it for the final product. The activity in this area is referred to as frontal processes because it is in this area that the culmination or grand finale of all that goes on below is produced. As such, it is dependent on the other areas for information. It does not act alone as a single or unitary process but is in concert with other areas.

The parietal is the sensory area and association where the information is processed and sent to the higher levels of the brain. Information is automatically processed at first entrance to the brain and then processed in a more complex fashion in this area. This is called secondary processing. For example, first impressions are automatically processed, such as the outline of an object. To give the object meaning such as "it is a lamp," requires more complexity, which occurs in a portion of the parietal area. Association cortex means that there are a number of functions it can do. We call this multimodal or several modalities. Modalities are the sensory systems such as taste, touch, sight, sound and smell.

The temporal lobe is the memory area and auditory system where memory, balance and the hearing system are housed. This area is one of the most vulnerable areas of the brain and is highly susceptible to injury and aging.

The occipital lobe is the visual cortex, where the visual system is located. It is the job of this area to direct all visual processes and to define vision to see the outline of things as well as details and colors. If someone is color blind there is a problem with this area. Some key points are as follows:

1. The only areas of the brain that are involved in attention disorder are the frontal and parietal areas.
2. These are the areas that primarily use the neurotransmitters dopamine and norepinephrine.
3. The frontal and parietal lobes would be affected by the loss or decreased availability of dopamine and norepinephrine. Negative impact on these areas of the brain would prohibit people from working at their potential. These areas would be sleeping and not working to their ability and not able to do their job.
4. These areas function as integral components in information processing by taking information from the environment and learning how to use that information to function successfully in the world in which the person lives.

1.9 How the Brain Takes in Information: A Step by Step Procedure

The brain works much like a computer.

1.9.1 Attention and Concentration

Basic attention and concentration are needed just to get information (or input) into the brain (Figure 1.2). It can be thought of as putting data into the computer; the information must be input before it can be used.

1.9.2 Information Processing

All of the information that comes into the brain must be processed in order to be used by the higher levels of the brain. The parietal area of the brain — the association cortex or multimodal cortex — is the area capable of performing a number of different functions. Information is *processed* here and then sent to other areas of the brain for use.

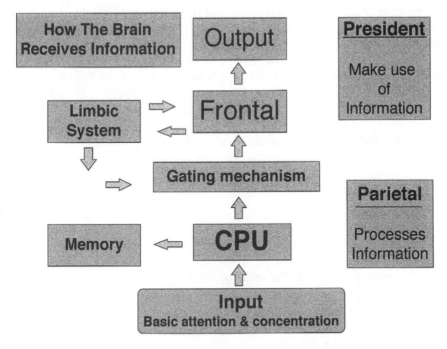

FIGURE 1.2

This next part is critical to understanding ADD. If the information is not processed the information simply drops out of the circuit. It never goes anywhere else. It does not get to the temporal area or memory area of the brain for short-term or long-term storage and retrieval. The person does not have the information at all. Further, the person cannot store the information to remember it at a later time. The information becomes lost after the automatic processing has taken place. ADD affects the higher-level functioning of the brain. The problem, therefore, occurs at this point and the information may be lost during this higher-level or more specific processing.

In summation, all of the information that comes into the brain must be processed in this central area, which can be called the central processing unit or "CPU" of the brain. It is similar to the control center Captain Kirk used to control the spaceship on *Star Trek*. Everything has to go through this central area to be used by the brain.

What happens if the information is not processed? It just drops out and is never sent to the areas of higher functioning to be utilized by the brain. As a result, a number of ADD individuals will seem to have a memory problem. Some common statements from ADD people include "You never told me that" or "You never told me about that time, date, or event." ADD individuals don't give credit for the possibility of having said something similar or having said part of whatever the topic is. The statements can be a very clear "no!" or denial that someone has said anything at all to them. This appears to be a memory problem, yet is truly an information-processing problem. The information does not get processed, and, therefore, does not get into the memory area of the brain for short- or long-term storage and retrieval, it just drops out and is gone. Therefore, the person may say, "You never told me," which means, "I do not have the information." If it were a true memory problem there would be more vagueness associated with it, such as, "I think maybe you might have said that but I am not sure." It would not be a very clear, "You never told me that!" which tends to cause one to doubt one's own reality and to wonder, if, in fact, the information was given. It's very difficult to declare that the information was delivered to that person, particularly if that person is your wife, husband, or child. This is how blaming and arguments begin; the classic miscommunication, the frustration, the pain of missed appointments or misunderstood directions and instructions.

1.9.3   Frontal Processes

If the information is processed it goes to different areas of the brain. Eventually the frontal processes intervene. Because the frontal processes are responsible for executive decisions and functioning, the area is called the president of the brain. The final response after the president pulls everything together is the output: think, walk, and talk.

It is the job of the frontal area (executive functioning with its integrative abilities to put things together with a perspective) to provide the appropriate output, response or behavior. When this area is not operating properly the hand can reach for a napkin and instead pick up a coffee cup, words may say one thing and behavior show something else. The person's actions are inappropriate. They do and say the wrong thing for the situation. The basic rules for social behavior are off balance. Something minor happens and the person overreacts and attaches all kinds of significance to it. A plate drops and breaks and the person acts like a crime has been committed or someone has died. It is the job of the frontal area to integrate with other areas and attach significance to events being processed that involve the emotional center or limbic system.

The limbic system, whose main outpost is the hypothalamus (which regulates hormonal balance) works with the RAS, which provides energy for the whole operation. Therefore, hormonal imbalance can also impact emotions as well as decisions and reactions to things happening in the person's life. The combined efforts of the frontal lobe and the limbic system (known as the emotional center of the brain) are responsible for appropriate behavior. If either area is damaged or not operating correctly in some way, there is evidence of inappropriate behavior. This irrational or nonsensical behavior is characteristic of stroke victims or people who have had a head injury.

Imagine what would happen if emotions existed by themselves without this regulatory system. The rational frontal area of the brain is needed to help make sense of feelings.

EXAMPLE

People may find themselves angry or in tears and have no idea why they are yelling or crying. As they think about it, they realize that they are angry and yelling because of this or crying because of that or maybe something that happened earlier that day or the day before or at another point in their lives. That is often the essence of therapy; to help them understand their feelings, why they respond as they do to certain events or stimuli in their environment. It is the frontal processes working with the emotional center that allows them to understand and regulate their emotional responses. When the processes are operating properly, they are able to process their emotions as information. Rather than acting emotionally, getting angry or upset, overreacting to others in their home, at school, or at work, they understand the reasons for their feelings and respond appropriately.

For example, a man who works with two women gets along with one very well and fights constantly with the other one, who has many of the habits and indiosyncracies of his mother — with whom he does not get along. In a similar situation, a woman feels very comfortable with one male supervisor while another intimidates her. Both of the cited office workers overreact in countless situations because of turmoil they thought they had gotten rid of long ago.

The frontal area has strong connections with the RAS, which is involved in arousal, alertness, and sleep. Its job is to keep the brain activity steady and stable. The RAS is a multisynaptic system that allows lots of connections to the neurons that run down the center of the spinal cord and into the brain stem area, which is the lower area of the brain that serves to pass information into the higher-level thinking or cortical areas. It is here that this multisynaptic system (again meaning that it has numerous connections) called the RAS exists to provide energizing necessary for the whole system. The RAS serves as a relay channel for the frontal processes and is not operating properly in ADHD people.

1.9.4   Regulation of Appropriate Behavior

The frontal area of the brain in connection with the emotional center serves to regulate appropriate behavior and responses to the environment. The limbic system in conjunction with frontal processes employs a gating mechanism to gate out information and to focus. There is agreement pointing to the limbic system as the vehicle to attach emotional significance to events and stimuli in the environment. This agreement enables the individual to gate out certain noises, sounds, sights, feeling, thoughts that are not relevant at the time and to focus on information that is more appropriate at that particular moment in time. The flow of information, like the flow of traffic, needs to be regulated and it is this gating mechanism that gives the frontal processes the ability for selective attention; the ability to select what the individual will or will not attend to at a given moment in time. This allows people to be in tune with the current setting, to attend to the teacher when in class, to attend to the book they are reading or the person with whom they are speaking, and to block out distractions, such as the movement of the trees or the wind. At other times, when it is in tune with the setting, they will attend to the wind and the trees and not to another person.

This is the brain's way of coping with the vast amount of information that is always available at any given point in time: only so much information is allowed in at one time, otherwise the brain goes into overload. People are able to gate out certain information and focus in on other information. They can snatch that piece of information, focus on it, make sense of it, use it, and then let it go to focus in again on another piece of information, gate out other information, snatch another piece of information, make sense of it, use it, and let it go, etc.

If this gating mechanism is not working, then the person will be overwhelmed by stimuli (noises, sights, and sounds) in this environment. He would be highly vulnerable to distractions from his environment; hearing all of the little noises and sounds around him.

EXAMPLE
Certain individuals can fly off the handle, screaming about chaos, when in actuality there are just too many "moving parts" or too many noises and they are overwhelmed. Others cannot carry on a conversation if there is too much background noise. They may need to move to a different setting. Sometimes, they cannot maintain eye contact as the act of looking at someone's face presents an overload of visual stimuli. They are distracted by the expressions on the person's face and cannot look at them and think at the same time. Instead of being able to study, they are distracted by the floor creaking, the sound of the dog barking, the sound of the telephone, the clock ticking and so on. They might drive down the highway paying attention to all the sights and sounds around them and not focus on the road in order to drive defensively and anticipate accidents. Some individuals are so sensitive to all of the sights and sounds around them that just walking into a shopping mall or large department store overwhelms them. They walk into the store and promptly forget what they came there for.

This happens to easily distracted ADD individuals on a continual basis. They can't always stop what they were thinking or paying attention to, and shift their focus to what is needed at that point in time.

EXAMPLE
This is similar to being lost in your own thoughts while someone else is talking. You suddenly realize that while "wool gathering" you missed what the person had to say. You then regroup, stop your internal thoughts, and refocus on what the person is saying. This happens more often to ADD people, and they can't stop their thoughts and they can't shift their focus.

These are all examples of how one can be distracted by one's environment resulting in forgetting things or missing information, whether that is by being distracted by all the noises and sounds around or by the thoughts in one's head. The vulnerability to being distracted can become so problematic that these people are literally overwhelmed by all of the sights and sounds around them.

Another kind of distractibility, in addition to being distracted by the environment, is more behavioral — going from one unfinished task to another or from one thing to another. Individuals may show distractibility in their daily lives in their inability to complete tasks. They wander from one project to another or zip around from thing to thing. An example of this is described by Bill Cosby in his book entitled *Time Flies*. He talks about old age and being distracted by describing what he calls the "Living Case." Cosby is talking about turning 50 years old. What he describes, however, is often similar to the "fog" of the ADD person, which is not related to age.

> One morning, you start the old routine of packing your attache case before leaving for work. On this particular morning, however, you also have two shirts that are going to the cleaners and a can of insect spray in case you're attacked by killer bees. And so, you pick up the fully packed attache case, the two shirts and the insect spray and there you stand, a well-organized man of mature years, who is ready to meet the day. But not this day, for suddenly you remember that you have forgotten to put something into the case.... So you open the case, and close it, and then you pick up the two shirts and the insect spray and the case and you look down to discover that something that was inside the case is now outside, a letter from the Internal Revenue Service, inviting you to the upcoming auction of your house. Now you open the case again, put the letter back inside, and close it. You pick up the shirts and the insect spray and then you discover that your new Whiffle ball that had been inside the case is slowly rolling across the floor. You are the owner of an attache case that belongs in a Stephen King movie.... After putting the Whiffle ball back, you decide to get a drink of orange juice. What you really need is a drink of grain alcohol, but you take the orange juice because you want to keep a clear head in your battle with your possessions. And so you go to the refrigerator and pour out a glass of juice. While drinking it, you hope that the vitamins will go directly to your brain. Then you pick up the case, pick up the two shirts, and are on your way back to the front door when your refreshed brain says, "Just a minute, pal. What did you do with the insect spray?" With growing despair, you begin a hunt for it. There is no point, of course, in also hunting for your mind: it is permanently lost. After a while, you drift back upstairs and are about to start the day again when your eye happens to fall on your desk, where the can of insect spray is sitting.

Distractibility is the one ADD symptom that everyone identifies with, and the reason that everyone thinks that they have a "touch of ADD." Distractibility and stress go hand in hand, and many people are overstressed with the demands of today's fast-paced environment. There is a continuum for looking at this gating mechanism. At the extreme degree of vulnerability to distractibility, the individual is continually overwhelmed by the environment and as a result cannot tolerate any excess stimuli. To the opposite degree, there is only mild vulnerability to being distracted by environmental noises, sights, and sounds as well as one's own thoughts. Behavior can be highly distractible and confusing or only mildly seen. The person controls such tendencies to not finish a task by using lots of structure to move to the next task only if the last one has been completed.

1.9.5 The Frontal Area Coordinates Efforts

It is the frontal area of the brain that coordinates efforts of all of the thinking areas of the brain to formulate an internal value system, goals and direction, and overall appropriate behavior for a given situation. The frontal processes also operate as inhibitory processes to block impulsive actions and provide a means of control over the behavior of the individual. This is the "stop sign" that every person needs to get along in society. It is when this "stop sign" is missing that people operate in an uncontrolled manner. They cannot delay gratification, they want things now, they can't wait, they have no system to make them aware of the consequences of their actions. There is no internal rule system to guide their behavior, to allow them to fit in and "do the right thing."

The frontal area of the brain, the supervisory system, is responsible for such things as

1. Time sense — the perception of length of time, 1 hour vs. 10 minutes
2. The ability to learn from one's mistakes — the ability to learn what when wrong, work to correct it the next time and to do things differently
3. Planning and organization — the ability to plan something and organize things into a cohesive whole
4. Sequencing — the ability to see things in a sequential order, first this and then that
5. Cognitive flexibility — thinking that is not rigid; the gray as opposed to either black or white, this idea or that, and the ability to be flexible enough to consider lots of alternative solutions to a single problem
6. Preservation — getting stuck like a needle on a record, inability to take an idea and apply it in different ways and to different settings. When one is stuck, one can't generalize from one experience to the next and use what has been learned in one situation to apply it to another)
7. Problem solving — to solve problems by thinking of different solutions and to not keep applying the same ineffective solution to the same problem

1.9.6   Summation

The frontal area of the brain is the most complex and the largest area of the brain. It is also the last area of the brain to be formed. The frontal area of the brain employs an inhibition system and thus provides what is socially and sexually appropriate. When this area is not working the individual has no sense of appropriate space or distance in relationships. The frontal area is connected with the executive functions, effective self-control, self-monitoring, and use of feedback. If it is not working properly, there is perseveration (one gets stuck) and low frustration tolerance (need for immediate gratification). One does what one wants when one wants to. The lack of time sense creates no concept of a future. The time is now and only now.

1.10   Summarizing ADD

To truly understand ADD we need to see attention as a global process and not just an issue of being able to attend, focus, and sustain attention to task. This has been a primary mistake in truly understanding just what ADD means to children, adolescents or adults and how it impacts their lives. Therefore, we see attention as a combination of events that are both cognitive (thinking) and behavioral processes. Attention is the ability to control and select stimuli and responses, take in some information, gate out other information, select and control how that information is utilized, and select and control the outcome or response. Attention is therefore not seen as a single process that can be specified to any one area of the brain. This conclusion is confirmed by a vast amount of research, experimental, and clinical findings. Those areas of the brain that are involved vary and change depending on the demands of the task involved. Different processes are used for different functions and what is needed determines what area of brain functioning is involved. Only the parietal and frontal areas of the brain are involved with ADD, because that is where the neurotransmitters, or brain messengers, dopamine and norepinephrine predominately operate.

ADD, affects everyone differently. There is a wide range across specific areas and the disorder occurs in varying degrees. Thus, two individuals may share the diagnosis of ADD yet exhibit distinctly different problems, patterns, and coping skills in the way they handle certain tasks. It is important to remember that there is a great amount of diversity in examining the ADD population as a whole.

There are legal issues emerging regarding ADD that range from medical malpractice (charging physicians with negligent misdiagnosis of ADHD and failure to obtain adequate informed consent for stimulant medications, and inadequate information about side effects) to coercive use of the school system in the absence of parental consent in medication of a child. There is the issue of differentiating an attentional disorder without hyperactivity from an attentional disorder with hyperactivity. Finally, there is the issue of providing appropriate educational needs for the ADD child and determining who is responsible for funding the specialized educational services offered by private facilities in both college and high school.

Using the model presented (how information gets into and is used by the brain), it is critical to have a clear diagnosis and comprehensive method of assessment to identify problem areas. It is imperative to know the assets and liabilities specific to the individual. This allows the ADD individuals to begin to develop coping skills based on their strengths and weaknesses.

Once problem areas are known, they can be targeted for help by using the strengths the person has to buildup the weaker areas. We always say, "Are we going to run the disorder or is it going to run us?" To understand what ADD is and to clearly diagnose the problems that exist using the model described is to begin to compensate for those problems and work with the disorder.

It is important to address the idea of grief and loss and the feelings that occur when someone is evaluated for and diagnosed with ADD. One man described it as feeling as if he had learned he was an "impaired plant." He would rather have found out he had a problem that he could treat and be done with, not one that is lifelong and does not go away.

The purpose of spending so much time understanding how the brain works and how ADD impacts these functions is to develop a clear picture of the disorder and create workable solutions to help individuals promote coping skills to conquer the disorder and not allow their lives and the lives of those around them to be run by symptoms of the disorder. They do not have to see themselves as impaired. Despite its lifelong presence, ADD (much like diabetes) can be controlled. Adolescents and adults in particular, once they understand the impact of this phenomenon on their lives, will require a grieving process to come to terms with the impact, make their peace with it and start anew. Thus, a grieving period will often follow diagnosis. Significant others, family members, and the ADD individual need to be aware of and prepared for the seemingly sudden onslaught of emotions that accompanies both diagnosis and treatment. This book will focus on understanding this disorder clearly, how to evaluate it, what its impact has been, and how to treat it.

2

The Two Subtypes of ADD: ADD Without Hyperactivity and ADHD

2.1 Understanding the Brain and the Differences Between ADD and ADHD

ADHD is often over-diagnosed. ADD (without Hyperactivity) is often under-diagnosed. The result is a lot of confusion and the disorders' being called the "yuppie condition" and not being looked at as medical disorders.

In our clinical practice we have found it extremely critical to be able to separate out the two disorders. The two represent very different issues for treatment and very different relationships with family members and other significant individuals in a person's life. There are different expectations related to each disorder based on different abilities and different ways each disorder has an impact on thinking and performance. Diagnosis and separation of ADD with hyperactivity from ADD without hyperactivity allows for treatment that is designed specifically to address the problems related to each individual disorder.

The ADHD individual may lie, display manipulative and secretive behaviors, and resemble more of the behavioral profile characteristic of delinquency, addictive personality, and oppositional defiant disorder. These behaviors arise not from an attempt to defend and protect oneself as in the case with ADD without hyperactivity, but as part of the manifestations of the disorder itself. Aggressive individuals may be seen with this disorder, especially when it is severe in nature and the impulsivity may be truly there and also involve another neurotransmitter, serotonin, in addition to the dopamine imbalance. ADHD tends to involve the RAS, the frontal areas of the brain, and, primarily, dopamine. It is more associated with learning disabilities for reading, writing and spelling due to the inability to learn as related to problems of the frontal processes.

ADD without hyperactivity involves a capacity problem, slow cognitive thinking, thalamus as the relay system, and parietal areas of the brain. Difficulty in school with reading, writing, and spelling tend to be related to spatial problems, characterized by a visual neglect, an inattention to the whole, problems at the phonemic level and not seeing words in a holistic manner to develop a sight vocabulary. The spatial area or the parietal area is more impacted and other spatial problems would appear such as gauging distances while driving, anticipation of consequences in terms of visualizing the whole and the impact of a specific action on the whole situation. Norepinephrine tends to be the neurotransmitter most involved with ADD without hyperactivity and these individuals will benefit from medications targeting that system.

The task is to try to distinguish one disorder from the other as much as possible. There is controversy as to whether the two disorders can overlap each other. It is believed that they do not and the overfocused subtype of ADD without hyperactivity may best fit that behavioral criteria. The picture is much clearer with adults in seeing the behavior and how it fits with the way the brain works associated with each disorder. With children, the picture is more cloudy; children are unable to support the findings of how the brain works and to explain their behavior.

Children will often appear oppositional and defiant, which may not be a behavior related to ADHD, but instead a means of defending against feeling insecure due to inabilities caused by symptoms of the attentional disorder. There are different correlated or comorbid disorders that result from the different combinations of neurotransmitter imbalances and medication that may or may not be different, depending on the diagnosis. The disorder will appear in different ways and through different behaviors. By understanding and knowing the difference, we can begin to reach these individuals and help them cope with symptoms of the disorder.

Finally, it becomes so important for those who are close to the ADD individuals to know what to expect and why they react the way they do, not only to help them but also to avoid being injured by them. We consistently hear the utter pain and exhaustion in the voices of spouses and parents of ADD individuals and these relationships tend to be very painful and disappointing.

2.1.1 Defining ADD without Hyperactivity

ADD without hyperactivity has as its most predominant general trait the issue of inattentiveness. Other behaviors observed are excessive daydreaming, "spacy" appearance, cognitive sluggishness, hypoactivity, lethargy, excessive confusion or mental "fogginess," and apparent problems of memory retrieval. These individuals tend to have considerable degrees of anxiety, be socially inept, shy, or have diminished social involvement. They are rarely aggressive, oppositional, or impulsive. These individuals will often think that they cannot do something and doubt their confidence when in fact they are quite capable of task performance. This misconception leads to a high degree of avoidance and procrastination. ADD without hyperactivity is a true sustained, focused-attention problem, and is seen as the less severe of the two disorders. The primary problem of this disorder is the inability to sustain attention over time and maintain focused attention and concentration to task.

Inherent to this disorder tends to be a capacity problem that produces a limitation on available energy whereby the individual cannot sustain effort. As a result, the individual only lasts for so long, like the engine that sputters and sputs. ADD without hyperactivity individuals lose their focus, get it back, lose it again, get it back, and so on. Sometimes, they are able to recover and continue on down the road and sometimes they can't and lapse into total confusion. It can be easily observed in task performance that these individuals can only sustain focus and attention for a limited amount of time. As a result, they do not follow through very well or complete things from start to finish due to the capacity problem.

ADD without hyperactivity individuals tend to forget what they are doing and then become confused. These are the dreamy, out-to-lunch, appearing-spacy, as-if-they-were-living-in-Tahiti individuals.

ADD without hyperactivity is often misdiagnosed as ADHD due to the extreme degree of anxiety these individuals have in both their family history and through their lifetime. These individuals are fear based and the disorder of ADD without hyperactivity is highly correlated (meaning it goes hand in hand) or associated with anxiety and depression (one does not cause the other, they just tend to travel together). There is a clear history in the family of anxiety and anxiety-related symptoms. These individuals seem to be hyperactive due to being so anxious and it is not uncommon to see both children and adults so anxious that their foot or leg moves continuously, or they constantly change positions and move. Sleep problems are prevalent and the sleeper constantly moves and shifts throughout the night, contributing to what may be called a "restless leg syndrome."

EXAMPLE
ADD children always need to be playing with something. Something is always in their hands. They tap on the cup they are holding or break apart the styrofoam cup they are finished drinking from. They tear tissue into tiny bits. I was meeting with a mother and her son, who was continuously playing with the strap of her purse. He was beginning to do untold damage to the purse when I interrupted, and, for lack of anything to give him, presented a packet of sticky notes. He began to play with the sticky notes and was having such a good time that before I knew it both he and his mother were tearing apart and re-sticking the packet of notes as we proceeded to discuss the emotional issues impacting the family. As anxiety increases, so does this type of nervous behavior.

Other diagnoses, hyperthyroid, hypothyroid, or hypoglycemia (a low-blood-sugar condition) are also associated and found to exist to a large degree in this population. There is a subclinical hypothyroid condition that is not easily diagnosed however is responsible for the person being constantly fatigued. What is important about this is that oftentimes behavior that can be interpreted as hyperactive, aggressive, low frustration tolerance, fits of anger, snapping behavior, high degree of emotional reactivity, easy to upset, quick to anger, impulsive, and irritable may in fact be due to the presence of a low-blood-sugar condition. Sometimes correcting these additional problems provides changes in behavior that is then misdiagnosed as ADD and/or treatment of ADD.

EXAMPLE
A man we treated was diagnosed with an attention disorder, ADD without hyperactivity, and came back a few weeks later with his wife, who stated that he had improved in his relationships with his employees and was much easier to live with in the work setting. Now, this man was taking only a minimal dose of Ritalin that in all probability was not taking enough medication to cause a change in his thinking.

What did happen in the above example was that he had begun to eat regularly, was no longer experiencing low-blood-sugar reactions and it was thus easier to interact with him. Something as simple as blood sugar can make such a difference in an individual's life. In addition, when an individual prone to hypoglycemia begins to take stimulant medication, sometimes the medication will stimulate or result in an increase of low-blood-sugar reactions and it becomes important to be aware of this and compensate for these possible effects. These effects also may contribute to a person's experiencing difficulties with taking stimulant medication that could in fact be corrected with simply eating every few hours, rather than changing to a different type of medication. If someone who is taking Ritalin complains of fatigue, the first thing to address is blood sugar. We have found that low blood sugar produces test results that are worse than they normally would be when the person is recovered. When blood sugar is normalized, one's scores improve.

2.1.2   Specific Thinking Problems of ADD Without Hyperactivity

To discuss ADD without hyperactivity, refer back to the brain model presented in the prior chapter and look at the symptoms that create this thinking disorder.

2.1.2.1   *Information-Processing Problems*

These individuals may or may not tend to have an input problem, however, they usually have an information-processing problem (meaning they do not understand things because they are always missing little pieces of information from their environment). They will miss small bits of conversation, communication, instructions, and directions. Problems due to missed information impact performance at school, work, and home. Often, someone will come up to the individual and say, "don't you remember" and they have to admit they don't. The details are absent. Hence, they miss the punchline of the joke, and socially miscue. They don't know what to do or how to respond in social situations. These are the individuals who will still be sitting there when the fight breaks out and everyone else has left the bar. They missed the events leading up to the fight that alerted everyone else to leave.

This probably occurs often to ADD individuals where they have to "fake it till they make it" and continuously attempt to keep up a conversation in which they become totally lost on a rather frequent basis.

As a result of the information-processing problem and missing information, ADD without hyperactivity individuals don't always fit in or know how to dress or act or know the social code (unspoken, but known anyway), especially if there is an input problem as well.

When there is an input problem and an information problem as well, this may lead to what we call a "double indemnity," meaning the information may or may not get in and then it may or may not get processed. The person is hit with the first problem, which can then be compounded into the next and the impact of both issues creates a more severe problem in general. Social information is learned by simply existing in the environment, "hanging out"; no manual is provided on how to be social. If there is a problem of missing information, these individuals will be at risk for not knowing how to act and interact socially and often they become overwhelmed by the socialness of their environment and retreat. Characteristics of this population are withdrawal and shyness.

ADD without hyperactivity can cause great confusion and continue to cause the sufferer to"not get it." By missing information, which is how we learn to be social, ADD individuals have difficulty saying the right thing at the right time and often find themselves in embarrassing situations. As a result, they tend to withdraw further and create their own internal world of fantasy.

2.1.2.2   Distractibility

ADD without hyperactivity individuals also tend to be vulnerable to distractibility in their environment and possibly, but not necessarily, can become distracted in a behavioral manner. This means that they will hear all of the little noises and sounds in the environment and not be able to focus and concentrate on what is going on.

These individuals can be distracted not only by all of the noises and sounds around them but also by the thoughts in their heads. Often these thoughts continue to race in their heads much of the time and they will miss information because they are thinking of something else while someone is talking.

An example might be ADD without hyperactivity individuals in a restaurant setting. They may look around and have difficulty concentrating on the conversation at the table because they are distracted by the stimulus overload.

Sometimes these individuals cannot maintain eye contact because they are overwhelmed by the stimuli of the other person's facial expression. They are unable to gate out to focus on the facial expression in order to hear what the person is saying unless they look away. People describe situations such as attempting to clean a house. They leave a room they are cleaning to go to another room to get something they need, get involved in something else and never return to the original room.

EXAMPLE
There is the story of a man who was washing dishes at the kitchen sink, looked up through the window and saw that the bushes were not trimmed, left the dishes and began to trim the bushes, whereupon he noticed a spot on the side of the house. He left the bushes and began to paint the house and so on. He is left with dirty dishes in the sink, partially trimmed shrubbery, and a spotted house.

Very bright individuals develop obsessive compulsive tendencies to compensate for symptoms of the disorder by trying to be perfect at whatever they do. Thus, everything becomes a major issue and tasks don't get completed because something simple becomes overly complex and involved. The person becomes overfocused and fixated on being structured and overly controlling in efforts to maintain structure and not be distracted.

EXAMPLE
In preparation for a change of residence, a man was supposed to clean his basement, which was full of many different objects and materials (because he never threw anything out). According to this man, to clean the basement he needed boxes. However, he needed special sturdy boxes of similar sizes. These boxes needed to be organized and labeled. He then had to decide what to label what, and what to keep, and what to throw away. Finally, the process became so complex that he avoided it until he could not longer remember that he had to do it and forgot it altogether. The day of the move to the new house, a separate moving company had to be hired just to move the contents of the basement..

2.1.2.3 Thinking Speed

Highly characteristic of ADD without hyperactivity is what is called a slow cognitive speed or slow thinking speed — as if the information is slowly moving through the brain like sludge. This makes conversation difficult. Imagine conversation is like a tennis match, someone speaks and then the other speaks and so on. The speaker has to wait and wait for a response from the ADD person. This can become very frustrating, can lead to the ADD individuals' not being able to carry on a social conversation in a comfortable fashion, as others become impatient with them.

Most importantly, on timed tests, the ability of the person is not measured. Instead all that is measured is time. With ADD individuals, consistently poor scores are obtained on timed testing and are well below the person's potential. Such an evaluation is often not a measure of the person's knowledge or ability but all that has been measured is time. Incidentally, this is changing in the school systems, particularly in college, where the student is often afforded untimed evaluation.

2.1.2.4   Difficulties in Understanding

ADD without hyperactivity individuals have a problem in understanding but once they "get it" they can use it. The frontal area of the brain is fine and their use of logic and problem-solving skills tends to be excellent once they are able to figure situations out. These problem-solving skills can be used to compensate for other deficits associated with the disorder. Often problems will not be seen due to the use of logic and strategy as a means of compensating.

EXAMPLE

Rather than attempt to read and understand directions, ADD individuals will put something together using logical analysis from a problem-solving approach. Thus, they will put mechanical things together without reading the instructions and directions, and using just the illustrations. They will use whatever pieces of information they have to attempt to solve the situation. The result can be the missing of information and often the miscueing of a situation, which can lead to miscommunication.

ADD without hyperactivity individuals who are very bright and use logic to compensate to an extensive degree for a problematic information-processing deficit will often formulate a conclusion based on the information that they have. To them it makes logical sense even though, due to some missing information, this conclusion may be at odds with the thinking of those around them or the reality. However, these individuals will steadfastly maintain that their position or view of the situation or event is the correct one.

2.1.3   ADD Without Hyperactivity and Associated Symptoms and Problems

- Anxiety — There is a high degree of anxiety in this group, which can result in the misdiagnosis of hyperactivity. What is important to note is that the anxiety is often unknown to them because they have lived with it for so long. It pervades them, runs through them and is a normal part of their lives. They are so used to it they are unaware of its impact on them. An example of this is an individual who said that he was nervous all the time and could not sleep. Amazingly, he was unaware that this was anxiety. These same individuals are then susceptible to difficulties with all of the illnesses impacted by stress, such as colitis, spastic colon, irritable bowel syndrome, ulcers and other disorders including:

- Depression
- Schizophrenia
- Obsessive compulsive personality or obsessive compulsive disorder
- Allergies and asthma
- Hypertension
- Hypothyroid, hypoglycemia
- Substance abuse

2.2 Defining ADHD

ADHD involves the traits of impulsivity and overactivity. Characteristics are hyperactive behavior, motor excessiveness, social inappropriateness, interruptive behaviors, aggressiveness, oppositional behavior, failure to conform to rules, lack of an internal value system, and the need for external motivation and structure.

- ADHD tends to be more pervasive than ADD
- It tends to involve the frontal area of the brain
- The person tends to be out of control in various ways
- Behaviorally, it is highly associated with conduct disorder, oppositional defiant disorder and antisocial personality
- Not reachable with values or conscience
- Emotionally out of control
- Cannot control thinking

The frontal area of the brain is down, is sleeping, and not available. As a result, there is no stop sign and no president to control things. ADHD individuals have little frustration tolerance and once they become upset or frustrated in any way, they are done with the task. It becomes virtually impossible to coax them to continue; they have already made up their minds and "that is all they have to say about that." The supervisory system is not in operation and therefore guilt does not impact them. They appear to others as if they don't care and, more often than not, they don't. We once tested a 5-year-old boy who, while in the testing room with his mother, father, and aunt, simply said "No" and that was the end of the testing.

This explains why we are generally unable to talk these individuals out of things and also helps to understand why ADHD individuals are unable to use the cognitive control strategies. They can't will themselves to stay on task or pursue a task if there is no will. Research shows that these individuals don't use private speech or an internal language to talk themselves through tasks. The motivational center is also impacted. This explains why ADHD individuals require and crave constant stimulation, novel situations all the time.

2.2.1 Thinking Problems of ADHD

ADHD individuals may or may not have a problem "getting" it but even if they do manage to get it, they can't use it. So this disorder is more pervasive with poorer statistics. This is also the reason that most of the research is directed at this resistant disorder.

ADHD individuals have learning problems. This is not the individual you can punish and discourage from doing it again. They tend to have difficulty learning from past experiences. The feedback system does not work so they do not learn based on feedback, nor do they use that information to modify their behavior.

This group truly has learning problems and disabilities. Recent research is beginning to confirm that the brains of ADHD individuals are different in very basic ways that impact the structures related to learning. As a result, they do not learn from their mistakes and can repeatedly apply the same solution that did not work the first time to the same problem time and again. There are learning disabilities for reading, spelling, and math.

There is no sense of time. The ADHD individual can be gone for 2 hours and swear it was only 20 minutes. This is a task of the frontal processes and the ADHD individual has no ability to sense time. They also have difficulty with delaying gratification due to this problem. Because they cannot feel a sense of time, 5 minutes seems like forever and they cannot wait because waiting seems endless to them.

Sequencing is a problem. There is no idea of one thing leading to the next in a sequential order. The idea of a sequential order is a concept that the ADHD does not have due to frontal processes being down. They cannot see the steps to reach their goals nor can they see how to organize those steps in some kind of order.

They have difficulty with the task of switching sets and maintaining a set. The cognitive flexibility to problem solve is absent. Thus, perseveration can occur and these individuals repeatedly try the same solution for the same problem even though it does not work.

Similar to the learning problems discussed, this issue relates to the rigidity of the brain. With the frontal processes not available, these individuals do not have the capacity to be flexible in their thinking. Things are black and white; there is no gray. It is their way or the highway. They are always right due to this rigid way of seeing things and their ability to only see things one way. Problem solving cannot occur because there is no capacity to generate alternative solutions when the first one does not work. These individuals do not have the ability to rethink a situation and devise a different approach. They also tend to be very rigid in relationships, which can result in poor communication and their not necessarily being a part of a group.

It is due to these issues that ADHD tends to be seen with true alcoholism. The tendency to become abusive is also an issue because of their intolerance, quick temper, and inability to see any alternative approach for coping with the situation at hand.

Planning and organization is a problem. The frontal processes that are responsible for the ability to plan and organize are not available and therefore ADHD individuals truly cannot plan and organize time, tasks, their desks, their rooms, or their lives in general. They have no concept of how to organize. Even if someone does that for them, they are unable to maintain the organization. There is no idea of a future, due to a lack of time sense, consequently they have no ability to plan things. The absence of sequential skills also prevents the individual from planning tasks in an orderly fashion.

ADHD individuals do not have a slow cognitive speed, they are fast, and this can lead to their being impulsive, which further adds to their problems. ADHD individuals may be both distracted by their environment and distractible in and of themselves. In other words, not only do they hear all of the noises and sounds but they cannot restrain themselves from being distracted and moving from thing to thing and place to place as well. They can be described as being "all over the place."

ADHD is often associated with (but not caused by)

- Hyperthyroid
- Conduct disorder
- Oppositional defiant disorder
- Antisocial personality disorder
- Alcoholism, gambling and so on
- Addiction: cocaine is often the drug of choice for its stimulating properties.

2.3 Common Misperceptions in Looking at Behaviors of the ADD Individual that Provide a Means of Separating ADD Without Hyperactivity from ADHD

2.3.1 Lying

2.3.1.1 ADD Without Hyperactivity

They will often lie because they are so concerned about anyone being angry with them. These individuals are overly concerned with the opinions of others and desperately want to please. The degree of anxiety over doing something wrong promotes lying, meaning that their fear becomes so great they lie at the time even if in the end it will come back to them in some way.

EXAMPLE

Dr. Fisher recounts: My son once spent the whole day with me carrying in his back pocket his latest progress report indicating a number of D's and E's. Knowing that I would be upset, he kept this hidden in his pocket. I found it while I was doing laundry several days later. When I asked why he had done that, he indicated he was fearful of my being angry (which I would have been), which would have impacted our day together. I then asked how he had managed to keep this hidden all day and his reply of, "It wasn't easy," indicated that his fear was more important than anything else. Due to fear, these individuals lie very well.

2.3.1.2   ADHD

ADHD people may lie just because they feel like it. There is no fear involved because they really don't care what anyone thinks. So they may lie one day and not the other, it just depends on how they feel. When you catch them in a lie, their response will probably often be, "So what?"

2.3.2   Stealing

2.3.2.1   ADD Without Hyperactivity

If they steal it will generally be to cover up something else without the clear intent of attempting to rob someone else and without the intent of trying to hurt anyone. One girl we saw in therapy had stolen some bonds from her parents and cashed them. She took the bonds because she was in real financial trouble and feared that if it was known, there would be a lot of problems in the household.

The girl felt very guilty about this for a long time afterward. This incident is revealing of the cycle of the ADD individuals who can't get to work on time due to being distracted, and so lose their jobs, can't pay their bills, and worry about others being angry. Low self-esteem then prevents them from getting another job, they feel worse about themselves and then become desperate to solve the situation any way they can.

2.3.2.2   ADHD

These individuals don't tend to become desperate. They don't care enough about their lives or those around them to get that upset. They basically live day to day, moment to moment. Due to frontal processes being down, they act outbecause they want something. There is no delay of gratification and they want it now. There is no connection so they don't care where they get it from or who gets hurt.

2.3.3   Manipulation

2.3.3.1   ADD Without Hyperactivity

ADD individuals can be excellent manipulators, however, again, this is due to their extreme fear of someone getting angry at them. Also, because of their guilt they don't tend to ask for what they want in a straightforward manner and therefore have to manipulate the situation to get it. Finally, there are classic issues of self-esteem in this group. Since they believe they don't deserve anything anyway, they rely on manipulation to get what they need rather than asking anyone for anything. These individuals are also very secretive for the same reasons.

2.3.3.2   ADHD

Manipulation is a means to get what they want and often a game or sport to see how far they can shift and move people. There tends to be a need for dominance due to the low self-esteem that is a consequence of symptoms of the disorder, and a consistent need to prove themselves better than others. Due to their need to be right and to their rigid way of thinking, they are forced to manipulate others to bend to their will as they do not see any other alternatives. They also have no idea or capacity, due to the loss of the frontal processes, of how to negotiate or bargain.

2.3.4   Reading and Math Problems

2.3.4.1   ADD Without Hyperactivity

Reading or math problems are generally due to an inattention to the whole, which is characterized as a spatial problem, not a learning disability. This means that the ADD individual has difficulty developing phonemic skills of approaching words and learning language as they cannot sound it out and then put it together as a whole. Often there are mispronunciations and the tendency to memorize words. Bright individuals typically start off reading quite well, however, as things become more complex, the words get longer and they can no longer memorize the word. Reading begins to falter. As a result, they read less and the problem becomes worse due to lack of interest. Typically, these individuals mispronounce words and see a word differently; a word such as "heir" is seen as "hair." Math skills also present problems when there is a spatial component, such as adding in one's head, which requires a visual–spatial whole. Geometry poses a specific problem for the same reason.

2.3.4.2   ADHD

Reading and math problems exist due to the presence of a true learning disability and an inability to learn from one's mistakes and to use information as feedback. Research indicates that there is a difference in the brains of the ADHD individual that results in learning problems.

2.3.5 Hyperactivity and General Restlessness

2.3.5.1 ADD Without Hyperactivity

These individuals are very anxious and tend to always be moving and seldom sit still. They appear restless or hyperactive due to the consistent moving of a foot or hand. Many of these individuals literally shake. The body movement is the consequence of a high degree of anxiety that results in this movement. The individual is unaware of the movement until it is pointed out. The base of the apparent "overactivity" is anxiety and not the motor issue related to ADHD.

These individuals are described as Type A. They are driven; they can't relax; they can't sit still for long. They easily feel trapped if something takes more than 20 minutes. They are often mistakenly viewed as ADHD because of their outward agitation and constant movement.

2.3.5.2 ADHD

This is where the true motor activity can be seen and it is crucial to separate this from anxiety. As children, these individuals move constantly whether they are in calm or anxiety-provoking situations. The RAS is underdeveloped and at overarousal that does not shut down. The ADHD children keep going all day, running on energy that remains unexplained. People wonder how these children can keep going all day and all night and not appear tired but have energy to spare. They run instead of walk. They move fast all of the time, there are no situation-stimulating anxiety reactions. As an adult, remnants can be seen in their fast movement and pace, and their cravings for excitement and stimulation.

2.3.6 Planning and Organization

2.3.6.1 ADD Without Hyperactivity

These individuals do not truly have a problem in this area. They may appear, however, to have difficulty with planning and organizing due to issues of distractibility, confusion, and slow completion of tasks. They look unorganized because they can't complete tasks, they get distracted and move from one uncompleted task to another until everything becomes overwhelming. Avoidance makes problems worse. They tend to plan less due to low self-esteem.

EXAMPLE

These individuals tend to be late and be poor planners of time due to distractibility and always having to finish one more thing. Inattention to the whole and the spatial problems result in their inability to size up a job and estimate how long it will take them and then to put that together in terms of how much time they have and if it can all be done. Also, they think they have time to travel from Point A to Point B when they don't. They grossly overestimate what they can do in the time allotted.

2.3.6.2   ADHD

The frontal processes that provide the mechanism for planning and organization are not available. The ADHD individual does not have the ability to plan and organize. Those skills are simply not available.

2.3.7   Impulsivity

2.3.7.1   ADD Without Hyperactivity

These individuals are not truly impulsive but may display impulsivity only after they have been working on a task for some time and become frustrated with their inability to perform. In later years, after coping with symptoms of the disorder, self-esteem can be quite low and the person may give up on a task at the first sign of trouble. This can appear to be impulsive.

2.3.7.2   ADHD

These individuals also may not be truly impulsive. Impulsivity by itself involves the neurotransmitter serotonin. What does happen is that their frustration tolerance is virtually nonexistent due to frontal processes being down. Therefore, at the first sign of trouble, they are done with the task and impulsively quit. Impulsivity is also noted because ADHD persons do what they want when they want. The frontal processes that work as a stop sign are down, so if they think of something, they just do it. These individuals appear impulsive because they live in the moment and do what they feel. This is due, however, to the lack of a value system and an effective feedback system. Otherwise, they would become aware of the consequences of their behavior. So, as a result, in their thinking there are no consequences, they just think of it and then do it. ADHD individuals are genuinely surprised to hear of the results of their impulsively decided behaviors.

2.3.8   Social Skills

2.3.8.1   ADD Without Hyperactivity

These individuals tend to be neglected, seen and not heard. They are shy and withdrawn and remain on the periphery. They don't bother anyone and blend into the woodwork. Due to problems of information processing they often do not know how to act, what to say, what to wear and what to do socially. They may use their skills of logic to think "streetwise" to compensate for their lack of knowledge or they may develop overlearned knowledge of appropriate social behavior, e.g., when in this situation or if this happens do this. This allows them to appear more intact than they are, and to attempt to fit in with their peers. These individuals tend to be immature and be with people who are younger than themselves, which is where they feel most comfortable.

2.3.8.2 ADHD

These individuals are the ones who are rejected due to their inappropriate social manners. Frontal processes are down and they do as they please, which often means violating the borders and boundaries of others to get what they want. There may also be problems of missing information and therefore they do not know how to be appropriate, i.e., how to do and say the right thing. In addition, with the frontal processes being down, they have no inherent ability to understand the need to be appropriate relative to a given situation.

2.3.9 Lack of Follow-Through

2.3.9.1 ADD Without Hyperactivity

These individuals do not follow through with tasks. This can be due to the problem of sustained focus, attention to task, distractibility, or a combination. They can be distracted or tend to move from one unfinished task to another as a behavioral pattern, a capacity problem, or both. The capacity problem is a result of limited brain energy at any one time. ADD persons can become distracted and not follow through, lose their focus and not follow through, cannot sustain attention to follow through, and can lose energy and not follow through. They can also develop low self-esteem, which results in avoidance and procrastination of tasks that become difficult. The person will start out great with all the intention of success and then be unable to finish. Task completion, as well as avoidance and procrastination, are major issues.

2.3.9.2 ADHD

The lack of follow-through tends to occur when they lose interest. ADHD individuals require high energy, highly motivating settings. They need external motivation to replace the loss of internal motivation due to the frontal processes being down. They also crave crises and turmoil. This need for stimulation results in a need for chaos and does not lend itself to the efforts required for task completion. There also may be a period of boredom while finishing what was initially exciting.

2.3.10 Aggression, Anger, Irritability

2.3.10.1 ADD Without Hyperactivity

With these individuals, when anger or aggression develops, it tends to be the result of several issues. These individuals often feel very overwhelmed much of the time. They are desperate to succeed and unable to do so due to symptoms of the attention disorder. The resulting despair or depression is displayed as anger. In addition, there is often an associated disorder related to hypoglycemia. Low-blood-sugar can easily produce irritability and anger that becomes more of a surprise to the ADD individual than the spouse who wonders why this person is angry all of a sudden.

2.3.10.2 ADHD

These individuals feel that their life is not going as expected. Not having what they want when they want it makes them angry. There is no capacity to wait (very low tolerance for delay of gratification) and it does not take much to send them into a rage. Anger may be a means of coping with the frustration for which they also have a very low tolerance. This relates to the symptoms of the disorder. They blame others rather than themselves and are angry and irritable at others when they cannot get what they want and think they should have. For example, anger can result following the loss of some physical item, a place in line, or a job they thought they ought to have.

2.3.11   Low Frustration Tolerance

2.3.11.1 ADD Without hyperactivity

These individuals will appear to have low frustration tolerance, but this is not the case. If anything, they will keep trying for too long, wear themselves out and then quit. If it seems as if they are getting it, it may be because of they have tried over and over with little success due to the impact of symptoms of the attentional disorder.

2.3.11.2 ADHD

There is low frustration tolerance and when the going gets tough, they leave. There is little tolerance for problems or any task requiring an exertion of effort beyond what they are willing to provide. Tolerance increases if there is a substantial reward for their efforts that is desired and valued by them.

2.3.12   Delay of Gratification

2.3.12.1 ADD Without Hyperactivity

When it appears that they cannot wait it will tend to be due to the fear that they will not get whatever it is they are waiting for. This is very common for the overfocused, worried child or adult who is fearful of not receiving something or not being able to do something and as a result must have it or do it now. If a fear issue related to not receiving is not a factor, usually these individuals can wait.

2.3.12.2 ADHD

These individuals just cannot wait. They have no sense of time, so a few minutes could be forever and they can't tolerate the wait. The frontal processes are down and they have no idea of *how* to wait. So they want it *now* and are determined to *have* it now, no matter what.

2.3.13 Poor Communication

2.3.13.1 ADD Without Hyperactivity

There is poor communication due to missing information, being distracted, and not being able to provide all of the information at one time in a clear, cohesive fashion. Something may be forgotten, the individuals may appear scattered, or a piece of the whole picture can be missing. They are anxious or too fearful and can't calm down long enough to say all they need to say. ADD individuals tend to have more conversations with themselves than with anyone else. They have private conversations much of the time and are not particularly skilled in communicating their feelings due to their tendencies of shyness and withdrawal. These individuals are quick to feel guilt, are sensitive, react to the opinions of others, and are so vulnerable they tend to withdraw.

2.3.13.2 ADHD

These individuals do not tend to connect with others and people tend to be viewed as objects. There is no "hook" with the ADHD person, who will tell you to go fly a kite at the drop of a hat and who really does not care how you feel or think. The result of frontal processes being down is a lack of connection to one's own vulnerability and need of people. It is this lack of vulnerability that establishes a lack of need for closeness that would be promoted by good communication skills. The lack of ability to differentiate what is appropriate and what is not does not foster good communication skills.

2.3.14 Poor Sustained Effort

2.3.14.1 ADD Without Hyperactivity

There is a true problem with sustained effort, i.e., an inability to maintain focus to the task at hand. The presence of a capacity problem, i.e., limitation on the availability of one's energy, results in the problems with sustained effort and attention to task that are inherent in this disorder.

2.3.14.2 ADHD

Problems with poor sustained effort may well be due to distractibility and an inability to focus on the task at hand or due to a lack of motivation to sustain effort. The need for immediate gratification and low frustration tolerance may also be factors in the lack of sustained effort.

2.3.15   Inconsistent Performance Pattern

2.3.15.1 ADD Without Hyperactivity

Problems of inconsistent work performance may be due to a variety of factors
from distractibility to a capacity problem to problems with sustained attention. Emotional factors may also intervene, resulting in inconsistencies in
performance. ADD is based on a biochemical process — the brain is not hard
and fast. Therefore, sometimes the brain may be aroused, which allows it to
function to its potential and, at other times, it will not be as aroused, based on
the inherent variability of the brain. Then there may be times when there is
more of the neurotransmitter substance than at other times. Finally, if something is externally stimulating, then symptoms of ADD may not be seen at all.

2.3.15.2 ADHD

Inconsistencies in performance may be due to the variability of the brain or
something externally stimulating. In addition, if performance is tied to something that is extrinsically rewarding, performance will have some consistency. If not, performance is tied to the impulsive decisions of ADHD
persons, how they feel and what they decide to do at the moment. Due to
frontal processes being down, the absence of the ability to plan does not
allow performance to be consistent over time and is tied to the internal value
system and, thus, is not subject to external influences on a continual basis.

2.3.16   Oppositional and Defiant

2.3.16.1 ADD Without Hyperactivity

These individuals, particularly children, can have all of the symptoms of
Oppositional-Defiant Disorder, yet this will not be the correct diagnosis.
Both children and adults may attempt to defend this newly diagnosed disorder and appear more intact than they are or feel that they are. Thus, they
may feel it is better to present themselves as obstinate and defiant of authority, rather than have others find out they're really incompetent and incapable of the simplest task. Defiance becomes a means of covering up
symptoms of the disorder.

2.3.16.2 ADHD

These individuals can be truly oppositional and defiant. This disorder tends
to be associated with ADHD as a correlated disorder due to the impact of the
frontal processes being down. Defiance seems to be a part of this disorder, in
that this individual appears to be able to say "no" to anybody. They do as
they please and get what they want when they want it. No one is going to tell
them what to do. For example, they drink because they feel like it, they lie
because they feel like it, they work or don't work because they feel like it. If
anyone attempts to trap them into a corner and tell them what to do they will

become defiant. They are not connected to those around them, thus there is no "hook" to obtain compliance.

2.3.17   Talkative, Out Of Seat, Always Moving

2.3.17.1 ADD Without hyperactivity

These are common descriptions of those highly anxious, possibly active, children who, due to the levels of anxiety, feel the need to be constantly moving. They have discussions while standing, eat while walking, rarely relax, show signs of Type A personality, and usually pair one activity with another to do two things at once. Unfortunately, this appears as hyperactivity.

2.3.17.2 ADHD

There is the presence of a motor drivenness that propels the person into a state of continual and constant activity. The involvement of the RAS results in the desire to always be moving.

2.3.18   Alcoholism, Drug Abuse

2.3.18.1 ADD Without Hyperactivity

These individuals tend to be characterized as people who drink or take drugs to self medicate. Usually they are self medicating the anxiety that increases in intensity with years of the attentional disorder and severity of its symptoms. ADD individuals will begin drinking during social years to allow them acceptance and to not be so anxious in the company of their peers. They tend to become more addicted to marijuana, which provides a sense of relaxation and probably helps the ADD symptoms. Not knowing the disaster of its effects, they use this drug for long periods of time, which results in a pervasive and all-inclusive state of lack of motivation. This only increases tendencies of avoidance and procrastination.

2.3.18.2 ADHD

These individuals tend to be the true alcoholics who start drinking early in life and drink to get drunk, excited, or whatever. The drug of choice tends to be cocaine, which is known for its intense properties to satisfy continual cravings of excitement. If they quit drinking, they may practice other extremes such as smoking, eating, gambling, or any of a number of dependent or addictive behaviors. The lack of a stop sign in their frontal processes results in continued abuse of alcohol or drugs until they are stopped by some force outside of themselves, such as a spouse or parent.

2.3.19 Criminal Activity

2.3.19.1 ADD Without hyperactivity

These individuals make poor criminals. They are usually the ones who get caught because they end up in the wrong place at the wrong time. There is an unawareness that the impact of events, because of either their behavior or an event, will lead to another event, which becomes part of a larger framework. There is an inattention to the whole or an inability to grasp this concept. Therefore, the ADD people cannot get themselves out of a situation in time to avoid being caught.

2.3.19.2 ADHD

Because the frontal processes are down, if they feel like it they do it. This disorder is highly associated with Conduct Disorder (delinquent behaviors) Oppositional-Defiant Disorder (defy authority, disregard rules) Antisocial Personality Disorder (often stated to be the criminal personality). People with any of these associated diagnoses are able to commit crimes due to a lack of an internal value system and a lack of connection to others. Therefore, they don't care who they hurt or how they get what they want. There are no internal rules to govern their behavior. Adults with ADHD are not usually seen by therapists, especially in a clinical practice. An abundance of this disorder, however, can be found among the prison and repeat-offender population.

2.3.20 Distractibility

2.3.20.1 ADD Without Hyperactivity

With this type of disorder, wandering distractibility may be most common. This is when they are working on one task, then think about something else, leave that task to work on another task, and so on. It is not a racing movement from one task to another but rather a wandering, meandering shift without focus or completion. It is common for this group to have numerous piles of things not completed. Although ADD individuals are highly susceptible to being distracted by their environment, more often it is by the thoughts in their head. They are always thinking of something. The thoughts race all day and all night, sometimes disturbing sleep because they can't shut off the thoughts.

2.3.20.2 ADHD

The distractibility seen with this disorder is the racing movement going from one thing to another in a fast-paced-momentum motion. They propel themselves from one task to another. They quickly become bored or lack stimulation and just keep moving. ADHD individuals are highly vulnerable to all of the external noises around them and notice everything from the bird chirping to the fan system to the fish swimming to the funny person over there to the fly, and so on. They move with their eyes from one thing to another in this fast-paced momentum.

2.3.21   Impatience

2.3.21.1 ADD Without Hyperactivity

These individuals tend to become impatient only after they have been trying unsuccessfully for a long period of time. They then become tired, worn out, disheartened and upset. Impatience can also be seen if their blood sugar is low or if there is anxiety operating. When they are fearful, they are impatient to get whatever it is over with.

2.3.21.2 ADHD

This population tends to be impatient on a continual basis without any underlying logic, but due to low frustration tolerance, inability to delay gratification, and simply wanting it *now*. Thus, overall and on a constant basis, they are impatient to get started, to leave, to go somewhere, to go home, and so on. They don't last anywhere for too long unless the situation is highly stimulating. The impatience occurs as a result of this.

2.3.22   Interrupting or Intruding on Others: Blurting out Answers before the Question is Completed

2.3.22.1 ADD Without Hyperactivity

The problem of information processing and the tendency to become distracted due to the constant stream of thoughts racing through the person's head causes ADD individuals to forget what they are going to say. As a result, they tend to interrupt, not to be rude but because they will forget what they wanted to say. They will blurt out the answer for the same reason — because otherwise they will forget. If you make them wait, often they will say that they forget what it was they wanted to say.

2.3.22.2 ADHD

These individuals do not like to wait for anyone, nor do they think that they should have to wait. Consequently, if they have something to say they say it and they are either unaware (issue of lacking in the appropriate) or don't care if they interrupt conversations. They will blurt out answers. Again, this is due to being unaware of the appropriate social rule that one needs to wait and to their lack of connection with others. Their lack of connection results in a lack of understanding of how to relate to others in conversation as well as how to be accepted. They are out of control and have no idea of how to blend with others.

2.3.23   Not Listening to Others and Losing or Forgetting Things

2.3.23.1 ADD Without Hyperactivity

This is a common occurrence with this disorder due to problems of absence of information that results from information-processing difficulties. Therefore, because these individuals are always missing pieces of information, others around them do not think they are listening. They often forget things or lose things either due to the distractibility (one man found his glasses in the refrigerator) or simply because they missed the information. While it is described as forgetting, what really happened was that they did not know they were supposed to do something in the first place. Rule of thumb is to ask these individuals for only one thing at a time and not chain a number of requests together. The memory abilities in this group are excellent but the issue of distractibility or missed information is crucial.

2.3.23.2 ADHD

This group also tends to forget things or lose things for the same reasons: distractibility, or missing the information in the first place. They are moving at such a fast pace that it becomes difficult for them to ingest the information, for others to get their attention, and to get them to stand still for a moment. They don't tend to listen to what others have to say because they are either too busy making their point or they really don't care what others have to say.

2.3.24   Engaging in Physically Daring Activities

2.3.24.1 ADD Without Hyperactivity

This group really shows very little of this type of behavior. If it is seen at all, it is a means to escape from the constant anxiety, constant fearfulness, and constant thinking. They may ski down a hill or drive fast, because for a few moments in time, they don't think. It is not the thrill for which they are searching, but the relief from anxiety and constant thinking that plague them.

2.3.24.2 ADHD

This group craves excitement. They crave stimulation. The more frightening the event the better. External stimulation wakes them and gets them excited, otherwise things are perpetually boring. The more dangerous the better. This can be a valuable asset in that this population takes risks because they will do things others are afraid to try. They are not afraid to try something new and, in fact, thrive on the novelty of things.

The downfall is that this population is drawn to chaos, crises, and problems due to the sheer drama of such situations. As a result, their lives reflect this need for constant stimulation and they are uncomfortable when things become too comfortable for them.

Note: These categories are not fast and rigid. There is overlap. The idea is to simply identify the problems and begin to work with them.

3

Looking at ADD Without Hyperactivity

3.1 What is it?

ADD without hyperactivity is that true sustained attention disorder, one that describes an individual as dreamy, out to lunch, and not always operating on all four pistons. These are the individuals who have more conversations with themselves than with anyone else. ADD without hyperactivity tends to involve more of the parietal areas of the brain, as well as some of the subcortical areas. The frontal or logic processes, however, are intact. Thus, these individuals have difficulty understanding or "getting it," but once they do, they can use it and can truly rely on logic to function as well as they do. Skills of logical reasoning and ability to analyze a situation are the assets they are missing to figure out and survive in a world that is constantly confusing to them.

ADD without hyperactivity is the less serious of the two subtypes of ADD and not always recognizable. Thus, this disorder is often overlooked. This can be seen in the child, adolescent, or adult who does not cause problems but, instead, just about fades into the woodwork. They don't bother anyone or call attention to themselves, and, if they are bright, they will be able to compensate to the degree that they can perform within the work or school setting to an adequate level. Performance generally will not match their abilities. It will, however, suffice and they manage to get by. The key issue about this disorder is that they "get by." They don't maximize themselves and they don't operate to the level of their potential but they perform adequately.

3.2 What to look for

These individuals are hidden and not easily seen, noticed, or understood. Very often, adults who are diagnosed complain that they were working with someone in the mental health field — psychologist, social worker, or psychiatrist — and are upset that they were not diagnosed earlier. Instead, they were seen as merely overly anxious or depressed. The reason that this disorder is so difficult to diagnose is that these individuals, by their very private nature, tend to hide problems associated with the disorder and strive to appear intact. Consequently, when someone is working hard to appear "okay" it is difficult to see the problems they suffer. The brighter the individuals, the more they hide symptoms and work to "look good." Sometimes they do this to the point of avoiding or procrastinating a situation just so they don't fail. Children will often appear defiant as a means of avoiding a task they feel incapable of performing because of the attention disorder and would rather be seen as a failure than stupid. When we do finally see symptoms of the disorder, it is not always enough to suggest to the person that they should be evaluated. As a result, the ADD individuals themselves are the ones requesting the evaluation after talking to someone, reading a book, reading an article in the newspaper, having their child evaluated, and so on. They recognize the symptoms in themselves and ask for help.

3.2.1 Signs and Signals

- Failures on the job
- Failures in school
- Failures in the marriage
- Problems within the family
- Depression that cannot be explained
- Inability to make decisions
- Difficulty choosing a career
- Increased stress
- Inability to handle activities that could previously be handled
- Confusion and a sense of feeling constantly overwhelmed
- Loss of short-term memory
- Forgetting and losing things
- Development of temper outbursts
- Increased impatience
- Increased irritability
- Not being able to relax
- So tired at night that it is difficult just to turn on the TV and press the clicker
- TV and computer addictions
- Overall fatigue and loss of energy

- Dependencies or addictions increase: marijuana or cigarette smoking, eating, drinking, shopping, etc.
- Bedtime gets later and it is harder to wake in the morning
- More avoidance and procrastination on the job, school, house projects
- A poor attitude about everything

The key thing to remember is that these individuals appear to be doing fine and then there is a slow, gradual process whereby they are unable to function as well as they used to and gradually they become more upset. This upset does not tend to focus on one thing but is due to a lot of things that build over a period of time.

3.2.2 Anxiety — Why This Disorder is Misdiagnosed as ADHD

These individuals tend to be underdiagnosed as a whole and often overdiagnosed as ADHD. Generally this is due to the great amount of anxiety they have. It is the type of generalized anxiety disorder that acts as a substrate; it is there all of the time as a kind of underbelly to the individual. One can trace the family history and see signs of anxiety in other family members, whether it be problems with the digestive system, illness related to stress, hypertension, and so on. The anxiety is so much a part of these individuals' lives that they no longer even notice that it is there.

3.2.2.1 *Panic Disorder — They Think They are Having a Heart Attack*

The anxiety is always there and, at times, it can increase to the proportions of a panic disorder. When anxiety moves out of control, much like a car going into a spin, a panic attack can take place. Panic attacks tend to occur when these people experience anxiety and become so fearful that they panic. Using the previous example, it is as if, rather than going with the swerve of the car, they put on the brakes and go into a spin. If a panic attack occurs this can be extremely uncomfortable: the individuals may feel short of breath as if they are going to have a heart attack, or they may feel very nauseated and may in fact become physically ill or have diarrhea and end up at the emergency room of a hospital.

3.2.2.2 *Phobias May Develop*

The panic attacks seem to occur all of a sudden, as if out of nowhere. The anxiety, however, has been building within these individuals for some time, unbeknownst to them, and then erupts. The panic attack, if one does not understand it, is highly unnerving and frightening. Thus, a phobia develops, around the location where the panic attack occurred; the person becomes fearful of going to that place in case it will happen again. This is common.

EXAMPLE
One woman had a panic attack while riding in a car as a passenger. She developed a phobia of being a passenger in a car. She could hardly drive herself yet always needed to be the driver. She became fearful to go anywhere in the car or anywhere that was not near a bathroom. Nothing actually occurred to indicate she would have actually needed a bathroom but she remains fearful of this almost 1 year after the incident occurred.

This is also what happens to the child with a school situation. They arrive on their first day as fearful as all the other 5-year-olds around them. Something happens to heighten their fear. They then become more scared and move into the panicky feelings. This frightens them more and the panic attack itself begins. This same child now develops a phobia toward school, going to school, thinking of school, and so on. Any phobia can develop when in a given situation the individual suddenly has symptoms of panic (a high degree of anxiety). There are feelings of a *loss of control* associated with the automatic or autonomic nervous system. Symptoms of being unable to catch one's breath, the heart beating faster and faster and the stomach feeling tied in knots. The idea of the situation creating those *out of control* physical symptoms then creates panic attached to the given situation or place and the belief that it has the power to recreate the whole scenario again. It is this type of thinking that then creates a phobic response or phobia about everything connected to that place or situation as well as any precursor action that will result in the individuals being in that situation or place. People who are fearful of flying will become fearful of going to the airport, walking into the airport, purchasing an airplane ticket, and so on.

3.2.2.3   Anxiety May Occur on a Continual Basis

These individuals will tend to fidget in their seats and move around on a continual basis, appearing hyperactive.

EXAMPLE
Tommy was so anxious as an infant that he broke his first crib and had to go to a second crib before he graduated into a bed. This child rocked the crib across carpeting and his mother would constantly hear this thump, thump back and forth as he was soothing himself rocking back and forth in his crib.

These children present with a "moving around and fidgetiness" that is characteristic of ADHD. It does not, however, have the motor quality that ADHD has. It is more anxious in nature. Instead of moving their whole body around they tend to move one leg or one foot and it goes up and down almost in a shaking motion. I continually place my hand on my son's knee as his leg goes up and down, up and down. Symptoms of restlessness and the inability to sit still can be the consequence of anxiety. Some people may never eat a meal while not walking around the table.

EXAMPLE

Elizabeth's mother indicated that beginning at 18 months Elizabeth would "zone out" on a rocking horse for 10 to 20 minutes and would not want to be disturbed. She completely wore out two rocking horses. Then she progressed to a rocking chair. Currently, she gets up in the morning with a strong need to rock and, so, rocks for 30 minutes before getting ready for school, and also rocks in the chair from 15 to 30 minutes before going to bed. She will rock for hours if allowed. She rocks with headphones with music playing, and will rock even if her music has been taken away from her. Her rocking is very intense the week prior to report cards and appears to provide a means to calm herself. This is a means of self-stimulation that, through its repetitive motion, becomes calming. There may be additional issues attached to something like this related to another disorder such as head banging and rocking related to sleep disturbances.

3.2.2.4 Stress May be a Risk in Later Years

It is this anxiety in ADD individuals that results in a high risk for stress-related disorders in adulthood. It is due to their continued state of tension and their body's being constantly alert. As a result, they wear out their internal organs because they are always functioning at three times the normal rate, and tend to have serious health problems early in life.

When an ADD person takes stimulant medication it can result in a great amount of anxiety that needs to be counteracted in some form. Calcium is a nutritional supplement found to help. General vitamins or a good vitamin program is necessary since these individuals are so vulnerable to illness.

One individual who had a great amount of anxiety developed psoriasis, a skin disorder, and eventually developed arthritis related to the psoriasis, which impacted his career as a professional golfer. He was diagnosed with ADD without hyperactivity. When on the golf course, he would become confused and distracted. Then he would become angry at himself. This, in combination with being warned about his performance, served to increase the anxiety to a higher proportion. This same individual would consistently play poorly in tournaments, starting well and finishing terribly as the anxiety mounted. Issues of anxiety in combination with the confusion and inability to sustain attention to the task created a frustrating experience. Near the end of one tournament, he chipped over the green, chipped back over the green *again*, and then he chipped over the green one more time. At the end, he wrapped his chipping iron around a tree. When working with this specific population, it is continually amazing to see the degree of anxiety that is present.

Finally, there is a sleep deprivation that haunts this population. Due to racing thoughts, these individuals keep thinking throughout the night. They never fall into 4th stage, REM sleep, due to their anxiety and continual thinking. Thus they never totally relax. The sleep deprivation can result in irritability and further thinking problems and confusion.

In summation, the presence of anxiety only contributes to the avoidance and procrastination. Thus, it becomes critically important to separate the ADD without hyperactivity from the ADHD because these children can easily be traumatized if someone in authority is overly parental and too strong a disciplinarian.

3.3   Comorbidity

ADD without hyperactivity is often seen with several disorders. There is the constant theme of symptoms creating more symptoms.

3.3.1   Hypoglycemia–Low Blood Sugar

The presence of hypoglycemia can create stress, more problems with a drop in blood sugar which, in turn, creates more symptoms of ADD. There is a condition called hypoxia that occurs when the blood sugar drops and not enough nutrients get to the brain. The result is damage to the brain that can look like symptoms of ADD. So the question becomes what is caused by low blood sugar and what is caused by ADD? A good evaluation needs to question this. It is important that the individual maintain good eating habits to avoid low blood sugar and its impact on the brain as well as the worsening of ADD symptoms, which can create more upset for the individual. Finally, when taking stimulant medication, sometimes hypoglycemia can be triggered. It is, therefore, important to watch food intake very carefully.

3.3.2   Depression

Symptoms of depression impact ADD individuals' lives and, over a period of time, they become more sad and helpless, and less in control. The depressed feelings create more negativity toward symptoms of the ADD disorder and decrease the tendency, on the part of ADD individuals, to do anything about their situation. Depression does not tend to affect ADD thought patterns. It does, however, decrease the motivation to change the impact of the ADD on one's life. It can also create a very deadly cyclical pattern whereby avoidance and procrastination become everyday events and continue until such people lose their jobs, careers, and families.

3.3.3   Anxiety

Anxiety tends to be genetically based. It can be in the family history. Symptoms of anxiety can be described as hyperactivity, especially if the person is anxious and active in temperament. Anxiety is a constant state. It is always there and has ups and downs, peaks and valleys that constantly cycle and react with symptoms of the disorder. The ADD gets worse, therefore anxiety gets worse, which makes the ADD worse and so on. People cannot think when their anxiety increases past a certain point. A little anxiety is all right because it works for us and keeps us alert but a lot of anxiety stops the thinking. For example, have you ever made a decision or said or done something while anxious only to wonder later how you ever arrived at that conclusion? That is the power of anxiety.

3.3.4 Hypothyroid

A thyroid condition results in tendencies to tire easily and have little energy, This can be confused with symptoms of ADD. It can also make things difficult for the ADD person.A certain depression and fatigue are associated strictly with the condition of hypothyroidism.

3.3.5 Schizophrenia

This is a very fragile person who tends to withdraw and then loses touch with reality. The condition of schizophrenia tends to be genetic and has a family history. If seen, it usually occurs in young adulthood as the stressors mount. ADD is a contributing factor to the stress that can build to cause this condition to burst forth with symptoms of nonreality. The fragile, vulnerable state of these individuals would tend to make them more secretive and guarded. Thus, they would cope with symptoms of ADD by themselves and try to solve problems alone, which would create more stress and more fragility. ADD then goes undiagnosed in these individuals and only the symptoms of the schizophrenia are seen.

3.3.6 Post Traumatic Stress

When a stressful event occurs that is traumatic and produces symptoms of this disorder, the brain changes on a cellular level, the neurotransmitter balance changes and symptoms of ADD become common. It becomes important to separate out the ADD. It's important to know if it exists at all, if it existed prior to the stressful trauma, if symptoms are due totally to the trauma. History as well as a detailed evaluation help to answer this question.

3.3.7 Hypertension

This is a constant condition due either totally or in part to stress or a family history and predisposition. What also happens is that, as a result of this condition, the brain changes. Changes occur at a cellular, biochemical level and plaques that cause arteriosclerosis are formed inside the arterial wall. All of this can lead to damage to the brain and symptoms of ADD. Again, a thorough history is critical to rule out ADD as a condition that may have existed before the changes that are due to hypertension or to determine if all of the symptoms are the result of changes in the brain due to hypertension.

3.4 Symptoms Specific to ADD without Hyperactivity

3.4.1 Capacity Problems

ADD without hyperactivity is a true sustained disorder that involves a capacity problem whereby the brain has limited energy. The result is that the person will understand something and forget it —get it and lose it. This can result in confusion. What can happen is they lose the understanding or focus and then recover and go back to what they were doing or they may lose it, not be able to recover, and lapse into total confusion. ADD individuals continually lose their energy. This is evidence of the capacity problem of having limited energy at one time.

You can clearly see this capacity problem in task performance as well as in the follow-through of projects. This is why oftentimes ADD individuals cannot complete tasks and do not follow through on their goals. It can become very frustrating when dealing with an ADD person because you think something is going to get done yet it rarely does.

When lack of completion of tasks happens on a repeated basis, the individual can become depressed and unmotivated to try again. A pattern of avoidance and procrastination sets in. To avoid getting stuck in the cycle of losing focus and then lapsing into confusion from which they cannot recover, they simply avoid goals and task completion altogether. This can be devastating to the individual, especially for one who is very bright.

Others who know very bright individuals with ADD think they should go to college and become a doctor, lawyer, dentist, or entrepreneur, and are surprised that they end up working in a nonprofessional capacity because they are absolutely terrified to go to school. The depression sets in because of the feeling and fear of failure. It's as if one continues to climb a mountain only to fall down, climbs the mountain again only to fall down again, and so on. The capacity problem can be extremely discouraging to this individual. This frustration from failures is so prevalent that when asked to do anything or invited to complete a task or a new endeavor, such as school or employment, they will become fearful and react with some defensive maneuver (such as getting angry that you would suggest such a thing) to end the conversation.

3.4.2 Confusion

These are the individuals who are dreamy, don't get it, and are often confused. As a result, they will miss information due to either an information-processing deficit, an input problem, or distractibility. Have you ever been thinking and totally missed what someone said? This goes on all the time with the ADD person. Problem-solving skills of the frontal processes, however, are intact. They therefore attempt to logically work their way through the confusion and make up for the missing pieces. Imagine having only part of the puzzle, part of the sentence, or a portion of the information and trying to bring meaning and relevance to one's experience.

If individuals are continually missing information, they can appear to have "forgotten." This is why ADD individuals can appear to have a memory problem when really the information has not been processed or they have simply missed its getting in. There is a wonderful book by Mercer Mayer, *I Just Forgot*, that describes some of the daily sequences in the life of the ADD individual.

> Sometimes I remember, and sometimes I just forget. This morning I remembered to brush my teeth, but I forgot to make my bed. I put my dishes in the sink after breakfast, but I forgot to put the milk away.

One man had to come back to the house four times before proceeding on to work because he kept forgetting things. This happened on a regular basis. ADD individuals are notorious for saying that they forgot whether it is the papers you asked for, the forms to fill out, or whatever. They forget where things are and misplace things. Like that man who found his glasses in the refrigerator. One man lost his wallet and had replaced all of the contents before he found the original in the laundry basket. This is why I tape record all of the sessions in which I explain the results to both the ADD adults and parents of ADD children. So often these individuals call me and ask "What did you say?" Notoriously, they forget instructions or suggestions and, at times, they lose the tape or the report.

These individuals forget to wash their hair, clean their clothes, brush their teeth, cut their nails, and so on. It is not that they do not want to keep themselves clean, they just forget.

When people are highly vulnerable to distractibility and also have problems with information processing, they can become overwhelmed in a social situation. This can be especially difficult at a party and the more people present, the worse it becomes. Not only are they overwhelmed by all of the stimuli, but at the same time, they're trying figure out what everyone is saying so they feel part of the group. Thus, they tend to avoid social situations and not like parties or groups of people. Socially, these individuals are isolated and neglected. They tend to say little and think a lot more. This can be extremely disturbing for anyone involved in a relationship with them. They listen well but communicate little and don't tend to respond. So you never know their feelings or their thoughts.

Having a conversation with an ADD individual is much like waiting for the bus to arrive. You speak and then you wait for them to respond. It is almost as if you can watch the information going into their brain in slow motion. It simply takes a period of time for them to "get it." This is why they are the last to get the punchline of the joke.

The major problematic issue that occurs between spouses is with communication, including missed communication. Common problems are the missed dates and times; one spouse thought something was going to happen but the other didn't. After a while this can become frustrating. It is this issue in particular that results in the high divorce rate as well as in strained relationships, whether they be between parent and child, spouses, or friends.

These individuals can be very fearful of expressing their anger. They can get angry, but they don't want anyone angry at them. So they say little, and keep their feelings to themselves. As a result, so that others do not get angry, they keep things inside, which only adds to the stress.

These individuals also tend to be passive–aggressive. Instead of saying they are angry, they will get back at you later. They don't get mad, they get even. With these individuals you may find yourself doing most of the talking and entertaining until eventually you get frustrated, angry and feel alone. This is how the spouses of ADD people feel—as if they don't know their husband or wife and how they think or feel.

3.4.3 Distractibility

The behavioral distractibility is more of a wandering distractibility in that ADD individuals tend to go from one uncompleted task to another. They do not finish things. This can be due to the capacity problem as well as to the vulnerability to being distracted by their environment both external and internal (the thoughts in their heads).

EXAMPLE

A familiar scenario is a person working on some project. He needs an additional item, goes to get it, and never returns to the project as some idea, a phone call, or whatever, waylays him.

House cleaning takes forever as rooms are never more than half cleaned. Going into another room to either take an item or get an item may mean never returning and the task remains half finished.

EXAMPLE

Bill Cosby in his book, Time Flies, *talks about thinking that his children have taken his glasses only to enter his bathroom, glance into the mirror and find them on his head. In another incident, he describes looking for his car, which he has parked in a parking lot.*

"And so, you start to wander around the wilderness, trying to conceal that you are looking for a car whose make has become foreign to you; it's on the tip of your mind, that pointy little place. Just as in looking for your glasses, you have to conceal that you are looking for something you handle every day; and a car, of course, is generally harder to misplace than glasses, especially a four-door. When you parked the car, you had said to your mind, 'Okay now, take this down; we're a blue Valiant parked in A2'. And your mind had replied, Got it, Have fun shopping. ...You even make up a little poem to fix the picture in your mind:

> Roses are red
> My Valiant is blue.
> An A1 car is
> In row A2.

For the next few minutes or hours, you keep interrupting your shopping to reassure yourself that nothing is simpler to remember than A2 blue Valiant. When you leave the mall, however, you find that this verse has taken wings and in its place is a less-winged one:

> Roses are red,
> My car must be near.
> Am I insured
> For losing it here?"

3.4.4 Slow Thinking Speed

The slow thinking speed results in conversations taking a longer period of time and performance in general being slower. ADD individuals tend to avoid and procrastinate. The brighter they are the more they want to do things perfectly, hence the more they avoid. Therefore, they take an even longer time on the things they can't avoid, which results in an even slower performance. Movement is slow, response is slow. This can be very frustrating for anyone involved with an ADD individual.

3.4.5 Perfectionism — Avoidance and Procrastination

There is a tendency for those individuals who are very bright to attempt to compensate for deficits of this disorder by doing *perfectly* whatever they can do well. The idea being that by doing things perfectly when they can, no one will suspect or see their deficits. Thus, compensation for this disorder can easily turn into traits of obsessive compulsiveness because the individual becomes overly concerned about doing things just so. There is an obsession with doing things just right and a drivenness to do things just so. Thus, the defense mechanism of being obsessive compulsive serves to work with the perfectionism by cultivating it and thereby allowing individuals not to feel their own inadequacies due to deficits of the disorder. The greater the deficits and the brighter the person, the greater the tendency for obsessive compulsive traits and perfectionism. This can become highly problematic in that these individuals work only to their strengths while totally neglecting their weak areas. Thus, by older ages, although they may appear to have damage to the brain, it is simply a result of some areas being overdeveloped to the detriment of others. These individuals rely so heavily on logic and logical analysis that they are often out of touch with reality.

Frequently, we will see individuals who have been diagnosed with Obsessive-Compulsive personality and what is missed is that underneath that personality lies an attention disorder that may have created this type of personality as part of the compensatory process. The OCD personality is quite different from the true biochemical genetic OCD disorder involving the handwashing, check and recheck and so on. These individuals have very poor task performance because they either avoid things or because the job has to be so perfect and becomes so involved that it is easier not to do it at all.

Due to the perfectionism and continued feelings of inadequacy, they may tend to give up and thus appear impulsive or unmotivated. They will say they are "bored," but they have lost interest due to feelings of hopelessness and inadequacy. They can easily detach themselves, retreat, and become "couch potatoes," which characterizes the avoidance and procrastination. There are a million excuses why they cannot do something, or why something will not work, and therefore they cannot do it. There is such fear of failure that they will avoid things at all costs and/or put things off until they have to finish them under a deadline. Somehow, with that deadline, there is no longer a choice, and it must be done NOW, so they get it done and usually do well. Thus, it is quite common for these individuals to wait until the very end, a crisis is created, their brain is stimulated, and they will say they work better under crisis. So things tend to be done at the last minute and thus they avoid all of that fear related to not doing something perfectly or, God forbid, failing.

3.4.6   Language Problems — Reading, Writing, and Spelling

Language problems of the ADD without hyperactivity individual are more related to a spatial issue. They truly have spatial problems almost to the point of visual neglect and this can be seen when using a page on which to write something. There is a loss of attention to the whole. Handwriting becomes problematic because the spatial consistency is poor and the letters are not all the same size nor are they even. Without lines as guidelines, handwriting tends to go downward. When they attempt to read, it becomes difficult to read the whole word because they can't see how the letters form the word. Problems are at the phonemic level. This also results in spelling problems because they can't look at the word and just see that it looks wrong and is not spelled right. Comprehension is intact but they literally do not know the word and how it compares with the sound of it, again due to a spatial issue.

As a result, these individuals do not tend to read very much and, in fact, avoid reading, hence they do not develop an extensive vocabulary. The brighter they are, the more they are able to compensate by memorizing everything, spelling, vocabulary, and so on. However, there is a limit to how much one is able to memorize while retaining the information. One individual told me that he reads by looking at the sentence and using pieces of the sentence to conclude what is being said, even though he cannot read a number of the words on an individual basis. Such "contextual" reading can lead to many errors in comprehension. The reading becomes work, and thus, boring. Avoidance becomes easier.

3.4.7   Internal Guidance, Private Speech

ADD individuals were found to be able to use private speech or self-talk to guide themselves internally through a task. This was because the frontal processes remain intact. Thus, ADD individuals can utilize self-talk to get through something and to cope with the distractibility. They are also able to self-regulate in this manner. They can feed in messages such as "keep going," "don't stop," "okay, we are doing this next and then this," and so on.

Private speech is highly significant in allowing ADD without hyperactivity individuals to compensate in their lives. This is one of the reasons that this disorder is not always diagnosed and they are able to get by and function. Not to their potential perhaps, but enough to exist comfortably within their world.

ADD without hyperactivity individuals can use private speech to feed in new thoughts and ideas about themselves and for this reason cognitive therapy works quite well.

EXAMPLE
One woman was working on coping with the release of all of her emotions. Upon starting medication, she finally was able to recognize that the depression and downcycling she had experienced as well as her thought patterns, speech patterns, and actions were born of a very poor diet of negative, harsh input from her mother. She did not want this belief system anymore and was determined to replace it with better "stuff." Finally, when the hurtful stuff from the past would rise within her and demand attention, she would sing "Zip-a-dee-doo-dah" meaning it's in the past and concentrating on that is not going to fix things, especially if she constantly runs in fear. Consequently, she is going to remember and sort through all of the input she receives, re-adjust the thought, speech, and actions, reflect on the good stuff and then proceed forward.

3.4.8   Substance Abuse

These individuals often use alcohol to self-medicate and may tend to use marijuana to increase the sensory systems and to calm themselves. There is a consistent pattern with this population whereby, on reaching the social years, they begin to drink. When asked what the alcohol does for them, they respond that it calms them down and allows them to interact with others, be friendly, and to fit in socially. For those anxious individuals, alcohol may be the only thing that helps them to finally experience a degree of peace. Thus, these individuals develop into what I term "co-dependent alcoholics," people who depend on alcohol to self-medicate the anxiety and shyness. They drink for a reason in a specific environment but not necessarily on a daily basis. Drinking can develop into daily intake. This, however, is usually if there is an influential external environment. Rarely do these individuals drink alone.

Marijuana helps them to calm down as well and they report being able to think better and more clearly. The problem with marijuana, however, is that it stays in the system much longer than originally thought and contributes to an overall, pervasive amotivational syndrome. These individuals are not interested in anything, their hygiene, themselves, their job, school and so on. It is easy for the ADD individual to become addicted to marijuana, again in a self-medicated perspective and to turn usage into a habit and a means to get through the day.

3.5   As They Get Older...

ADD without hyperactivity tends to be the unrecognized disorder. Individuals who are very bright will not come to the attention of anyone as a problem because they will get by. As they get older they have kids, the job demands increase, etc. and they can no longer continue to compensate. Thus, they appear more stressed. They don't tend to go to college or technical/vocational school for an extended degree. Problems escalate as their lives become more complex and then the disorder becomes more apparent as they can no longer compensate as they did in the past.

Unfortunately, as they get older, they lose brain cells and thus the brain cannot compensate as well as it once did, especially when there is so much dependence on frontal processes to compensate for the deficits of the disorder. Adults who are seen in their 40s and 50s do not need medication for the ADD, they have been compensating for 40 or 50 years. Medication is needed, however, for the stress that exists to compensate for the deficits. All too commonly, these adults are so tired that by the time they get home they are exhausted and can only watch TV, eat, and go to bed. Thus, their lives become going to work, eating, sleeping, and going to work. Relationships suffer and they retreat.

Allergies and asthma are common with this disorder and exacerbated or increased with stress and anxiety. These individuals do not get the REM sleep needed and they suffer from sleep deprivation. REM sleep occurs four or five times per night beginning approximately 90 minutes after falling asleep. REM episodes become longer as the night goes on and eventually occupies

20% of our sleeping time mainly in the early morning hours. People who are kept awake for a week become irritable, disoriented, and uncoordinated, have difficulty concentrating and may develop hallucinations and delusions. REM sleep is an especially constant and inflexible need, meaning its presence is critical to our health. For these individuals, sleeping is filled with constant body movement, which results in their being tired when they awaken, and generally feeling as if they had not slept at all.

4

Over-Focused Subtype of ADD Without Hyperactivity

4.1 Defining the Over-Focused Subtype

There is a subtype of ADD without hyperactivity that can look like a combination of ADD without hyperactivity and ADHD. The two disorders are generally seen as separate, and we do not sustain the belief that there is a combination of ADD without hyperactivity and ADHD, but rather that there is a subtype of ADD without hyperactivity.

The reason this is described as a subtype of ADD without hyperactivity, is that the clinical picture — how the brain operates — shows ADD without hyperactivity. The frontal processes are highly intact. Problems seen in an evaluation are information processing, distractibility, slow cognitive speed and all of the symptoms characteristic of ADD without hyperactivity. So the symptoms of the disorder fit the classic pattern of an attention disorder without hyperactivity, but they look hyperactive from what we call a *behavioral pattern* — their behavior appears to be that of an individual with the classic pattern of an attention disorder with hyperactivity. This is why professionals in the field arrived at this combination disorder; it explains why both types of symptoms are seen in one person.

In light of how the brain takes in information and the clear differences between the two disorders, it seems virtually impossible to have such a combination disorder exist. The two disorders use different biochemical systems and to have an effect on different structures in the brain. It does not make sense that a combination disorder would exist when the two disorders appear so different in nature. Regardless, a certain subtype emerged in children and adults diagnosed with ADD without hyperactivity. The group of individuals had similar characteristics that seemed to have a more severe attention disorder and also have more severe emotional and behavior problems both at home and at school. They were also more susceptible to having other issues such as allergies, tics, asthma, and eating and sleeping problems. Overall, they seemed "fragile." They appeared highly sensitive, very overreactive to all of those around them and to the settings they live in. They are emotional and overly dramatic (adolescence seems to be elongated throughout the lifetime).

4.2   Signs and Symptoms

4.2.1   Over-Focused

What makes this over-focused subtype look like ADHD is that they appear to perseverate, they get stuck on one thing and think about nothing else. Perseveration occurs when someone gets stuck on an idea or thought and then ends up repeating that idea or thought over and over even though the time, setting, or issue has changed. Therefore, in a new situation, they are still repeating the thoughts of the old situation. Usually, this is seen when frontal processes are decreased as in ADHD or any injury to the brain resulting in the frontal processes not working as they should. When the frontal processes do not work properly, individuals are unable to be flexible in their thinking or to entertain new ideas and thoughts and as a result, the repeating of the past occurs, or perseveration. In the case of the Over-Focused Subtype, this over-focused behavior or thinking occurs not due to perseveration but instead an individual will over-focus on something that they really want to have or want to happen. It is the fear of its not happening or their not being able to get what they want that results in the thinking and behavior pattern of over-focusing. Thus, the over-focusing is due to the high level of anxiety that pervades this group. So it is the anxiety and the fear of not getting or not being able to do what they really want that causes the over-focusing and thinking or talking of nothing else to occur.

EXAMPLE
A family arrives at Disney World. The over focused child has a specific ride in mind, the rocky mountain ride that is a recent addition to the theme park. He had been promised by his parents when he visited the park he would be able to go on the ride. The ride is about 2 hours into the park, located pretty much at the end of the route one takes through the park. For 2 hours all the child talked about was this rocky mountain ride and how he had to go on it. He literally steered the group to this ride that he was determined to go on.

Unfortunately, there was no way the ride was going to be worth all of the energy he had expended prior to arriving at the ride itself. Although it was fun, the ride could not possibly meet the expectations of all the energy that had come before it. This happens over and over again with the over-focused individual: whether it be to purchase a game or an activity or worrying about a test, exam, or whatever. Whatever the issue is, it becomes larger than life, the total focus in the person's life, and nothing else is as important at the time this is happening. The build-up is great and the letdown is always there. Nothing can match the build-up, so the person is always disappointed.

EXAMPLE

The following is about the over-focusing of an adult ADD without hyperactivity individual who wanted a compact disc (CD) player. At the time, there was not enough money in the family budget to afford the player. So he talked about this CD player for approximately six months. Finally, he began to purchase CDs without having purchased the player. By the time he had accumulated CDs that were worth far more money than the player, his wife decided that he had definitely lost control of his logic. This man was so determined to get the CD player that her best bet was to buy him the player just to stop him from buying all of the CDs and thereby attempt to place a limit on his spending. He was so over-focused on the CD player that she couldn't stand it any longer and went out and bought it for him.

Usually, these individuals will get whatever it is on which they are over-focused simply because no one can say NO to them, they will not take no for an answer and they won't stop until they get what it is on which they are over-focused. Thus it is this excessive determination of the over-focusing that results in their getting what they want. The problem becomes the impact this has on those around them in addition to perhaps making poor decisions, appearing stubborn, and being overly rigid in their thinking processes and decision-making skills.

4.2.2 Sensitive

These individuals are very sensitive and as a result can easily take things personally. Comments made by those around them are taken literally and they are easily hurt. For instance, someone teases them about their looks, clothes, or actions saying something like, "Boy, was that stupid!" and it becomes a major deal. They can worry about it, feel terrible, question themselves and on and on. Then they think about whatever they did, analyze it, and then analyze it again and again, until they drive themselves crazy. "Well, I could have done this, and why didn't I do that" and on and on. The questioning continues, which causes the self-esteem to go lower and these individuals to feel awful. They question everything. They have a need to be perfect due to their sensitivity and because they want those around them to think they are wonderful.

4.2.3 Always Worried

The anxiety in this group is tremendous. They are always worried (and I try to never say "always") or always fearful about anything and everything: *worry, worry, worry.* There are stories of these individuals as children being worried as young as 3 years of age, worrying if everyone will come out of the water and not drown, worrying if the rain will ruin the day, if it is okay to leave the house and it won't burn down, always worrying about something bad happening. They have a persistent and consistent tension to the face, the brow is furrowed, the face looks worried and afraid. They are afraid to try new things because someone might be hurt or it won't work. There is always the anticipation of the worst and a constant conviction that the worst will happen. This is probably the most limiting aspect of this disorder and results in these individuals, whether in childhood or in adulthood, not trying new things, not stretching their limits and not reaching their goals. They can't have fun and they can't relax. The worry runs them and it runs those around them.

4.2.4 Dramatic

Along with the sensitivity, there is a tendency to be dramatic at times overly dramatic. Everything is a major deal. They cry at the drop of a hat and the littlest thing easily becomes a big thing. If something does not work out or someone gets angry, they cry. They tend to be melodramatic, which is like living in technicolor on a continual basis. Emotions fly all the time. You think that you are having a nice conversation and all of a sudden things turn and the person is in tears, is upset, and distraught. The conversation is over and the emotions have begun. As a consequence of all these continual emotions, issues do not get addressed. It is difficult to communicate, set rules, borders, and boundaries, or discuss problem issues in general when the person is continually reacting emotionally.

4.2.5 Emotional and Reactive to Others

This is again similar to what was discussed regarding the individual being overly dramatic and making everything a major emotional issue. The Overfocused Subtype, in addition to being generally dramatic, is emotionally reactive, continually reacting to those around them. Someone says something and they react or someone teases and they react. Due to the continual reaction, conversations are difficult and it is also difficult to address household issues, rules, and behavior issues, whether that occurs with parent to child, spouse to spouse, teacher to child, peer to peer, sibling to sibling and so on. Eventually these people are avoided due to the emotional reactions. Significant others come to expect this emotional reaction and prepare for it even when it does not happen. Due to the expectation of their emotional reaction, they have fewer conversations and say less. Eventually, they are left alone.

4.2.6 Stubborn

These individuals appear very stubborn. It is not a true stubbornness because they do not intend to be stubborn and it is not as if they must have their own way. It is not the stubbornness and the "I'm right and you're wrong" characteristic of ADHD, which is caused by frontal processes being down so these individuals are unable to be flexible in their thinking. They cannot shift sets or think in different ways. They appear stubborn on the surface because of their tendency to become over-focused and then they get stuck and cannot refocus. The over-focusing makes them stuck; they only see one thing, one idea, or one solution and they cling to that thing, idea, or solution without consideration of anything else. This results in the appearance of being stubborn. If it is suggested that they are stuck on one track and are then asked to consider another track, this will release them from over-focusing and appearing stubborn.

4.2.7 Rigid: Stuck Like a Needle on a Record

This is similar to the discussion of being stubborn and the rigidity, described as being "stuck like a needle on a record," appears to be due to being over-focused and, consequently being stuck in their idea. It is not a true rigidity such as what would be seen in ADHD or any time the frontal processes are down and there is a lack of flexibility of thinking. This is more because of being over-focused than anything else.

The tendency to over-focus that results in appearing stubborn and rigid creates a drivenness and an inability to put on the brakes and stop. There are negative consequences to the person who is driven in this manner. These individuals tend to drive people crazy because they don't know when to stop. You can say "stop" and they keep on going past the point of other people's frustration. They are unaware of their impact and miss the social nonverbal cues and again don't read the signs of when to stop.

There are positive attributes in the rigid, stubborn behaviors of these individuals. Even if something appears that it is not going to work out, these individuals will keep on trying, they will keep on plugging and not give up until the job is accomplished. They don't take *no* for an answer, they keep going until they get *yes* and something works. As a result, they can accomplish the impossible; they make the business happen; they make the school project work; they make the impossible physical happen; they walk when told by medical doctors that they can't. This *driven* quality appears as obsessive-compulsive tendencies. They are productive and often quite successful. As the underdog, the long shot makes good.

4.2.8   Dislike of or Sensitive to Touch

These individuals are very sensitive and as a result they dislike being touched. A tap on the shoulder feels like a slug.

4.2.9   Intolerance of Transition or Change

Transition is awful. There is no tolerance for change. Change means something new, something different. Something new or something different spells trouble because there is more room for something to go wrong or for something bad to happen. They are also used to what they have, therefore, the idea of having to get used to something new all over again can feel frightening. I talked with one adolescent who by the age of 17 still remembered a house move that took place at the age of 9 and took her 6 years to recover from.

4.2.10   Colicky at Birth

We have found that these individuals, as infants, are easily upset, cry often, and cannot be soothed. Parents report their babies crying for hours and hours and nothing they do will relieve their child. This can create very difficult years, depression on the part of the primary caretaker, and, sometimes, eventual resentment of this new child. Digestive systems are problematic, food cannot be contained, different formulas must be tried, spitting up and projectile vomiting are common, everyone becomes tired and spent. Early infant years that are supposed to be filled with joy are filled with hours of trying to relieve this upset child, of being tired, and of feeling incredibly hopeless and helpless.

4.2.11   Eating Problems and Food Allergies

These infants, colicky at birth and experiencing difficulty with early feeding, develop food allergies. They become finicky eaters, eating only certain foods. Some parents report that their child will only eat peanut butter and jelly sandwiches. Often this population is allergic to milk products or is lactose intolerant. When there are eating problems, medication will tend to increase that problem and steps must be taken to ensure regular eating habits to avoid the stimulant medication causing significant weight loss.

4.2.12   Allergies in General

Due to the fragile nature and sensitivity of their systems, allergies are generally quite common and can be anything from allergies to stimulants in the environment or allergies to animals and so on. The definition of allergies is a basically harmless overreaction of the immune system to stimuli in one's environment. The immune system believes that these "harmless" stimuli are threatening and sets off the reaction that results in the "histamine" effect with runny noses, coughing, sneezing, and so on. Often, these allergies come and go throughout the lifespan, sometimes decreasing in adolescence and early adulthood, and sometimes increasing with the stress of productive adult years or with menopause. Anxiety does appear to be a factor that increases allergies and the tendency for the allergic reaction to occur.

4.2.13   Sleep Problems

Sleep problems are common to this subtype because their systems are always going. This group is phenomenal for always having that running conversation in their heads. They are always worrying, analyzing the situation, and consequently always talking to themselves. They are very busy in their heads and this pattern does not stop just because they want to sleep. So with the continual internal conversation that does not stop, they lie awake for hours before finally falling asleep. Once they do, this group is subject to waking in the middle of the night or long before it is time to get up. They wake up worrying. They are also very sensitive, so the slightest noise wakes them. As infants, they wake so easily things have to be totally quiet to get them to sleep and then must remain quiet or they awaken and the whole process begins again. As a result of intermittent sleep patterns, broken choppy sleep, and difficulty getting to sleep, there is chronic sleep deprivation. This is a great way to make someone mentally disoriented. With such sleep deprivation these individuals have dark circles under their eyes, are cranky, easily angered, and irritable, in general. And to top it off, they are less able to think and even more confused, which can add to the symptoms of the ADD.

4.2.14   Can Be Subject to Seizure Activity

These Over-Focused Subtypes appear to be a highly sensitive group, described as "fragile" and thus more susceptible to seizure activity. They are susceptible to mild seizure-like activation that results in tics and to the appearance of a mild seizure activity that occurs without the presence of any overt motor signs. Research is beginning to document a genetic type of seizure disorder. Seizures can occur at night with the individual moving all over, kicking off the covers. Sometimes children awaken on the floor. Sleep-walking is being seen as a form of seizure disorder. Babies are found at the foot of their crib. Children awaken just as tired as when they went to bed because, unbeknownst to them, they have actually been moving all night and never truly rested. There are mood swings, aggressiveness, and emotional over-reactions that make no sense. Often the presence of undiagnosed seizures results in the misdiagnosis of Bipolar Disorder. In other words, it is common for this group to develop symptoms of tics once placed on the stimulant medication, or often, these individuals will fly into an emotional speech, stop, and then not be aware of what just occurred or what they just said. It is as if they awaken up after being asleep for a few seconds and have no idea of what just took place. For a few moments in time, they are disoriented and seem very confused. Within the brain, a blip in the electrical balance has occurred. Remember, the brain communicates with itself in two ways; electrically and chemically. This involves the electrical communication system, and, during a seizure, everything stops for a few seconds. The result is this odd behavior without the memory of it and a loss of nutrients to the cells that eventually will cause damage to the brain if allowed to continue over a period of time.

Researchers have found that this subtype does tend to be more susceptible to seizure activity that is *awakened* by the stimulant medication. Parents often report that, once on Ritalin, their child turns into a different person. Once it is awakened, it is active and usually does not stop unless the stimulant medication is discontinued and, sometimes, it does not stop then. Therefore, with this population, it is important to determine a thorough family and individual physical and health history to make an informed decision about the use of stimulant medication. Everything is carefully considered, but often the stimulant medication is so critical to the functioning and needs of the individual that it will be utilized despite the knowledge that seizure activity may be stimulated or activated.

People report to me that they think the stimulant medication *causes* tics or evidence of seizure activity. This is *not* the case, the stimulant medication only stimulates what is there below the surface. If the problem is not in existence before the use of stimulant medication, then the stimulant medication cannot cause its existence. Therefore, tics will occur only if a tendency exists prior to use of the medication.

The last point from a clinical point of view, is that, generally more often than not, stimulant medication can be given with just about any medication (provided it does not load on the same neurotransmitters and does not have similar effects on the stimulant medication within the brain). It becomes a matter of identifying the underlying diagnosis, e.g., mild seizure-like activation, and treating the problem with antiseizure medication. Then the use of the stimulant medication can be resumed and taken with the new medication that has been identified to treat the underlying disorder.

4.2.15   Sensitive to Medications

Generally, these individuals are very sensitive to any type of medication and will over-react physically to them. So, taking a very minimal dosage of medication would impact the person with physical symptoms characteristic of a much higher dose. Very often, the person can be taking a mild dosage of the stimulant medication and it will create a physical reaction that results in immediate discomfort. The person blames the medication and discontinues use. Instead, we suggest that these individuals begin with a much lower dosage than the norm and then increase the dosage very slowly, in very minor increments.

For example, adults generally begin with 10 mg of Ritalin and then increase by 5 mg to their proper dose. For individuals sensitive to medication, it is suggested that they begin with 5 mg and increase by 2.5-mg increments to get to the proper dose. It is also suggested that a longer time span exist between the incremental increases in dosage. The usual time span is several days to a week but with this population, a week time span between each of the smaller increments is suggested instead.

Finally, this sensitivity does not occur with just the stimulant medication but also occurs with most medications these individuals take. The same dosage pattern is therefore suggested. This is one population for whom the use of nutritional supplements is strongly suggested to address the underlying issues that exist in addition to the attentional disorder. As a result, before suggesting any further medication in addition to that of the stimulant medication, it may be wise to try a nutritional supplement first.

4.2.16   Prefer to Chew Pills, Can't Swallow Pills

This group is highly sensitive as stated before and therefore they have a hard time swallowing pills. Very often pills need to be mashed and put into applesauce or chopped into little pieces to be taken orally. There is a discomfort about things getting "stuck in their throat." They, therefore, can only eat soft foods and can't swallow large pills. It is this issue that influences the description of finicky and particular eaters for this population.

4.2.17   Dislike Tight Collars and Cuffs

They feel something uncomfortable with anything tight against them. They like loose clothing and like things to fit loosely against their more sensitive areas such as the neck and wrist. Things that do not appear tight to others feel tight to them. They also can easily find clothing itchy and uncomfortable.

4.2.18   Combinations with Other Disorders

- Obsessive Compulsive Disorder
- Obsessive Compulsive Personality
- Borderline Personality Disorder
- Panic Attacks
- Phobias

- Depression
- Schizotypal Personality Disorder
- Schizoaffective Disorder
- Dissociative Identity Disorder
- Post Traumatic Stress Disorder

4.2.19   Summary

As infants these individuals have difficulty and become adults who are cranky, irritable, poor sleepers or short sleepers, colicky, finicky eaters and highly sensitive to touch, sometimes not even allowing touch. They overreact to change and see transition as terrible. It can take them years to recover from changes. They are sensitive to certain types of clothing, smells, climate, weather changes, and so on. We have found that they do not like anything touching their necks or wrists and prefer loose clothing. They can't swallow pills and need to chew them instead. Many are found to be overly dramatic, as if everything is a big deal. There can be a consistent emotional reaction that takes place. It is like adolescence expanded throughout the life span. Asthma or allergies are often present. This is where restricted diets are helpful. To help this population, we look to nutritional supplements in addition to the use of stimulant medication.

This is a group that demands creativity and the use of lots of ideas and resources. They tend to have many unexplained symptoms and prove very perplexing and frustrating to both the professionals who treat them and family with whom they live. There is a fragility to them and again lots of sensitivity. They tend to persistently invade other people's personal space and are very anxious. They, therefore, appear to be ADHD and are often misdiagnosed as such. Yet they think like the ADD without hyperactivity individual. The combination disorder of ADD without hyperactivity and ADHD has been proposed. It is our contention that what appears to be the combination disorder is truly the Over-Focused subtype of ADD without hyperactivity.

5

ADHD Revisited

5.1 Where Do We see It?

This is a more severe disorder than ADD and therefore makes up a smaller percentage of the overall population. In following the medical model, the more severe the disorder the less it exists in the population. The common cold is generally thought of as a milder illness and it happens very often. There are billions of colds occurring every day as opposed to something like strokes and heart attacks (although unfortunately they, too, are becoming far too common). Strokes and heart attacks represent a more severe disorder and so are seen less often than the common cold. ADHD is often seen in the criminal population but is less visible in a private-practice clientele. ADHD individuals have difficulties in maintaining employment and, as a result, have neither medical insurance nor a stable income. These individuals are impacted by symptoms of the attentional disorder to the degree that their lives do not recover. Their lives can become a series of endless failures, more trials and tribulations.

5.2 A Severe Disorder

This disorder is pervasive and involves more of the areas of the brain that are not operating as they should. Thus, these individuals may miss information, not be able to grasp information, or may become confused. Once they do manage to comprehend, they don't know how to use it. Frontal processes are nonfunctioning, and, therefore, the integrative processes are disabled. They can't understand pieces of information, they don't see the whole picture, nor do they think of the consequences of their behavior. The inhibition system is disabled and there is no stop sign. So they want *what* they want *when* they want it and they want it *now*. They operate out of the inappropriate because there is no appropriate regulation. They have no "stop" for the emotions because the frontal processes that work closely with the emotional system of the brain are not functional. So they get mad at little things and their anger is exaggerated. The punishment does not fit the crime. There is no tolerance. There is no hook to get them back. When things are overwhelming they leave and that is that. They don't care about the consequences or the impact of their behavior on those around them. They are not aware of their behavior nor able to process what it will mean in the future.

5.3   The ADHD Brain is Different

Research has shown that the ADHD brain is different from that of non-ADHD brains. The presence of this disorder has been found to be highly associated with what is called structural changes in the brain. This means that the sizes of certain brain structures are different from what has been seen in individuals without this disorder. Changes are in certain areas of the brain and can result in the presence of learning disabilities, dyslexia in particular. These specific areas are smaller in size, which has been thought to mean that there are fewer cells, thus fewer connections and a decreased ability for thinking. Areas targeted are the parietal area, parts of the frontal processes, and a watershed area where the primary lobes meet, entitled the *angular gyrus*. The presence of brain abnormalities also supports the notion that this disorder is more severe in nature.

5.4   General Problem Areas for the ADHD Individual

5.4.1   Time Sense is a Problem

With ADHD there is a skewed time sense. They cannot see that what they do now will impact the future of others and/or themselves at a later date. There is no delay of gratification due to disabled frontal processes and so they want it now. There is no time sense to allow any sort of wait. They therefore can't wait in lines and so on. This is the individual likely to cause a problem if waiting in a line for a long period of time. They blow up and explode. Due to a complete lack of time sense they can be late for appointments or miscalculate how long things will take. They justify tardiness, for example, by saying that the show won't start until they get there, or everyone will just have to wait. They are attempting to make sense of their experience for themselves.

5.4.2 Rigidity

Thinking is rigid or black and white with no gray due to the loss of the integrative functions of the frontal processes. Life is looked at from one perspective, i.e., tunnel vision, and therefore it can be difficult to get them to look at things differently or to take in new information. There is no argument — if they feel they are right, that is how it is. They also have excuses for their behavior, whether they make sense or not. They state their case so convincingly and feel so strongly that they are right, that one can't argue with them. These individuals do not work well with a team, cannot participate in teamwork, and constantly go out of their way to be the leader because they feel they know best and are right. They tend to do better at their own businesses. They like to have others working for them. These individuals tend to feel they do not have to go through the proper channels and will attempt to cut corners when possible. This can be a wonderful asset or a serious detriment if not used properly.

Interpersonal and significant relationships are highly affected by this rigidity. The inability to shift their thinking makes it difficult to see the other person's point of view and to see the whole picture. As a result, they are not willing to listen to significant people around them.

5.4.3 No Internal Stop Sign

Individuals with ADHD do what they want when they want to because their impaired frontal processs do not interjet the stopping to "think it through." There is also no hook and when they decide to leave, quit, or whatever, you have nothing to use to get them back. Guilt does not work. There is no anxiety and no reason to feel anxious, due to the "stop sign" of the frontal processes not being available. Anything goes and this is okay. These are the individuals most rejected because they will tend to do the unthinkable or the inappropriate. They stand too close or too far away. They are totally unaware of the impact of their behavior on others. They are missing the whole picture and missing the standards and value system with which to operate. With this often more serious diagnosis, these individuals are often the ones with the poor statistics, i.e., they get into trouble with the law, they get fired, they get into car accidents, they have numerous and overwhelming problems, and truly wear out the ones with whom they live and who try to take care of them. Outcomes are negative, there are many lost marriages, lost jobs, and lost opportunities. They are rarely seen therapeutically in a private-practice setting because they can't afford the treatment due to consistent job loss, and no medical insurance.

They don't know the word "no" and basically do what they want. On the plus side, these same individuals might create a million dollar business out of nothing because they would not take "no" for an answer and they keep going despite all odds. They may not quit a task as long as it is challenging, because it is exciting for them. When they do quit, it is due to low frustration tolerance and the tendency to give up as the going gets rough. The going gets tough and they get going. If someone else is upset it is not a problem or if someone says "no," they keep bothering them anyway, until they say "yes." This is a very powerful means that ADHD people use to get what they want.

5.4.4   Apathy

The ADHD person appears to not care about things ouside their own interest or self. This again is due to insufficient internal structure. It becomes difficult to discipline ADHD children, because they don't care, and if they truly want something or want to do something, they are going to do it regardless of your approval. It becomes difficult to think of things that might have an impact on them and create the desire within them to respond to your wishes as a parent. As spouses, ADHD adults tend to rationalize their behavior and to always have an excuse and, thus, do not respond to the feelings of others. Overall, this is a tough population to reach, impact, or convince of any way other than their own. To reach ADHD individuals means to create something that they find interesting — otherwise, forget it.

5.4.5   Moment-by-Moment Lifestyle

There is a need for instant gratification — *now* is the password. Due to the inhibition center being down there is no mechanism to allow waiting to occur. Instantaneous is the only way. There is no brain mechanism to allow them to see anything in the future and thus only the moment is an issue. Things that take a long time to complete don't get completed, due to the inability to see or visualize something long range. It becomes easier to quit and start something else. The continual "giving up" only serves to increase feelings of negativity and low self-esteem.

5.4.6   Fast-Paced Lifestyle

They are hyperactive and fast-moving, craving stimulation, and engaging in lots of risk-taking behavior. Frontal processes are down, there is no monitor, no gate, everything and anything goes. These individuals are not slow. They are quick in everything. It is not, however, the quickness of anxiety. There is a motor quality to their fast-paced movement. You don't see symptoms of anxiety. You see craving for stimulation instead — easy boredom and the need to be aroused. These individuals play hard and live hard. Those with ADHD are often more addicted to cocaine and heavy users of alcohol (possibly binge drinkers). In general, they tend to excessively over-drink, over-spend, over-gamble, overwork, and overeat. Overuse and substance abuse not so much to escape, but from the absence of the word "no" and without "no" there is excess.

5.4.7 Parenting Difficulties

ADHD children do not respond to consequences, which often can lead to parenting problems. There is a great amount of parenting stress with ADHD children. They are less likely to listen to their mothers, but will sometimes respond to their fathers, who have deeper voices and still retain some degree of novelty, as they tend to be home and with the child less of the time.

Many books available for parents detail working with the ADHD child. They suggest home programs and behavioral programs — e.g., tracking their child's behavior, making contracts with their child, and, generally, strong rule-based households. Consistency is a very critical issue. Parents of any child need to be consistent. Why? One, it ensures stability for the child and they can count on the rules to be the same time after time. Two, with the ADHD child it provides the much needed borders and boundaries. By detailing what they can and cannot do in a very explicit manner, it also clarifies consequences — what will happen if they don't perform the expected chore. Behavior and consequences are addressed.

With the ADHD child problematic occurrences will commonly happen when the parent most needs the child to behave. Talking on the telephone, in public settings, out to dinner, at the home of friends or relatives, riding in the car, while entertaining guests, mealtime, bedtime, and chore time become focal points in coping with the ADHD child who may or may not (depending on how he feels at that moment) behave, comply, or misbehave. The behavior of the ADHD child is not predictable. Finally, there is a good degree of sibling rivalry, jealousy of anyone who gets more attention or just more of anything. The whole family system tends to revolve around the ADHD child, who demands incessant attention.

5.4.8 Distractibility

Distractibility makes ADHD people veer off topic and not be aware of what someone with them might need or feel. Thus, they can appear highly insensitive. That is not the case, however; they are, in fact, very sensitive human beings. There is *constant movement* from one thought to another, one task to another, one place to another. They cannot sit still and need continual stimulation to remain in one spot. Anything stimulating or novel distracts them and will move them off task. They can easily shift from one activity to another without any sort of coherence or plan, rather it is just constant movement.

ADHD individuals will interrupt because their thought patterns just changed due to the distractibility.

The motor hyperactivity of the ADHD child is due to an additional system called the RAS which is not developed. By adulthood, what is left of the hyperactivity is overactivity, a constant state of movement. It is important to separate out anxiety symptoms from that constant movement and overactivity that has more of a "motor" quality. Adults are in a constant state of restlessness that contributes to their being impatient.

5.4.9   Planning and Organization: Sequencing Problems

ADHD people truly cannot plan and organize, frontal processes are down. They have absolutely no idea how to arrange things, whether regarding a sequential order or planning things in advance. They can't conceptualize — first we will do this and then that. They cannot organize their time and, therefore, do best on a constant schedule or routine with plenty of structure. The external structure provides the structure they are unable to create internally. They may have a million things to do and no idea of how to plan for all of those things to happen. Very specific steps must be provided for the ADHD individual. Tasks need to be broken down into specific steps with a specific order and setting priorities. They can't sequence to tell what should happen and when. They are unable to set priorities to figure out what they should do first, second, and so on. With ADHD, everything tends to be scattered "all over the place," e.g., their homework, their bedrooms, their bathrooms, and their lives.

5.4.10   Behavior Problems in School

The inability of the frontal processes to inhibit doing what they want results in considerable behavior problems. In school, they come to the attention of the teacher and those around them by being disruptive and again doing the opposite of what they are told to do. They don't listen and can be defiant. They are aggressive and don't always listen to reason. Again, this is because frontal processes are down. They see themselves as the most important people and can display arrogance. The egocentrism remains throughout the life cycle, rather than disappearing in childhood. That is why it is surprising to people that they are so sensitive; it's like they can dish it out but can't take it in return. Because this is so different a disorder and needs to be approached differently, it is important to separate ADHD from ADD without hyperactivity and clearly differentiate the two.

The behavior problems of the ADHD child result in the school not wanting to work with the child. The label of ADHD has come to mean something that produces a groan with school officials. As a result, they may act differently and, perhaps with a self fulfilling prophesy, wait for that child to become a behavior problem. This really was confirmed in a recent local issue involving a parent of an ADHD child who felt that the school administrators had not met the needs of her child. She took the case to the courts and a circuit-court judge ordered the school district to re-admit an ADHD student who had been accused of considerable disciplinary problems. The judge in this case did leave the door open for the district to return to court if the child's disruptive behavior continued. The supervisor of special education had wanted to send the child to a special school for the emotionally impaired and the parents wanted him to remain in the regular school setting. Unfortunately, it often happens that the child's behavior is so problematic that it becomes easier to label that child as emotionally impaired rather than cope with the symptoms of ADHD.

Thus, educators tend to give up on these children and parents feel abandoned and confused. It is hard to see one side or the other as being right. Teachers have too many children in their classes to continually address the behavioral issues of the acting-out ADHD child. If they do address these issues the rest of the children do not receive the same degree of education. The more time the teacher takes to discipline that child the less time she or he has for the other children and the more frustrated that teacher may become. In this particular case, the teachers argued that they wanted to be able to teach and not provide continual behavioral restraints. On the other hand, for the parents their child is not emotionally impaired or sick. They are ADHD, which is a genetic condition they cannot help and they should not be labeled as sick or refused needed help. If children are continually being pulled out of the normal classroom, how will they learn how to behave and exercise the appropriate restraints? The debate continues.

5.4.11 Learning Difficulties

ADHD people struggle to use feedback as information to modify their behavior or learn from their mistakes. They have true learning problems or learning disabilities. This disorder is highly associated with learning disabilities due to the frontal processes not functioning at level. What researchers are now finding is that there are actual measurable differences in the brains of those with ADHD from those diagnosed with learning disability. These are what we call structural differences, which means that some of the structures in the brain are actually different in size and makeup. The findings point to the frontal areas of the brain and to the watershed area that connects to a number of other areas and is more of a central location in the brain. QEEG showed frontal findings with abnormality. Therefore, when attempting to teach the ADHD individual, learning needs to be clear and short not overly long and involved. Explanations are best kept short and to the point.

Unfortunately, ADHD has been severely over-diagnosed and ADD without hyperactivity individuals, who are so easily traumatized, end up being treated improperly. With ADHD, consequences need to be swift and without warning. Because they don't learn from their mistakes, it's important to catch them off guard, lower the boom, and attempt to make an impact to get through their wall of indifference.

5.4.12   Impulsivity

ADHD individuals think of a behavior and do it. Most people think of doing something and then another thought comes into their heads and reminds them of the consequences or what will happen. So they don't do it. ADHD people think of it and do it before going through the rest of the process and considering what the results of "doing it" will mean. With ADHD, behavior is characteristic of true impulsivity, which involves the absence of the neurotransmitter serotonin. When tasks become more boring, there is more non-conscious processing and poorer inhibitory control. ADHD individuals cannot use private internal speech to learn. As a result, they don't have the self-regulation necessary to either talk themselves through a particular task or stop a behavior. This is the reason those cognitive or thinking strategies do not work with the ADHD person. They cannot have a conversation with themselves and say, "This is not a good idea to do" or to use cool-down statements like, "I will not take this personally," "I will not react to what is going on," "I am in control," "I can handle this," "I can make this happen," and so on. By the same token, they have difficulty taking in the positive, and in using and remembering positive statements from others or positive reinforcement. So they can't say to themselves, "I can do this, I remember doing this before," "I can make this happen as I did before."

5.4.13   Irritating to Others

The ADHD individual does not know when to stop doing something that is bothering someone else. The lack of an internal "no" and "stop sign" can make them irritating to others. The child irritates and agitates both siblings and peers. The adolescent alienates others with an "attitude." Adults are totally unaware that they might be offending others with their behavior. Even when told of the offending behavior, they still continue. If you ask why they would continue in a behavior they know is offensive, with an angelic smile they will respond, "Oops! I forgot," and indeed they probably do and did. The lack of the stop sign makes the ADHD person who may have the best intentions continue to be aggravating to those around them. They easily become identified as the bad child, the defiant teenager, and the pain-in-the-neck adult. They can be ones to be avoided at all costs and the ones with whom no one asks to play or do things.

5.4.14   Low Frustration Tolerance

There is a very low frustration tolerance, meaning that when they are done, they are done. And again, there is no hook to get them back, because they don't care. When things become difficult there is no mechanism to make them stick with the task and to keep going until they learn or until things become easier. As a result, they give up after little tolerance and that is that. This is a considerable problem that creates numerous difficulties for the ADHD individual and results in a lack of follow through, poor task completion, inability to meet goals, loss of job position, failure to advance in job setting, and lack of career advancement overall. It becomes easier to just live day by day. As money becomes harder to earn, crime might become more appealing and looked at as a means to resolve the financial problems that have accumulated over time.

5.4.15   Cannot Delay Gratification

There is no mechanism to delay gratification. The internal "stop sign" is down and there is no available apparatus to inhibit one's desire or allow one to wait. It simply has to be *now*. Also, due to a lack of time sense, they don't conceive of a future and cannot delay what they want because it could mean they won't get it. These individuals have to be taught the concept of time and continual practice of waiting for things with the consistent idea that they will have what they want in time. Practicing waiting a little bit more and a little bit more improves this problem and allows the person to get used to the idea.

5.4.16   Abusiveness with Significant Others

These individuals are easily agitated and their sensitivity makes them vulnerable to criticism, so they *react*. They get angry and can take out that anger on others. There is projection of their responsibility on others; others are to blame for their behavior or the problems they have created. It is not their fault, but the fault of others. As the reaction continues, they can strike out at children, spouses, or anyone who comes in contact with them. Abuse also takes place because there is no stop sign available to say *no*, so anything is okay. Finally, when abuse does tend to occur, more often than not there is a family background for it. Abuse is not approved of by society and when the family or mini society accepts, then it is more likely to occur. Thus, children raised with abuse go on to abuse, they marry spouses who abuse and it goes on and on. This is the only way they know to resolve problems and express anger. Interestingly enough, along with the abuse that is passed down to family members comes also the attentional disorder of ADHD. As a result, very often abuse goes hand in hand with ADHD; they feed off each other. Due to the problems associated with the attentional disorder, the person becomes frustrated and takes it out on family members.

5.4.17   Lack of Follow Through or Poor Task Completion

They do not complete what they start. They can't see the end. They don't know and can't follow the steps. Everything is overwhelming and it is easier to quit and give up. There is little tolerance for difficulty or discomfort. Tasks do not get completed, follow through does not occur and it is usually someone else's fault.

5.4.18   Lack of Connection to Others

Connection to others does not usually occur. It would only be an intense need for something that would make this individual pursue any "connectiveness." This is primarily based on the generalized tendency to avoid connection and the lack of a value system — they do not care how they affect those around them. Due to the frontal processes not being available, there is a lack of caring that is necessary for a connection to occur. People tend to be seen as objects around which to move and to manipulate to get what they want.

5.4.19   Angry and Insensitive to the Feelings of Others

These individuals generally are angry, irritable, and insensitive to the feelings of others, again due to the lack of connection. In addition, people tend to get in the way of their wants and needs and are, therefore, seen as problems that intervene with getting what they want when they want it. Thus, ADHD people tend to become angry with others, especially when they are in their way. There is a lack of feelings and a lack of empathy due to the lack of availability of the frontal processes necessary to provide the whole picture, control the emotions, see things from someone else's perspective, feel things from someone else's perspective, and care about someone else's perspective.

5.5   The Future is Filled with Problematic Outcomes

There are worse statistics for this population than for the other subtypes of ADD. ADHD individuals tend to lose their jobs and become involved with the legal authorities. They are often convicted of criminal charges ranging from traffic violations to breaking and entering, assault, robbery and offenses related to either the possession of narcotic substances or the sale of narcotics. Substance abuse tends to be that of the most addictive drugs available as these individuals search for a new "high" in their desire for constant stimulation. Cocaine, heroin, and substances similar to these drugs tend to be the drugs of choice.

5.6   A Number of Other Diagnoses Will Look Like ADHD

It is very important with this diagnosis to rule out other factors such as Hyperthyroidism, Antisocial Personality, Conduct Disorder, or Bipolar Disorder to determine which factors are due to an attentional disorder and which are due to some other underlying disorder. There is a need to separate mania from ADHD symptoms. The symptoms of these disorders are interchangeable and symptoms that appear as ADHD may in fact be something else.

5.7   Other Diagnoses Seen With ADHD

- Oppositional Defiant Disorder
- Conduct Disorder
- Antisocial Disorder
- Bipolar Disorder
- Alcoholism
- Substance Abuse
- Addiction
- Learning Disability
- Hyperthyroidism
- Child Abuse
- Dyslexia
- Impulsivity
- Tourette's Syndrome
- Spousal Abuse

5.8   A Final Note: Let's Not Forget the Positive Attributes

ADHD individuals are exciting. They are the movers and the shakers and they don't stop. They keep going. There is no end to their energy. There is that drivenness but more from the need to be best or the craving for stimulation as opposed to escape behavior or over-focusing. In certain areas or occupations, having the symptoms of ADHD can pay off and produce very positive results. Certain occupations demand that aggressiveness, that forging ahead despite the odds or the feelings of others, that getting the job done and forget about the means. The ADHD person can work in some settings or job situations quite effectively.

6

Comorbid, Associated Physical Disorders

6.1 Differential Diagnosis The Importance of

Having an attentional disorder or ADD alone is usually not the case. If you think about the idea of disturbing the biochemical balance in the brain and creating an imbalance, then it would stand to reason that such an imbalance could result in other disorders besides ADD. ADD, being a biochemical imbalance, involves two neurotransmitters or brain messengers, dopamine and norepinephrine. The job of these two brain messengers is arousal and alertness. They arouse and alert the brain structures in specific areas so those areas function as they should. Given the decreased amount or capacity of these neurotransmitters, and that they specifically impact the parietal and frontal processes, it would stand to reason that those areas do not function as they should. Once you disturb the brain's biochemical balance with ADD, further difficulties will ensue. Neurotransmitters are like dominoes. Some excite and some inhibit, but they all constantly impact each other. Once this system has interference, other systems have interference. Further, the neurotransmitters dopamine, norepinephrine, and serotonin are the same neurotransmitters involved in just about any existing emotional or psychological disorder. It makes sense that the imbalance would not just create ADD but other disorders as well.

This is exactly what occurs. More often than not, ADD is not seen by itself but with a whole host of other disorders. Therefore, the diagnosis of ADD is often just the beginning, but certainly not the whole story. There are other diagnoses that accompany this disorder, both physical and emotional. This chapter addresses physical disorders that are commonly seen and some that are rarely seen in conjunction with the attentional disorders. Some disorders will look like ADD but in fact are the result of another disorder instead. Symptoms overlap and can easily confuse the diagnosis of the true disorder. There are often accompanying, unexplained behaviors that cannot be understood merely from the standpoint of ADD. The presence of these disorders can make the ADD person look *demented* or out of balance. Instead of seeing this behavior as due to the presence of some other disorder, it is seen instead as only ADD, which can be a grave mistake. A good rule of thumb is to expect other disorders to occur along with the attentional disorder.

ADD is the *substrate*, the *base*. There are other diagnoses in addition to the attentional disorder that exist in the everyday population. The idea is that ADD exists as the primary disorder that often results in layers (or symptoms) of secondary disorders. As such, ADD serves to further complicate things, especially if existing as an undiagnosed base. Symptoms that are thought to be connected to depression may well be the result of ADD. Reasons that treatment is not working, and the situation is not changing, may be due to undiagnosed ADD factors. Often, as clinicians, we diagnose the other disorders and miss the attentional disorder and attribute symptoms of ADD to something else.

For example, a common mistake is the diagnosis of depression without recognition that much of it may be reaction to the presence of the attentional disorder and its impact on the person's life. Depression is a common reaction to knowing that you *can* do something and yet often not being able to do it. Every now and then ADD individuals can accomplish the task, which confirms that it is *possible* but then it can be followed by a failure of some type. They are left wondering if they can or can't accomplish the task, or perform the job and so on.

This chapter and Chapter 7 look at the overlap and interference of the diagnosis and the syndrome of ADD as it relates to other disorders. ADD without hyperactivity generally will be co-related with

- Reading disorders
- Problems with the parietal and temporal areas of the brain
- Spatial problems
- Hypoglycemia/hypothyroid
- Asthma

Physical symptoms seen with this disorder are

- Eating problems
- Fatigue
- Stress
- Headaches
- Sleeping problems
- Irritability and nervousness
- Stomach upset

- Aches and pains
- Rapid heartbeat
- Dizziness–lightheadedness
- Nausea and vomiting
- Diarrhea
- Constipation
- Weakness
- Confusion
- Dry mouth
- Mental and physical restlessness

ADHD tends to be co-related to

- Hyperthyroid
- Learning disability
- Tourette's Syndrome

Overfocused subtype of ADD without hyperactivity has physical symptoms seen with this disorder

- Difficulty chewing and swallowing pills
- Upset stomach
- Colicky as an infant
- Cannot stand tightness at cuff or sleeve
- Easily stressed and frightened
- Sleep problems, sleep deprivation
- Fatigue, can't sleep, and can't get up in the morning
- Low blood sugar, hypoglycemia

All ADD/ADHD groups tend to be more vulnerable to allergies and asthma than the general population. Allergies and asthma associated with ADHD and ADD without hyperactivity often improve when diet and nutrition are properly maintained. Thus, the practice of withholding anything containing dye from the ADD child's diet produces some positive results. We thought at first that this was the answer and the cure to ADD. These results were temporary however, and did not impact the child's thinking abilities beyond the initial positive effects from the overall report of feeling physically better.

6.2 The Following Disorders May Commonly Be Seen With ADD or Appear as ADD

6.2.1 Dyslexia

Research indicates that those with familial dyslexia (meaning that this disorder was seen in the genetic history among several family members) have greater incidence or presence of prenatal complications, left handedness, right–left confusion, reading and spelling problems, and are more likely to report depression and anxiety symptoms. Studies show that the brain of the dyslexic is inherently different in a number of ways. For instance, there can be damage to the brain that results in difficulty with reading. ADHD has been found to be associated with learning problems such as dyslexia. Recent research indicates structural differences in the brain itself. There appears to be a problem in the connectivity between the neurons that results in less efficient or inefficient functioning. Researchers are currently attempting to determine which specific area of the brain is involved. There are differences noted in the striatal system (caudate volumes), corpus callosum, and an area called the planum temporale, where areas have been found to be smaller in the brains of those individuals diagnosed with dyslexia. The planum temporale is an area responsible for skilled reading and malfunctioning, which is why it can create the reading difficulty seen with dyslexia.

Because they display reading difficulties, many individuals with ADD without hyperactivity are often mislabeled dyslexic when really they suffer from a spatial problem that results in an inattention to the whole. Research shows that an inability to see the whole of something is due to the parietal or spatial area of the brain not functioning properly.

This differs from the brain of the ADHD individual. The problem for ADD individuals is not structural but instead the result of a faulty chemical-messenger system. This is not the same as the brain that is structurally different at birth, as is the case with ADHD. Therefore, with ADHD there is a structural problem and with ADD without hyperactivity there is a functioning problem. This is similar to a building being structurally sound but not operating as it should. Genetically at birth with A.D.D. without hyperactivity, it is the parietal area (or spatial area) and its connections that are impacted by the biochemical imbalance. However, by the time of 5 years of age the problem that originally was due to ADD is now the result of lack of use. ADD individuals while compensating for attentional symptoms over-build the logical reasoning area of the brain and the consequence is the under-building that naturally occurs with the spatial area. The need to remain focused on fixing the symptoms of ADD leaves the person little time to address naturally weak areas of brain functioning. It is the under-building of the spatial area that produces the inability to think from a spatial perspective. It affects reading in that the person cannot learn to read phonetically; they know the individual sounds, but cannot blend them into the word to be pronounced. In our testing process over the last 15 years we see the same problems of pronunciation with everyone who has this spatial difficulty, *meaning they all sound out the word the same way.* **Epitome** becomes *Epit-a-tome*, **paradigm** becomes *para-dig-em*.

One of the best ways to see if this problem is present is to hear someone read a paragraph out loud. With numerous omissions, substitutions, and additions, pretty soon that paragraph takes on a whole new meaning.

Oftentimes, it is the Overfocused Subtype of ADD without hyperactivity that creates the greatest gap between very poor reading skills due to lack of use of spatial areas, and evidence of well developed logical reasoning abilities. These are the individuals who are so determined not to fail that they avoid, in any manner possible, the task that is difficult for them. Often these individuals are excellent readers in early years, sometimes known as prodigy readers. They memorize their words and become contextual readers (using the words they know to determine what the sentence is saying, trying to understand the context of the sentence without knowing all the words). However, as words increase, demands of the academic environment increase, and the pace quickens, this method of compensation becomes a more difficult task. Reading begins to decline. These individuals report that they no longer like to read (they were avid readers before) and they avoid reading, which further exacerbates the problem. The brighter the individual, the more the gap and decline in reading in later grades.

EXAMPLE

I recently worked with the mother of a 10-year-old boy who could not read and was diagnosed with dyslexia. Having reviewed the testing, I saw no evidence of any problem with learning, therefore I ruled out a learning disability. I did find a severe ADD disorder with inattention to the whole and spatial problems. This diagnosis fit with what this mother knew about her son. Her son could sound out words, knew his letters, and understood words and word meanings but could not read because he could not put the sounds together. His word-attack skills were the problem. He could not visualize the whole of the word. This was a bright boy. When tested intellectually, however, he scored in the mentally retarded range, when, in fact, he had average to above-average potential. The severity of the ADD and the reorganization of brain functioning to accommodate the symptoms of ADD and to compensate for these symptoms had produced such serious spatial problems that this child was not learning to read. He, therefore, was seen as having learning problems and not as disabled or unable to learn. He had learning problems due to these severe attentional symptoms and spatial deficits. If this is not recognized, teaching cannot be tailored to meet his needs and he, therefore, cannot learn to read. This is why it is so important to separate out what is true dyslexia and the reading problems due to the presence of ADD.

Similarly, I recently met with a 25-year-old male who was absolutely convinced that he had learning problems. He exhibited learning disability symptoms and was diagnosed dyslexic early in his school years. He was told he was unintelligent, could not read, and that was the end of it. On further examination, I learned that his problem was solely a severe inattention to the whole: an inability to see the whole of the word, thus making it difficult to read. He was amazed to learn that he was not dyslexic but rather ADD. He repeatedly questioned the results of our battery, reviewed the findings over and over and still was not convinced, until attending a seminar. At that seminar, he asked Dr. Beckley, who is a specialist in dyslexia, why he had been diagnosed dyslexic if this was not the case. He was informed that at the time of his evaluation (some 15 years earlier) that his diagnosis was based on the way dyslexia was measured and understood.

Another child was unable to read as a result of more serious issues, damage to the brain, or brain deterioration. Seizure activity, often undiagnosed, will affect memory processes and result in memory deterioration. Memory processes are directly targeted as an area of brain functioning that is more susceptible or vulnerable to seizure activation. This child's diagnosis, ADD without hyperactivity, Overfocused Subtype, and seizure disorder, resulted in a combination of symptoms that caused him to be unable to use memorization to compensate for the reading difficulties caused by the spatial issues related to the ADD symptoms. Therefore, one of the two methods of compensation used daily by the ADD individual, memory and logical reasoning, was impaired. Without memory to learn, this child could not memorize information. This child could not visualize the whole word, after phonetically sounding out the individual sounds, and could not rely on memorization abilities to memorize the word instead. Learning, affected by memory loss, was substantially negated. Without the ability to purely memorize information, the information cannot be effectively recalled unless the person somehow can categorize the information into something relevant and attach meaning to it.

Memory processes of registration, storage, and later retrieval for both short-term and delayed recall cannot operate unless the material is logically formatted into some type of structure. Children often have reading difficulties that we expect them to grow out of. Difficulties are perceived as a lack of effort or lack of motivation on the part of the child. Children often show reading problems as early as kindergarten and continue to have problems from that time onward, particularly in the areas of reading comprehension, relating letters to sound out the whole word, learning phonetically, and often substituting sounds and words, thus changing the meaning of the sentence. However these are not learning issues, but issues either related to spatial problems, missing the whole of the word or sentence, or extenuating circumstances such as a memory problem. This illustrates much of the problem in the field. Many of the adults who are now being evaluated have been previously diagnosed with learning disabilities, specifically dyslexia.

Typically, the diagnosis of dyslexia is made by comparing intellectual testing with achievement evaluation. The Verbal IQ obtained on the intelligence assessment (generally the Weschler scales, WPPSI-R, WISC-III, WAIS-R) is compared with the reading standard score obtained on the achievement assessment (generally the WIAT, WRAT-R, Woodcock Johnson Psychoeducational Battery). If there is a 15-point discrepancy (in the expected direction, the IQ is 15 points higher than the Reading standard score), the individual meets the criteria for a reading disability or dyslexia. The average for this type of scoring is 100, and 15 points in either direction will yield above- or below-average performance (115 would be above average and 85 would be below).

The diagnosis of dyslexia in this manner can be problematic for several reasons. First *the Verbal IQ obtained using the intellectual assessment is incorrect due to a number of issues*. One, there are problems of spatial issues affecting the person's ability to view things from a whole perspective. Certain subtests composing this IQ value are particularly subject to this problem. Two, the person has not been able to learn due to motivational issues, giving up and the negative learning environment that has been created. Three, attentional deficits of information processing result in the failure to pick up information from the external environment. As a result, these people lack information. Four, they have memorized their words. Therefore, they have difficulty defining words to respond correctly to one of the verbal subtests in the intellectual assessment.

The achievement evaluation for reading is also incorrect. These individuals have experienced difficulty sounding out letters, putting the sounds together to sound out the whole word. They cannot recognize words correctly and generally word-attack skills are deficient as a result of spatial problems directly related to ADD. The expected 15-point difference may occur based on one or more of the above issues. When any of these are operating, the diagnosis is incorrect. A correct diagnosis of dyslexia can be made only when taking into consideration the issues of learning and the ability to learn, as well as the impact of my spatial issues.

6.2.1.1   What To Do

Clearly identify the dyslexia and exactly what problems are creating the reading difficulties. Address these issues. If there is a spatial issue — an inattention to the whole — then employ the computer for a whole-language approach. Teach memorization of words and specifically target the parietal area for remediation. Targeting the spatial area with different enhancement programs has proven to be quite beneficial. If there is a learning problem, it will be necessary to address those difficulties and develop and teach alternative reading methods. These suggestions are well laid out in learning-disability literature. If a seizure disorder is creating a memory problem that is negating the learning of reading, then medical management will need to be employed to stop the seizuring.

6.2.2   Learning Disability

The diagnosis of a learning disability can often be a rather convoluted and erroneous process similar to that described with the diagnosis of dyslexia. Current assessment involves comparing the IQ values obtained from the intellectual assessment with achievement assessment to determine the presence or absence of the 15-point discrepancy. However, the use of the intellectual assessment is subject to the following problems that can often result in incorrect conclusions.

1. A primary symptom of ADD is slow speed. The timed measurements on the IQ assessment will be affected and will not display the individual's ability. Instead, all that is measured is time as opposed to ability. Therefore, the potential is based on an incorrect assessment from the start.

2. The achievement assessment only reflects the learning difficulties these individuals have due to the attentional problems and not necessarily their inability to learn.

3. The entire testing becomes invalid due to the above-listed problems and, consequently, an incorrect evaluation can occur.

What we once thought was learning disability we now understand as problematic learning due to other issues. Learning disability was a blanket term simply used to describe a significant discrepancy between the potential and actual learning that one is able to attain in the academic setting. Evaluation tested one's potential by using an IQ assessment and then comparing that with scores on an achievement battery to determine the degree of learning. Based on the difference, the individual could be pronounced learning disabled in the specific areas where the problem occurred, such as reading, math, spelling, and so on. As previously explained, when diagnosing a learning disability, it is very important to have an evaluation that rules out the factors of an attentional disorder to determine if there truly is a learning disability.

Research indicates that learning-disabled (LD) children used a type of cognitive self-talk (private speech) as a means of allowing them to stay on task. Private speech is focused on and relevant to the task and is used by the LD group more so than controls. Interestingly, the use of task-relevant private speech increased in those diagnosed ADHD in addition to LD. Private speech is defined as externalized thought that is used as a self-guiding means to allow the child to remain focused on the task at hand. Discovered in this research was that this self-guiding function increased as the task or the conditions became more difficult and demanding. Even more interesting with this research was that ADHD children who had milder cases of the disorder and fewer symptoms were able to use private speech more as a means to self-regulate their behavior. It is also used as a strategy to alleviate the problems of the attentional disorder.

The issue of self-talk is important to consider when using cognitive control strategies as a means of controlling behavior, handling aggression, and problem solving. Using private conversations, these individuals talk with themselves about why they are angry and what they want to do about it. They talk to themselves about problem solving; how to define the problem and identify its solution. Finally, they talk to themselves to remain motivated, cheer themselves on, and remain on task. They tell themselves not to become distracted, finish what they start, and not quit.

ADHD individuals are missing this important tool. This is a very important tool in helping the ADD without hyperactivity individual to function well. It allows them to remain focused and to appear more intact than they are. By definition, ADHD individuals do not usually have this asset available to them. In all probability, those identified in the research as having mild forms of ADHD are probably ADD without hyperactivity because it is so rarely recognized and so difficult to define. Much of the research to date is questionable in its validity due to problems of identifying the "true" ADHD. Therefore, those individuals identified as mild ADHD who were capable of private speech were probably closer to the diagnosis of an attentional disorder without hyperactivity. ADHD, due to unavailable frontal processes, does not have the ability for private speech and cannot reason things. The lack of this asset is the reason that they typically experience increased difficulty and come to the attention of school officials earlier than ADD without hyperactivity.

6.2.2.1 Importance of Self-Talk and Its Use

Self-talk is an important concept because it can exist within people to help them in a number of situations. Whether self-talk is in the form of a cooldown, motivational, or encouraging statement, it helps them to analyze and talk things out rather than react. It is used as a strategy to stay on task and not become distracted. Think about all the times we naturally converse with ourselves and don't even notice we are doing it. This conversation can provide a number of different ways to handle oneself in a given situation and is a powerful tool to use in coping with life.

Persons with ADHD do not have access to this tool that others use so much they are unaware of its presence. As a result of the frontal processes being down, the ADHD children or adults are unable to use self-talk or "cognitive" strategies and, therefore, lose their ability to rationalize a situation and not react emotionally. Self-talk cannot be suggested as an approach for ADHD people because they do not have it available. This also explains their reactiveness and tendency to do as they please without interaction with or from others in their lives.

6.2.2.2 Statistics and General Information

Seventy percent of ADHD children investigated qualified for learning disability diagnosis and services due to poor language abilities. Just as in the case of the dyslexic, it is critical to distinguish a learning disability from an attentional disorder. LD simply means that the individual is unable to learn at his or her potential for some reason. ADD individuals are constantly misdiagnosed as LD when, in fact, learning problems are clearly due to the attentional disorder.

ADHD generally is associated with LD. With frontal processes unavailable, the person is unable to learn. ADD without hyperactivity, however, is not an issue of LD. The confusion and inability to process information often make them appear as LD. Much of the intellectual assessment conducted with ADD children reveals IQ levels that would clearly qualify as LD. However, these scores are often varied and differ from one another because of ADD. Thus, IQ scoring is not necessarily relevant or valid for testing the ADD population. For this reason, we do not administer IQ tests to ADD adults. Also, it's important to remember that very bright ADD individuals will tend to work with their strengths and neglect their weak areas. They will do this to such extremes that at later dates it appears as brain damage or LD. They score extremely high in some areas (strengths) and extremely low in others (weaknesses) that can appear as damage to the brain or the result of learning problems.

A recently isolated disorder, Social Emotional Processing Disorder, was indicated to impact nonverbal skills with severe spatial issues, missing of social cues, information-processing problems, and poor communication skills. We tend to find characteristics of this disorder with some adopted children, particularly from countries where there is a question of early deprivation. We tend to see more-involved and more-serious symptoms of the attentional disorder and, in addition, the seizure-like activation affecting the spatial areas that coincides with the description of this disorder.

6.2.2.3   What To Do

Clearly identify the presence of LD and rule out other issues that may be masking themselves as a learning problem. If a learning problem is identified, there are numerous ways to approach the condition using alternative techniques that have been well addressed in LD literature.

6.2.3   Autism

Autism is seen as having a defined and characteristic course, with symptoms of social deficits, communication abnormalities, and stereotyped or repetitive behavior. Causal factors are genetic, with a rate of occurrence of 6% to 8% in families with a diagnosed member and less than 1% of the general population. Social and communication problems are primary issues measured in the families of autistic children. Autism can be viewed as the result of sensory overload. The senses are inundated with stimuli bombarding them and are without the ability to gate out the stimuli and thus provide some sort of degree of regulation. A helpful picture is that of a person being attacked from all sides. Stimuli come rushing at them and they are unable to compartmentalize or separate them. Everything becomes a blur. These individuals become so sensitive that a light touch feels like a punch. As a result, they don't like touch. It unnerves and alarms them. Everything is just too sensitive. Noises above a whisper are too loud and upsetting. Too much noise easily results in overload and discomfort. Conversations are too busy and filled with too much activity to comprehend.

Several areas of the brain are currently under investigation as developing abnormally, thus producing the symptoms of autism. Research indicates a general abnormality in the limbic area and its connections. There appears to be an abnormal level of activity that consistently occurs in this emotional center of the brain. This results in the emotional sensitivity that becomes so heightened it is unbearable for the person. Autism can be correlated with or related to an attentional disorder in that symptoms are similar: vulnerability to distraction and inability to gate. It is difficult to define at this point whether this disorder is seen more with ADHD or ADD without hyperactivity. However, with improved evaluation, there is the probability that the latter disorder will become more typically related to the autistic individual. The general fragility and problems with the parietal areas are found to be more involved with autism, which is also the area more involved for ADD without hyperactivity.

There is the need to separate out one unique form of autism — Asperberger's Syndrome. This syndrome has symptoms that are highly characteristic of the Overfocused Subtype of ADD without hyperactivity and the Fragile X Syndrome. Often children are mislabled as autistic when there are memory problems or seizure activity that are producing the communication difficulties and odd social behavior in relationships. Recent research is identifying a disorder called Pervasive Developmental Disorder to describe a range of symptoms that are autistic in nature. The idea is that some degree of autism may be present but symptoms may range from mild to severe. The other idea is that often the child is diagnosed as autistic when there may be other issues instead, hence the term Pervasive Developmental Disorder.

6.2.3.1 Defining Asperberger's Syndrome

Asperberger's Syndrome is seen as a social isolation disorder characterized by

1. There is a tendency to be solitary.
   a. The person has no close friends.
   b. The individual avoids others.
   c. The person has no interest in making friends.
   d. The person is a loner.
2. Overall, there is impaired social interaction.
   a. The individual approaches others only to have immediate needs met.
   b. There is a clumsy social approach.
   c. There is a one-sided response to peers.

     d. There is difficulty sensing the feelings of others.

     e. There is a detachment from the feelings of others.

3. There is generally impaired nonverbal communication.

     a. They have limited facial expression.

     b. The person is unable to read emotions from the facial expressions of others.

     c. They are unable to send messages with their eyes.

     d. They do not look at others.

     e. They do not use their hands to express themselves.

4. There are odd speech patterns and abnormalities in the inflection of speech.

     a. They talk too much or too little.

     b. There is a lack of cohesion in the conversation.

     c. There is a repetitive pattern of speech.

     d. There is an idiosyncratic (specific to that person) use of words.

In our clinical practice we tend to see the presence of Asperberger's Syndrome with ADD without hyperactivity. This individual can also look like the dramatic, shy, Overfocused subtype. Autism as a whole can be paired with either ADD without hyperactivity or ADHD. It is *critical* to separate out the two disorders to understand how to cope with these individuals and their needs.

6.2.3.2   *What To Do*

Identify the level of autism. What is really needed is not a neurological evaluation but a full neuropsychological evaluation — the paper-and-pencil testing to evaluate the brain. Then, depending on the findings, the child should be referred to a physician. Rule out other issues and other diagnoses that may be confused with this disorder. When identified, suggest support groups and the large body of literature available to specifically address the problems of this disorder.

6.2.4   Mental Retardation

Mental retardation is defined as less than 80 IQ points. It is usually genetic but can be due to brain damage at birth, a disease of the brain, trauma to the brain in childhood, and more. If simply based on numbers and intellectual assessment, evaluation of an attentional disorder could yield scores that would categorize the child as mentally retarded. Mentally retarded people who also suffer from an attentional disorder tend to display fewer behavior problems than would typically be seen with ADHD. This indicates that the retardation may stunt the intellectual ability to become delinquent. The idea is that attentional problems and conduct disordered behavior may be associated with mental retardation on a general level, but are not necessarily related to ADHD.

Finally, one must question the validity of self-report measures as a means to diagnose ADHD in this group because symptoms may be due to mental retardation and an absence of knowledge as opposed to the disorder of ADHD. This points to the inherent problem of using self-report measures to diagnose an attentional disorder. Similarly, there is a question as to whether the mentally retarded population can be termed ADD at all as they would automatically have difficulty in attentional processes as a result of their impaired brain functioning. One must measure the symptoms of the attentional disorder against the individuals' specific level of functioning, then measure symptoms relative to the people themselves. Once the intellectual level is determined, all scores on attentional measures are compared to generate a measurement of the level of mental impairment.

6.2.4.1   What To Do

Diagnosis is critical and must clearly identify mental retardation as opposed to evaluation problems and misdiagnosis. There are specific support groups available, as well as large amounts of literature, to cope with this disorder. Finally, recognize that a low intellectual level can be due to a number of different factors ranging from neurological disorders to injury to the brain to seizure activity and so on. The list is endless. It is easy to say someone is mentally retarded. Determining why their IQ level is so low is the challenge. Adequate treatment will depend on a good, accurate diagnosis.

6.2.5   Tourette's Syndrome

This syndrome is defined as a chronic familial disorder that has symptoms of motor and phonic (sound) tics. These tics are said to wax and wane in severity, meaning that they come and go. In addition, these tics are accompanied by a number of behavioral and emotional problems. This was once thought to be a rare condition, but is now estimated to occur as often as one case per 1,000 for boys and one case per 10,000 for girls. The typical age of onset is approximately 7 years of age; however, symptoms can appear in those as young as 2 years or delay presentation to as late as 20 years. Onset tends to be gradual, with one or more transient episodes that are short lived and eventually followed by more-persistent patterns of motor and phonic tics. The pattern eventually becomes severe enough to diagnose as the disorder itself.

However, Tourette's Syndrome is being looked at as emotional or aggressive outbursts from an unidentified location, perhaps as self-injurious behavior or head banging. What can be seen clinically is attentional and overactivity problems. There are many characteristics of Tourette's and this disorder has typically been defined as present with ADHD. It is proposed that children have ADHD difficulties before the onset of their tics. ADHD-like problems can be classified as predictors of the earliest manifestation of the biological vulnerability to this eventual tic disorder. Therefore, it may not be ADHD at all but, instead, the beginning of the behavioral display of the tics (or seizure-like activations). In our research, we commonly see ADD without hyperactivity associated with Tourette's Syndrome as the true clinical disorder that is present when not measuring things from a behavioral perspective.

Research, however, remains inconclusive regarding the comorbidity or co-association of ADHD and Tourette's. There is however, a proposed relationship to a seizure disorder, as tics may represent seizure-like activation of a small group of cells. What we have observed in our clinic is that severe cases of ADHD or ADD without hyperactivity tend to carry a predisposition to develop tics or seizure-like behavior that presents as a mild seizure activity with an absence of symptoms (meaning the lack of motor symptoms). For example, the person stares and then seems to awaken or gets highly emotional and then stops abruptly. A child, adolescent, or adult may become aggressive for no apparent reason and hit someone, swear or over-react in such a way that the punishment does not fit the crime. The behavior does not make sense. They may be described as being overly aggressive with emotional outbursts and not subject to reason. The key factor is that they have no recall at all of the behavior that just occurred and will deny that it happened. The child hits another child, seems to wake up as if in a dream, and has no idea that he or she just created this major scene. The adult becomes angry, swears and is verbally abusive, stops suddenly and looks as if they have just lost a moment of time. Which, in fact, is the case. Stressful situations can induce seizure activity. The individual may overreact to the situation that was triggered by stress, then move into seizure activity followed by inappropriate, out of control behavior.

Those individuals with undiagnosed seizure activity or Tourette's Syndrome, either initially or after a period of time on stimulant medication will have the tendency to develop tics or tic-like behavior. It may become necessary to remove the stimulant medication, introduce an antiseizure medication and then reinstitute the stimulant medication. The two medications appear to work quite well together. There is a technique called the QEEG, a computerized EEG, or a SPECT scan (measuring how the brain utilizes its energy) that identifies abnormalities in the severe ADD population, which may be more susceptible to other disorders. Again, it is critical to separate ADD seizure-like activation from Tourette's Syndrome. It is common for individuals to first be diagnosed as ADHD and placed on medication only to later find that Tourette's Syndrome is underlying and becomes stimulated and brought to the surface by the medication. The mistake is that the person is placed on medication to treat the Tourette's and the attentional disorder is never treated. We have found, clinically, that these individuals can function quite well on a combination of stimulant and antiseizure medications.

As a final note, remember that, although this syndrome is tied to ADHD, this is not necessarily the case due to the problems of diagnosis and misdiagnosis of ADD without hyperactivity.

6.2.5.1   What To Do

It is very important to identify the presence of this disorder as well as the presence of an attentional disorder, because the two usually appear together and are closely connected. As a neuropsychologist, Dr. Fisher is able to clearly identify the pattern of characteristics significant of seizure activity, however, this becomes a rather difficult task to prove on some of the medical measures such as the EEG. The EEG only has a 15% detection rate (85% of those with seizure disorder will not show up). Sometimes, the video EEG, QEEG, 24-hour EEG or SPECT scan offer alternative measurement with positive results. However, we have seen parents who are very aware of and able to document this confounding behavior that is highly typical of Tourette's Syndrome or seizure but cannot prove it to their doctor to institute medical management. Many parents suggest that their physician or neurologist come to live with them for just one day.

In our contact with the support groups, we have learned it is important to medicate both the syndrome and the attentional disorder. Too often, the seizure activity is treated with the necessary medication but the attentional disorder is not. Often after ceasing use of the stimulant medication in order to introduce the dedication for the seizure activity the stimulant is not re-introduced. There are many new antiseizure medications available with minimal side effects, such as Gabitril, Tegretol, Lamictal, Neurontin Toparimate and Depakote. They have been used with both adults and children. For those children unable to swallow pills, there are now Depakote Sprinkles available. They can eat them plain or sprinkle them on something. Depakote has side effects that require special maintenance from the neurologist or physician. This medication, however, has proven particularly helpful in targeting the manic, aggressive outbursts. Nutrition can also be quite helpful in improving overall physical health. Stress reduction and development of a comfortable lifestyle are also important components in coping with the disorder. Finally, this diagnosis can coexist with a number of other factors. Accurate assessment of Tourette's Syndrome as well as other issues is critical for effective treatment.

6.2.6   Epilepsy

Epilepsy is a condition involving seizure activity that occurs on a sporadic, occasional, or continual basis. The problem with seizures is that, at the time of the event, there is a cessation of all brain activity. For that very brief moment when things come to a screeching halt, there is a loss of oxygen to the brain, a shut-down of the electrical messaging system because cell death or damage to the brain nutrients don't reach the cells. The key to clear diagnosis is the description "brief." There is a "brief" spurt of emotion or a "brief" outburst of anger or aggression. It is not long lasting. It is "brief," with a rapid shift of symptoms. The brief outburst can also look like a panic attack with a cluster of anxiety symptoms such as heart pounding, loss of breath, and so on. There is a blank stare. One young man with tumors and documented seizure activity put his head down mid-task, then raised it a minute later and resumed the task as if nothing had occurred that was out of the ordinary. However, he had lost all that he had learned prior to the seizure. He had forgotten what he was doing and had to start over, yet remained oblivious to the incident

Research is now viewing seizure activity as related to unnatural phenomena such as sleepwalking, restless legs, unexplained personality changes, and a general emotionality that remains highly unpredictable and not related to the event. There is more anger than necessary for the situation so things don't make sense to the objective observer: the crime does not fit the punishment. It becomes important to separate this over-reactivity from an overfocusing that may be occurring internally within the individual.

The brain communicates with itself both chemically and electrically. When the electrical system stops there is a seizure. Like a blip on the computer, for a brief period of time everything stops. It is during this time that damage to the brain can occur because the cells are not getting the nutrients they need to live. Epilepsy may be a condition unto itself or due to other factors such as

- Trauma to the brain
- Substance abuse and overdose
- Toxicity
- CNS (Central Nervous System) or brain infection
- Hypoglycemia (low blood sugar)
- Fever
- Alcohol withdrawal
- Anoxia—loss of oxygen

All of these issues can produce seizure activity. Most seizures last approximately 30 to 90 seconds. Seizure activity can be triggered by stress and psychological factors as well. Clinically, it has been found that sometimes people can have a full-scale seizure, i.e., a *grand mal* with all of the motor symptoms of the body thrashing about, and then never have a seizure again. They take medication after the seizure, discontinue it a period of time later and may never experience another seizure. Some have chronic epilepsy requiring constant medication. Sometimes it is not recognized that they are having seizures. They may actually have seizures at night (nocturnal seizures) or absence seizures that occur for years that no one knows about.

EXAMPLE
We saw a 40-year-old woman whose father had been diagnosed with nighttime or nocturnal epilepsy. She herself, without realizing it, had been having seizures as well. On evaluation, considerable damage to the brain was found, particularly in the memory areas that are often affected by seizure activity in a very direct manner. The woman began taking antiseizure medication and although she could not reverse the damage at

that point, she prevented further loss of memory, and she began feeling and thinking better. The brain attempts to rehabilitate itself when there is no longer a process of continuing damage to the brain to prevent new learning or to negate the positive effects of lifestyle and diet changes and nutrition.

EXAMPLE

A teenager had been beaten up by a gang of girls at the age of 12 years. By the age of 16 she was moody, alternating between being highly aggressive and argumentative, and then sweet and considerate. Her school work had declined considerably and, once an excellent student who attained all As and Bs, she spent the first year of high school failing most of her classes. She had been seeing a psychologist for the previous four years and although things had definitely improved, problems obviously remained. The teen had been on a number of medications and the only one that seemed to make a difference was Depakote, so she was diagnosed as Bipolar Disorder. Trying to make sense out of the situation, her psychologist referred her for ADD testing to see if ADD symptoms were responsible for the academic problems. Upon being evaluated , it was clear that she was ADD without hyperactivity. However, that was the least of her problems. She had a very poor memory and further neuropsychological evaluation isolated a head injury from the original incident when she was 12.

It has been a common belief that the brain has greater rehabilitative ability in younger people. Until the age of about 13 years, the brain is still differentiating itself. While all of the cells are in the right spot, they have not yet become fully developed, specialized, or differentiated. Therefore, if there is a death of cells, then there are plenty more cells to take over and adapt to the area. What was not factored into the equation was the element of new learning and just how much learning occurs in the early grades of first through third. Therefore, the new research is now showing that even when children are younger, the cell death that occurs with seizure activation has far-reaching consequences. New learning is disrupted, and, until the activation is stopped, new learning continues to be impacted. Once the activation is stopped and new learning can occur, these children then have to make up what they have learned while facing a high demand for new learning in their academic environment.

The brain can still make progress and improve in functioning past the point of 13 years. Wonderful success has been seen when specific brain areas are rehabilitated. Therefore, rehabiliation can occur at all ages. There are, however, specific factors that occur with each developmental age, whether that is early childhood, late childhood, adolescence, young adulthood, adulthood, late adulthood, or advanced age. Computer training is one such rehabilitative technique. Specifically, virtual-reality training allows for generalization of learning. That learning can occur in a specific environment and then be applied to other situations as well.

6.2.6.1 What To Do

It is critical to identify the occurrence of seizure activity and to treat this problem with medication *as soon as possible*. The difficulty occurs when seizure disorder cannot be identified using the measurement techniques that are available. One of the problems that I have observed in my clinical practice is that symptoms highly characteristic of seizure activity may be measured using neuropsychological evaluation that may indicate that the brain is deteriorating. Yet EEG measures that are available to determine seizure activity may produce negative results.

Neuropsychologists may find themselves in arguments with neurologists regarding the utility of the EEG and its ability to adequately measure seizure activity. When unable to identify seizure activity, neurologists understandably will not prescribe medication. Other forms of measurement such as PET/SPECT scans or QEEG may help with diagnosis. If neurological diagnosis cannot be achieved to warrant medication, nutritional supplements can be used to calm the brain and hopefully provide some relief from seizure activity. (This has been seen to be effective in our clinical practice over the past several years as a first line of defense, but never constitutes treatment.)

EXAMPLE
The best example we saw of this problem occurred with a 5-year-old boy diagnosed with ADD who was having so much difficulty in his daycare setting that they were no longer able to have him at the facility. Having been placed on stimulant medication, this little boy began to have violent outbursts of which he was clearly unaware and did not remember later. When not suffering these outbursts, he was the nicest child you could find. Certainly, he was not the type to engage in such violent behavior. These short outbursts were highly characteristic of seizure activity. Neuropsychological evaluation indicated similar patterns tending toward epilepsy, yet neurologists could not confirm the disorder using EEG assessment and therefore would not prescribe medication. This was one case when nutritional supplements were utilized as an alternative solution.

Recently, we worked with the mother of a child who appeared symptomatic of seizure activity. Her child could not read by the age of 9 years, and his memory was highly impaired, although he tested well above average in the superior range for skills of logical reasoning. The neurologist administered a 24-hour EEG while the mother prepared all kinds of stressful situations to attempt to elicit a seizure that could be recorded. This method was employed when the office EEG documented no abnormal activity. The 24-hour EEG did show abnormalities and the child was placed on medication that ultimately changed the course of his school performance. He was reading one year later almost equivalent to his peers.

Neurologists are beginning to use trials of anti-seizure medication (given the new medications available with fewer side effects; Lamictal, Gatitril, Topamax and Neurontin are now available) when EEG findings are normal, however specific neurological deficits have been documented with neuropsychological evaluation, realizing the inherent problems of confirming this diagnosis with the EEG and similar types of testing measurements. Recent research is presenting Vagus nerve stimulation as an alternative to medication for partial-onset seizures, but long-term research would be necessary to confirm the validity of this approach.

6.2.7 Parkinson's and Huntington's Disease

These disorders involve the premature death of selected neurons in the central nervous system characterized by a progressive clinical disability.

6.2.7.1 Parkinson's Disorder

This disorder is clinically determined and distinguished by symptoms of slowed voluntary movement and tremors that occur when the person is at rest. The classic age of onset is after 50 years of age. It is defined as a *complex neuro-degenerative condition involving a motor disorder with symptoms of rigidity and tremor, with later effects on thinking abilities.* This disorder is found to be related to reduced levels of dopamine in the structures that compose the limbic system. The prefrontal region has been isolated as the area primarily impacted by this disorder. In later stages of its progression, the disorder displays symptoms related to damage in the supervisory area of the brain. Attentional processes regulated by this area show deficits which, by their very definition, are symbolic of symptoms of ADHD and may masquerade as an attentional disorder. Research with this population has found evidence of deficits related to problems in the frontal processes characteristic of an attentional disorder. Symptoms increase with stress.

6.2.7.2 Huntington's Disease

This is an inherited disorder that loads on the autosomal dominant gene and, at present, can be identified in individuals at risk for the disorder. It has a very strong genetic base and is classically seen in families passed down from generation to generation. This is a degenerative disease with clinical features of motor problems that are characteristic of a choreiform, dance-like movement whereby the body jerks and moves without warning and not at the will of the individual. What we did not know previously is that very early in the onset of this disorder, a psychiatric disorder becomes progressively worse until the person is so out of control emotionally that confinement is necessitated. Early stages of this disorder produce symptoms that are highly characteristic of psychosis. The person appears insane, but, at first, only intermittently until, as things progress, they appear demented all of the time. Dementia, or the loss of intellectual faculties, is also a characteristic of this disorder and occurs somewhat later in its progression. Onset can occur generally between the ages of 30 and 40 years and have a duration of 17 to 20 years. This disorder has been found to impact the GABA neurotransmitter system. Research is in the process of identifying specific medications for treatment, and nutritional supplements aimed at impacting this system are being studied as well.

6.2.7.3 Misdiagnosis with ADD

What is important about both of these disorders is that they can be misdiagnosed as ADD or vice versa. The attentional problems and problems related to the frontal processes are exacerbated Disorder Parkinson's or Huntington's Disease rather than ADD, and can easily be misdiagnosed. Even the emotional symptoms related especially to Huntington's can be mistakenly seen as the lack of inhibition and impulsivity of the ADHD individual.

6.2.7.4   What To Do

Again, there is the issue of identifying the correct disorder. Determine whether there is a combination of these disorders or a premorbid attentional disorder and know exactly what the symptoms are and the reason for them. Once identified, address problem areas with specific treatment. Nutritional supplements are emerging as a possible viable means of addressing the progressive deterioration of the brain and may prove very important in treatment.

6.2.8   Closed-Head Injury

Closed-head injury is defined as trauma to an area of the brain that is enclosed by a covering called the meninges. This outer covering is designed to protect the brain and injuries that occur beneath this protection are called *closed-head injuries*. Closed-head injuries can range from mild to moderate to severe. One way to determine the degree of injury is by noting the length of time the individual was comatose after the injury occurred. Another method is determining if a concussion followed injury. Symptoms of concussion are headache, disorientation, general dizziness, vomiting, and nausea. It is difficult to assess the degree of damage to the brain in a closed-head injury because often these individuals will appear quite normal to the outside world and may function as they did before the injury. Those close to such injured people, especially children, will probably assume they are intact to move following the trauma that occurs with such injury. Consequently, if they appear okay, it is easy to assume that they are okay and that we can forget the matter, consider it a bad dream and move on. Those involved in lawsuits are often told that they appear fine, there is no identifiable problem and thus no reason to sue for damages.

There is a real tendency to assume that because a person measures with average intelligence that they are fine. We tend to negate the fact that someone may have been superior in intellectual abilities prior to the injury and post-injury average functioning represents a huge drop for them. This may result in fear of failure, fear of risks and new learning situations, and ultimately low self-esteem. Additionally, children of 5 years and younger often appear intact, with average intellecual assessment, only to show later that they actually sustained enormous deficits as a result of the earlier trauma that do not appear until the brain is taxed with the demands and rigors of academic learning in later grades.

Only recently has there been recognition that a mild closed-head injury can have far-reaching consequences for individuals by significantly altering their lives and efficiency in everyday functioning. The most common issue is the inability to identify ongoing seizure activity that eventually results in personality changes, aggression and unexplained emotional outbursts, sensitivity to noise, temperature and touch, and overall undefinable inability to function as they did prior to the injury. We now know that there is an excitotoxicity that occurs in the brain as a result of head injury. This is the process whereby the brain reacts to any type of upset in its ongoing activity. The chemical balance of the brain is disturbed, thus upsetting the electrical balance and triggering a state of imbalance and ultimately seizure activity.

A diverse pattern with diffuse and generalized deficits in both the frontal and temporal areas of the brain affect the executive decision-making processes and memory processes and are most notable in closed-head injury. Deficits are difficult to define; recent and short-term memory are impacted first. These areas are affected because they are the more complex areas of the brain and are the last to form. They are, therefore, more vulnerable to impact to the brain. Attention and concentration problems as well as short-term memory problems are classically associated with closed-head injury. Outwardly, these people can look fine, however, they report symptoms of forgetting things, being unable to problem-solve situations as they did before the injury, and finding themselves easily distracted and inattentive. What occurs commonly is that either there is injury to the brain that masks itself as ADD, or there is ADD and the problem is not injury at all, or there is injury on top of ADD (whether diagnosed previously or not). One differentiating factor is memory. Generally, there will be no evidence of a true memory problem with ADD. It is important to identify the existence of a premorbid attentional disorder in the case of head injury. Usually, if there is a premorbid attentional disorder, the attentional problems will be exacerbated and those areas most reliant on frontal functions will be affected to a greater degree post injury. The person can present symptoms that can be characteristic of either of the attentional disorders, depending on the specific area of the frontal region that has been affected. Finally, it is important to note that the impact of head injury on a person already suffering from symptoms of ADD can be particularly devastating as the injury to the brain tends to impact the memory or logical reasoning processes — the two methods on which the person has relied before the injury to compensate for symptoms of the attentional disorder. Symptoms of the "pre-onset" or "premorbid" attentional disorder will increase as a result of the lack of formerly used compensatory mechanisms.

A neuropsychological evaluation can indicate several common problems

- Sustained inattention
- Problematic cognitive processing speed
- Learning problems
- Specific personality changes of disinhibition, apathy, and general irritability with head injury

6.2.8.1   What To Do

It is important to determine if there was an attentional disorder prior to the trauma or if all the symptoms are related to the injury. This is important because with ADD, the brain is already vulnerable and the head injury will exacerbate the ADD symptoms. Medication becomes an issue due to the possibility of seizure activity. Generally, in the presence of injury to the brain, abnormal tissue, or cell death, the brain responds with an electrical reaction of seizure activity. This needs to be medically managed. Stimulant medication has been shown to be highly effective with the head-injured population (whether identified as premorbid ADD or not) but should not be introduced until seizure activity is no longer operating as a variable. Further, if ADD did exist prior to the injury, it will make a difference in the rehabilitation process as there are additional factors to consider.

Nutritional supplements provide excellent help in rehabilitating the brain by impacting the neurotransmitter systems. Research reveals that head injuries have an extensive impact on the functioning of the brain by altering cellular changes via changes/alterations in the chemical messenger system. This problem tends to ensure continued deterioration of the brain following injury. Nutritional supplements are providing evidence that they are helpful in addressing this problem.

A neuropsychological evaluation will provide a wealth of information to aid in rehabilitation, target the specialized brain areas, or arrive at coping methods to move around or compensate for problem areas. This specific type of evaluation should include administration of a full battery: the Halstead-Reitan, in addition to selected additional measures of memory assessment, attentional assessment, and assessment of logical reasoning processes; also the Wisconsin Card Sorting Test, the MAS, the PASAT (CHIPASAT) Bender Visual Motor Gestalt Test, WRAML, and Children's Auditory Verbal Learning Test (AVLT) Cancellation Test. Such a battery of tests takes between 6 and 8 hours to administer. A new neurodevelopmental battery, the NEFCY, provides a full range of measures assessing children ages 3 to 13 years. When they have been completed, the neuropsychologist is able to specifically delineate problem areas, strengths as well as weaknesses, degree of problem, and potential of the brain.

Finally, it is critical with injury to the brain to have absolutely no use of alcohol. We once evaluated a woman 1 year post-injury from a serious auto accident. On testing, it became quite clear that there had been little, if any, spontaneous rehabilitation of the brain. Usually, within the first year, the brain has some automatic or spontaneous rehabilitation of itself as adjacent healthy cells take over the functioning of dead cells. We learned that, for medicinal purposes, she was consuming one glass of wine per day and this small amount was enough to prevent the automatic process of rehabilitation.

6.2.9   Allergies

Although it is common to find allergies among the attention-disordered population, allergies and ADD do not have a common biological background. This means that one disorder does not cause the other. It was once thought that allergies caused ADD or vice versa, yet this has not proven to be the case. Oftentimes, ADD and allergies coexist; that is the reason that diet programs are used to show some sign of relief for the ADD child — they feel better but changing one's diet has not had a permanent impact on the symptoms of ADD.

6.2.9.1 What To Do

The first means of defense is diet. Identify specific allergens and remove them from the person's daily environment. Nutritional supplements also are proving to be a means of controlling this overreaction of the immune system.

6.2.10 Thyroid Disorder

At one point, a theory was proposed that the symptoms of ADHD were due to a thyroid condition and that the two disorders shared a common biological origin. Abnormalities found in the HPA Axis (Hypothalamic Pituitary Adrenal Axis) occurred in one half of the ADHD children who were evaluated as part of a research project. When this finding first emerged, it was sensationalized by the newspapers and, for a short period of time, ADHD was seen as being due to a thyroid disorder. This turned out to be a rather small study that had inherent problems and the research was dismissed as being premature. The overall research, however, has consistently found severe ADHD individuals to be highly associated as an at-risk population for thyroid dysfunction and, in particular, hyperthyroidism. This is more of an issue for the severest, as opposed to the mildly hyperactive child.

In conclusion, disturbances of the HPA axis may have some causal effect on some of the symptoms associated with ADHD, such as disorganized sleep patterns and other habitual patterns. Several other statistics are of interest. An evaluation of the thyroid function showed that the presence of ADHD was 3.2 times greater for male subjects with thyroid problems — generalized resistance to thyroid hormone. Overall, the presence of ADHD was 2.5 times greater in those identified with generalized resistance to thyroid hormone.

6.2.10.1 What to Do

Several years ago, when a newspaper article linking ADHD to thyroid problems appeared, it was thought that a cure had been found for ADHD while providing a cure for the thyroid problem as well. Now what is understood is that while there is evidence of thyroid problems in conjunction with ADHD, one does not *cause* the other. Simply bear in mind that when diagnosing one of these disorders, the other may be present. Finally, in dealing with issues of either depression or anxiety, ruling out problems related to the thyroid is very important.

6.2.11 Digestive Problems Due to Anxiety

The physical consequences of anxiety impacting the digestive system in particular present problems such as

- Colitis
- Ulcers
- Irritable Bowel Syndrome

Symptoms seen are

- Problems with digestion
- Bowel problems
- Frequent urination
- Inflammation or burning
- Agitation

These symptoms may eventually create social problems. With anxiety as the substrate or causal factor, symptoms related to these issues are going to be highly related to ADD without hyperactivity. The more severe the attentional disorder, the more it will affect the level of anxiety, and the greater the level of anxiety, the greater the number of physical symptoms.

6.2.11.1 What to Do

This is one area where better diet and nutritional supplements can greatly impact and improve physical condition. Something as simple as calcium has a wonderful effect in relief of symptoms of anxiety. In addition, exercise or any means to reduce stress is extremely helpful. Use medication to treat anxiety, especially when symptoms are severe, because anxiety can have a negative effect on one's physical health. Medications that address the psychological symptoms of anxiety currently in clinical use are Luvox®, Paxil®, Zoloft®, Remeron®, Wellbutrin®, Serzone®, Effexor®, and Buspar®. Other antidepressants or anti-anxiety agents may also provide good results. If there is a great amount of agitation, other types of medications may be employed, such as antipsychotics, e.g., Risperdal® or Zyprexa®. It is suggested that your physician be consulted on a regular basis to address the physical ramifications because often these illnesses are not followed by the patient and can worsen with time. Later they often cannot resolved with medical management and necessitate more-drastic surgical procedures.

6.2.12 Chronic Fatigue Syndrome

Chronic Fatigue Syndrome (CFS) has been found to be associated with immune abnormalities. Symptoms of the disorder are characteristic of decreased immune-system functioning and have been found to increase with stress. Further, the type of immune problems may lead to a viral reaction that results in individuals' contracting the latest viruses found in their external environment. If the person is already diagnosed with an attentional disorder, stress increases symptoms of both CFS and ADD. Although there is no research known at this time, it would stand to reason that this disorder would be found more in the populations of ADD without hyperactivity and the Over-focused Subtype, due to their relationship with stress.

6.2.12.1 Symptoms

- Excessive tiredness
- Headaches
- Muscle tenderness
- Sore throat
- Irritability
- Crying spells and overall depression
- Low grade fever
- Painful lymph nodes
- Myalgias
- Generalized headaches
- Neuropsychological complaints, e.g., short-term memory, confusion, slow psychomotor speed
- Sleep disturbance
- Excessive vulnerability to the development of continual colds and other viruses
- Fibromyalgia lookalike symptoms

6.2.12.2 What to Do

Physicians tend to suggest consistent rest and good use of nutrition and diet. Nutritional supplements have been found to be highly effective in treating symptoms related to this disorder and helping move it into remission. It is important to also rule out other disorders such as thyroid issues, depression, anxiety, and fibromyalgia as well as other neurological conditions that can mimic these symptoms. When diagnosed with an attentional disorder, more often ADD without hyperactivity, there is great benefit from stimulant medication. However, medication needs to be carefully titrated or increased due to the upset that occurs with low blood sugar (hypoglycemia is frequently a coexisting symptom) and to exacerbation or increase of symptoms of CFS. CFS symptoms are often mistaken for Lyme Disease.

6.2.13 Fibromyalgia

Diagnosis is difficult and depends on the cardinal symptom of pain. There is a minimum of 3 months of generalized aches or stiffness, which

- Involves at least three anatomical locations
- Has at least six typical and reproducible tender points
- Excludes other conditions with similar clinical pictures

Four of the following eight minor criteria are required for diagnosis.

1. Generalized fatigue
2. Chronic headache
3. Sleep disturbance
4. Neuropsychiatric symptoms: depression and anxiety most common
5. Subjective joint swelling but no objective swelling
6. Numbness or tingling sensation
7. Irritable Bowel Syndrome
8. Modulation of symptoms by activity, weather, or stress

Similar to CFS, this disorder would seem to associate more with ADD without hyperactivity although there is no known research to date.

6.2.13.1 *What to Do*

Diet and nutritional supplements are important, as is targeted treatment for specifically identified problems via medication or physical therapy. Again, it is critical to rule out other disorders that may mimic symptoms related to thyroid, neurological disease, anxiety, and depression. Similiar to CFS, when an attentional disorder is diagnosed, there is great benefit from stimulant medication. Such medication appears to relieve the stress that frequently increases symptoms associated with both of these disorders.

6.2.14 Hypoglycemia

This condition is brought on by low blood sugar. A loss of nutrients to the cells results in the decrease of sugar or energy levels in the brain to the degree that physical symptoms result. This condition genetic, often seen as can be the precursor to late-onset diabetes and, if left untreated can result in a loss of insulin-producing cells (often seen with gestational diabetes). Hypoglycemia can often be seen accompanied by hyperthyroidism. This is a rather common disorder, not always diagnosed by physical evaluation, but most often identified by the individual if they are aware of the symptoms and their bodily reactions.

Hypoglycemia can be a common disorder resulting from malnutrition, malabsorption, drug use, and liver dysfunction. It is commonly seen in the alcoholic population and can be particularly in evidence when these individuals stop drinking and maintain sobriety for lengthy period of time. It can result in brain damage due to cerebral hypoxia (a loss of glucose, the energy substance necessary for the brain to function).

6.2.14.1 *Symptoms*

- Fatigue

- Can't get up in the morning
- Late afternoon fatigue
- Confusion
- Profuse sweating
- Blurred vision
- Binge eating — eating without stopping
- Sugar craving
- Poor appetite
- Rapid heartbeat
- Dizziness/lightheadedness
- Vomiting/nausea
- Irritability

This condition is highly observed in the ADD without hyperactivity population and often contributes to their being misdiagnosed. There is an irritability or "snap" that occurs with the drop in blood sugar that is misunderstood and the person is seen as having temper outbursts and moody behavior. Although these symptoms seem to be ADHD, they may be due to blood-sugar issues and not necessarily the true persona of the individual.

EXAMPLE
For example, we saw a couple in which the husband was diagnosed with ADD without hyperactivity. As is commonly seen, there were symptoms to suggest low blood sugar. Because sometimes the disorder does not appear in physical testing, I suggested that he simply eat small meals every 2 hours. One month later he returned to discuss his progress. After changing his eating routine, he found that he was able to manage his employees without the frequent temper outbursts he had prior to diagnosis and was displaying a more even emotional temperament. This man was not taking a dosage of medication significant enough to produce this change in symptoms. The difference was simply that he was eating properly and often enough.

6.2.14.2 What to Do
It is suggested that the individual eat small meals every 2 hours and have a light snack before bedtime. This should alleviate the characteristic exhaustion upon awakening in the morning associated with hypoglycemia. We have found that ice cream is a wonderful treat just before bedtime, requiring little in the way of digestion and having a rather low glycemic index. The individual is subsequently not difficult to awaken in the morning nor unduly angry. In using medical management of the stimulant to treat the ADD, it is important to keep in mind that stimulant medication may increase the likelihood of low blood sugar reactions. Finally, nutritional supplements have been found to be extremely helpful in providing control over the blood sugar by stabilizing it. It is important to rule out other conditions related to thyroid, neurolog-

ical disease, anxiety, and depression as their impact on this condition is important as well.

6.2.15   Weight Problems

Obesity may be a problem with all of the subtypes of ADD. Obesity is currently seen as a heterogeneous disorder with multiple causal factors. It is a condition characterized by an excess of body fat distribution and generally has a distinctly genetic component that can be tracked through the family history. Body fat predisposes the individual to increased disease risk factors. Some of the causal factors suggested by recent research relate to the adipose tissue. One theory is that mild and moderate obesity may result from maintaining body weight at an elevated level and that lifestyle changes, not diets, will hold the key to treatment. There are medications that work to decrease appetite by acting centrally on biochemical systems and the hypothalamus as they are viewed as the integration center for feeding behavior. There is a family history of obesity, hypoglycemia, and stress reaction. Research and clinical observations do not tend to support the relationship specifically with any of the attentional disorders. There are, however, many eating-disorder problems among the attention-disordered population that may be a consequence of anxiety, low self-esteem, and need for approval by others. However, continual failure leads to more emphasis on one's physical features, which further promotes the eating disorder.

6.2.15.1   *Anorexia and Bulimia are Common Eating Disorders*

The symptoms of anorexia include

- Refusal to maintain minimal normal weight for age and height due to fear of obesity
- Distorted body image
- Amenorrhea (loss of menstrual cycle)
- Disturbed functioning overall due to loss of vital nutrients
- Cold intolerance
- Hair loss
- Sunken eyes
- Hypotension
- Edema
- Hypothermia
- Disturbance to brain functioning

Recent research identifies brain damage and cell death in individuals diagnosed with anorexia.

The symptoms of bulimia include

- Recurrent binge eating
- Fear of not being able to stop during binges
- Regular vomiting, laxative, dieting, or fasting to counteract binges
- A minimum of 2 episodes per week for 3 months
- Overconcern for body shape and weight
- Can result in life-threatening loss of body nutrients
- Dizziness
- Hypotension
- Dental problems

There are several Medical complications for anorexia and bulimia.

- Cardiovascular changes
- Hematologic changes
- Gastrointestinal complications
- Renal abnormalities
- Endocrine changes

6.2.15.2 *What to Do*

Individual psychotherapy as well as family therapy are badly needed as the eating disorder may represent a symptom involving the family interactions. Diet and nutritional supplements contribute greatly to treatment by addressing issues of metabolism and stabilization of blood sugar, an imbalance in which tends to result in cravings and subsequent binging, followed by the need to purge in some way. Hospitalization maybe required as the severity of this disorder can become life threatening. There are different medications currently enjoying success in this population such as antidepressants (Prozac®, Zoloft® or Paxil®), anti-anxiety agents (Xanax® and BuSpar®) and, in cases of agitation, medications such as Depakote® or Tegretol®. Finally, ruling out thyroid disorder, obsessive-compulsive disorder, or any underlying neurological disease is very important for successful treatment.

6.2.16 Stress

Stress is a major factor when working with attention-disordered adults. We have been evaluating a large number of individuals in their 40s and 50s who have found themselves under such a great amount of stress by this time that they are now discovering symptoms of an underlying attentional disorder. ADD without hyperactivity has been there all along but, until now, they have been able to cope with the symptoms and logically problem-solve their way around the issues of missing information and distractibility. As they age, it becomes more difficult to compensate for symptoms of the disorder and their lives become more complex and stress factors become more noticeable. By the time of evaluation, they do not need medication to regulate the attentional disorder; they have been coping successfully for 40 years. They may, however, need medication to manage their stress levels, which, at this point, have become detrimental to their physical health.

Chronic stress has been found to lead to extensive depression, low blood sugar, increased blood-sugar levels in diabetics, heart disease, stroke, and hypertension. It is found to exacerbate multiple sclerosis and cancer and to create or increase digestive problems such as colitis, irritable bowel syndrome, and ulcers. Sleeping disorders, and sleep apnea in particular, are beginning to emerge as more-frequent phenomena, as observed in our evaluations. Individuals might be ready to retire from a rather stressful career to play golf on a daily basis, yet they can't remember anything, particularly what club they used last or what their score was for that particular hole. Stress Disorder Syndrome is a disorder that eventually results in the wearing down of internal organs, as they are running at three times their normal rate. We now know that stress alone can create high blood pressure or hypertension, which can create arteriosclerosis, which can create strokes, heart attacks, and TIAs (transient ischemic attacks or mini strokes in the small branches of the arteries).

6.2.16.1 *Symptoms*

- Insomnia and sleep disturbance
- Exacerbated or increased physical illness overall

6.2.16.2 *What to Do*

Originally, we became involved in a nutritional program to address the growing number of stress-related cases we were treating. This particular nutritional program has been excellent in addressing all the aspects of stress in addition to reducing the risk of heart disease. Use medication as recommended by a cardiologist. Address emotional issues such as obsessive-compulsive personality, depression, and anxiety. Rule out neurological disease and mania. We now know from the research that stress can lead to hypertension, which can lead to eventual strokes and symptoms of TIA, with an accompanying loss of nutrients and oxygen resulting in cell death as part of the stroke process which invariably produces damage to the brain.

6.2.17 Hypertension

We are learning that the effect of hypertension on brain functioning is a complex and involved process that occurs over a period of time and slowly deteriorates and erodes the system. Problems occur as a result of increased pressure on the capillary walls (part of the arterial system), that leads to occlusion (closing-off of the system) and creates infarcts (areas of cell death or brain damage) due to the loss of oxygen and nutrients. Arteriosclerosis, the formation of plaque inside artery walls, causes a closing of the artery walls and can result in eventual bursting of blood vessels and substantial damage to the brain due to mini-strokes—large strokes, depending on the size of the artery that has burst.

Hypertension is proving to be a very potent issue, and new research indicates that both treated and untreated hypertension have an impact on brain functioning on a general level. Those who have hypertension are at continual risk and are highly susceptible to toxins in their environment. There are studies linking toxins in our environment to the development of cancer. Stress factors also create a response that is, in general, slower than normal.

6.2.17.1 What to Do

Aside from medication, a cardiologists strongly advise a healthy diet and consistent exercise.

6.2.18 Diabetes

Type I Diabetes has an early onset, usually in the teens, and is insulin dependent throughout life. Type II diabetes has the following symptoms.

- Late onset
- Hypoglycemia or low blood sugar disorder can be the precursor
- If symptoms persist, individuals can become insulin dependent

Diabetes is emerging as a very serious disorder. Statistics indicate it is the third-largest killer in the nation. Complications from diabetes are far reaching and can affect both internal organs and the brain. One issue is peripheral neuropathy. This is a general term to indicate that the neuron is not functioning as it should and peripherally involves the voluntary muscle system. These neuropathies can develop in both the upper and lower extremities and then spread throughout the system, thereby causing a great deal of pain, a burning sensation, and problems in overall motor abilities.

Diabetics are at risk for chronic blood pressure alteration, development of arteriosclerosis, acute myocardial infarction, microangiopathy, and retinopathy. There can be indirect effects from toxemia due to kidney failure. Lowered insulin levels result in the production of ketone bodies that are toxic or deadly to the neural or brain tissues, producing both peripheral and central effects (outside and inside the brain). A condition called ketoacidosis results from disregulated insulin production, which may also produce brain damage due to swelling of the brain or brain edema. Finally, with diabetics there can be increased incidence of cerebrovascular accidents that appear earlier in the adult's life and result in loss of functioning due to the effects of stroke.

When a diabetic is also attention disordered, it becomes a tricky business to regulate insulin levels and use stimulant medication. There are times when stimulant medication can help the diabetic regulate blood-sugar levels, while at other times (particularly in times of increased stress), the same medication can throw off the blood-sugar levels. Maintaining blood-sugar levels is critical for the diabetic. If they are too low or too high, there are both short- and long-term complications. So the task is always to remain at an exact level for absolute control. It is important to swiftly diagnose attentional disorders in the diabetic because often, before diagnosis, they forget to eat, forget to test their blood sugar, are unaware of insulin levels, and have overall difficulty maintaining effective and absolute control of the illness, which is critically necessary.

EXAMPLE
We once saw a diabetic individual before diagnosis with ADD. He was constantly sinking to such dangerously low blood-sugar levels that he frequently came close to passing out. He was unable to regulate his food intake, ate too much or too little, and constantly put himself into positions where he could not get what he needed (insulin or food). His lifestyle was very dangerous to his health. His diabetes was clearly out of control. Since his ADD diagnosis and subsequent treatment, he is a new man. Since on stimulant medication, his blood-sugar levels are exact, his eating habits are excellent, and he does not leave himself in precarious positions as he anticipates his needs on a continual basis.

We often wonder when we look at diabetics who are out of control if there is not an undiagnosed attentional disorder. In fact, recently we evaluated a child who had all the classic signs of ADD and, in fact, was diagnosed ADD. His father, who had been diagnosed diabetic 15 years earlier and was on kidney dialysis (treatment for kidney failure due to poor insulin regulation), had an ulcer on his foot that had not healed in 3 years and he had lost a toe. We casually asked the father about his health and capability to regulate his diabetes. He shrugged us off, commenting that other family members younger than him had already died of diabetes (and perhaps also the complication of unrecognized and treated ADD).

6.2.18.1   What to Do
Maintain an exact diet and excellent insulin regulation. Recent research indicates that the best control involves insulin four times per day while testing sugar levels as often as eight times per day. Nutritional supplements are proving themselves to be critical additions to prolonging the life of the diabetic. Diagnosis of the attentional disorder if signs are evident is also critical. Address other emotional issues that could interfere with good medical management, such as depression or anxiety, mania, psychosis or neurological disease.

6.2.20   *Candida albicans* (Yeast Infections)

This is the common yeast infection that is classified as a fungus. Normally, levels are in control, but there are conditions that foster overgrowth and are major risk factors.

- Excessive use of antibiotics
- Birth control pills

- Corticosteroids
- A diet high in sugar and fat

The symptoms include

- Acne
- Allergic reactions and symptoms
- Bloating and distention
- Blurred vision
- Chemical sensitivities
- Cold hands and feet
- Constipation
- Cramping
- Cystitis
- Depression
- Dizziness
- Earaches
- Fatigue
- Gas colitis
- Gastritis
- Frequent headaches
- Hives
- Hyperactivity
- Kidney and bladder infections
- Lethargy
- Menstrual irregularities
- Numbness
- Nausea
- Pain that travels from joint to joint
- Poor digestion
- Rashes
- Rectal itching
- Sensitivity to molds
- Yeast vaginitis

6.2.20.1 What to Do

These symptoms can easily mask themselves as an attentional disorder and diagnosis is the key to correct treatment. Also, addressing other emotional issues, particularly those of anxiety and depression, is very important.

6.2.21   Cancer

Cancer can impact a person and create symptoms that may mask themselves as an attentional disorder, especially in the case of cancer of the brain, which consists of tumors that press on brain structures. Studies are being conducted that suggest that stress and its emotional factors create an overall vulnerability that increases the risk of contracting cancer from toxins in the environment. New research is implicating a high-fat diet as being more conducive to the onset of cancer.

6.2.21.1 *What to Do*

The first step is always to obtain an accurate diagnosis. If an attentional disorder is left undiagnosed, it will contribute to the quality of care. Recent research has pointed out the benefit of stimulant medication. It is important to carry out any necessary medical procedures. Finally, nutritional supplements are having excellent results in both prevention and as an accessory to treatment. Address emotional issues and other neurological illnesses, and participate in support groups, self-talk, and any other method that helps the individual to "keep going" and "keep trying." There are many positive results relating to hypnosis and the power of suggestion in treating some forms of cancer. Further, there is a question as to the impact of emotional issues in the disease process in dealing with the fact that some individuals survive cancer and some do not.

6.2.21   Toxic Substances

We are now becoming aware that specific and naturally occurring environmental substances are actually neurotoxins, meaning that they can cause damage to the brain. Damage can occur at the level of the messenger systems, impacting both the chemical and the electrical systems. These substances are capable of damaging the cortical or brain transmissions that make up the central (brain) and peripheral nervous system. The loss of oxygen (anoxia) is being recognized as one of the principal mechanisms of damage to the neurons. Structural damage as well as damage to the transmission system is what makes this so deadly for the individual. Neurons that are more sensitive to the loss of oxygen or require more oxygen than other types of cells are at particular risk. The whole neurotransmission system can be impacted, including the release, storage, synthesis, and termination of the neurotransmitters. The communication system is then altered. Damage to these systems results in damage to the brain.

6.2.21.1 *Symptoms*

- Attention deficits
- Memory impairment — particularly short-term memory

- Impaired arousal, vigilance, attention, motor speed, and coordination
- Visuospatial and visuomotor impairments
- Impairments in cognitive (thinking) flexibility and efficiency
- Seizure activity
- Lowered IQ levels
- Dementia
- Hyperactivity
- Depression
- Hallucinations

Symptoms can easily mask themselves as an attentional disorder, in which case use of stimulant medication would only increase or exacerbate symptoms.

6.2.21.2 What to Do

Accurate diagnosis is critical. Address treatment based on diagnosis. Addressing other hormonal, thyroid, emotional, and neurological issues is very important for a whole-treatment approach. Nutritional supplements can be very helpful, especially in future protection of the brain.

6.2.22 Smoking

Smoking is often seen in the ADD population, particularly if the individual is anxious. Smoking creates physical symptoms that need to be addressed. It is difficult to give up smoking because nicotine operates as both an upper and downer, thus fulfilling many needs in the individual. There is a physical withdrawal due to the needs this substance fulfills. Nicotine has all the features of an addictive drug, both stimulant and depressant. It excites — provides energy — and relaxes and calms. It is highly addictive as a result. It is a cholinergic drug that stimulates ganglionic neurons.

Smoking is seen in the ADD population, particularly that of ADD without hyperactivity, as a means of self-medication to calm the high levels of anxiety. Smoking, however, only adds to the problems of physical health to which this adult population is subject. Smoking to excess is seen in the ADHD due to its "drug like" properties. It is fairly common to see alcoholics trade off alcohol for tobacco — both are used in excess and both are dangerous.

6.2.22.1 What to Do

QUIT. However, quitting does not have to be "cold turkey," but can be gradual. We have had excellent success using a method of hypnosis (breathing is directly tied to what smoking provides for the individual in terms of relaxation) and nutritional supplements carefully combined to avoid adverse physical effects. This method gradually weans individuals over a period of 6 weeks by altering their habitual patterns and allowing cigarette use when they need it most.

6.2.23   Lupus

Lupus occurs when the body becomes allergic to itself. Immune functioning breaks down, overreacts, and turns against itself. The body overreacts to a nonthreatening stimulus, makes too many antibodies or proteins, and directs them against body tissue. There are different types of antibodies, including one that affects the internal organs (heart, lung, kidney, or liver) and one that is limited to the skin. Lupus develops between the ages of 15 and 45 years. This is a difficult disorder to diagnose. It involves general nerve inflammation and can increase with stress.

6.2.23.1   *Symptoms*

- Pain on taking a deep breath
- Fatigue
- Weight loss
- Lack of energy
- Muscle ache
- Lack of movement of muscles due to intense pain
- Fevers
- Swollen glands
- Swollen joints
- Rashes

One individual diagnosed with ADD without hyperactivity indicated that her symptoms improved with stimulant medication that reduced her reactionary stress levels in response to the symptoms of the attentional disorder.

6.2.23.2   *What to Do*

The critical issue is to diagnose and treat the disorder. Rule in or out any attentional disorder. Also, addressing all other emotional or neurological issues is very important. It is important to ensure proper nutrition, rest, and reduced or limited stress.

6.2.24   The Aging Process

Those individuals who have fragile systems do not age very well. They can develop Alzheimer's or Dementia. Both disorders are the result of the degeneration of neurons in selected areas of the brain that present symptoms that can resemble those of an attentional disorder. For the individual with Alzheimer's or Dementia, statements have to be repeated over and over. They can become lost and have no sense of direction. They cannot make decisions and are confused and inattentive. Their short-term memory processes are clearly problematic. Neuropsychological evaluation is invaluable for specifically defining symptoms, strengths and weaknesses, and for differentiating the types of Dementia. This diagnosis, in turn, dictates the different types of treatment that will need to be implemented.

6.2.24.1 Alzheimer's Disease

Alzheimer's is a disorder of severe memory loss indicated by the presence of plaques and tangles on microscopic examinations of brain matter. There is a direct correlation or relationship between the extent of impairment seen in the individual and the number of these neurofibrillary tangles in the brain. Frontal and temporal areas are specifically targeted, which results in symptoms of problematic decision-making processes and short-term and working memory problems. Early in the disease, what will be seen clinically is memory problems — mainly of the short-term type as well as more-recent memories. Also notable will be spatial problems, right–left confusion, disorientation, problem with directions, handwriting changes, and blocks that can be detected medically as well as with a neuropsychological evaluation that can differentiate Alzheimer's Disease from Dementia. It is important to diagnose as early as possible, given the results of the preventive medication Aricept. When medical evaluation yields no conclusive information, yet there is clear impairment or loss of short-term memory and evidence of spatial issues, it is especially important to consider a neuropsychological evaluation that targets the memory and spatial areas. Problems can be clearly seen with the block design task of the WAIS-R, a measure of problem solving using block formation that requires intact spatial abilities, as well as the drawing of designs on the Bender Visual Motor Gestalt Test. There are memory measures using spatial designs such as the Brief Visuospatial Memory Test.

6.2.24.2 Dementia

This disorder tends to reveal overall impairment with no targeting of specific areas and reduces the person's overall intellectual facilities. Dementia can be present as a result of a number of causal factors usually involving some type of breakdown of frontal or logical processes. While with Alzheimer's there are memory and spatial problems (loss of direction, orientation, drawing, handwriting changes and so on), with Dementia there is evidence of very poor decision-making skills and an inability to understand what is being said in a conversation.

6.2.24.3 What to Do

The presence of either of these disorders can impact the functioning of the person and also mask itself as an attentional disorder. In addition, sleep apnea can cause similar symptoms. Therefore, the first step is an accurate diagnosis using a neuropsychological evaluation in addition to other testing currently available. Nutritional supplements are helpful. If an attentional disorder exists, its treatment can reduce the effects of stress, which can increase or exacerbate these disorders. Finally, it is the more-fragile subtypes of ADD that are at risk for developing either of these disorders. We now know that these disorders involve a number of different factors, produce a variety of emotional issues, and can be complicated by other neurological issues. A good assessment that takes into consideration a family history in addition to other factors involving the individual is of utmost importance. Medical management of Alzheimer's with Aricept has been effective and, during later stages, employment of antidepressants, as well as antiseizure and antipsychotic medications, are effective as the brain begins to decompensate.

6.2.25 Anger

It may surprise the reader that this is included as a category. I think we often fail to realize the extensive and far-reaching consequences of anger that can result in long-lasting, irreversible physical impairment to the individual. ADD individuals can become obsessed with anger, possibly anger over what was lost to them: e.g., the lost years, the lost income, the lost abilities; sometimes this translates into lost college, lost studying, lost opportunities. It is easy to become so upset with what was lost that these individuals cannot envision any positive attribute to finally being diagnosed. It is also difficult to understand how this can improve their future and provide a sense of hope, especially when this occurs with adults and adolescents. Anger is pervasive and eventually costs us our health. The positive results of anger occur when we use this emotion to take action, to confront a situation that we had been previously avoiding, or to make the changes we were previously afraid to make. Anger supersedes and comes before fear. It is when we do not use anger for action that we are in danger of becoming depressed and hopeless, because then the anger is turned inward against the self. People then become critical and judgmental, initially of themselves and utimately of those around them.

Anger results in the rise in the adrenalin system due to an increase of stress. Over a long period of time, it will lead to stress-related symptoms and illnesses.

6.2.25.1 What to Do

Increase problem-solving skills aimed at resolving issues of anger and anger-provoking situations. Use cognitive self-control methods to help these people learn to calm themselves in anger-provoking situations. Nutritional supplements, exercise, free time, and just plain fun are all stress reducers that can help provide some joy in these individuals' lives. Too much work easily creates tension, which is the breeding ground for anger.

Finally, address the possibility of an attention disorder that might be causing the frustrating experiences and producing continual anger. Generally, anger can be a component for all subtypes of ADD. It will, however, affect the more-fragile and anxious person mostly on a physical level. Medication to treat the agitation or stress effects may be helpful. Finally, rule out any neurological disorder, especially seizure activity, that may account for this intense emotional reaction.

6.2.26   Substance Abuse

6.2.26.1 Drugs

Substance abuse is common with all of the subtypes of ADD for various reasons. It is more a case of self-medication for ADD without hyperactivity while ADHD individuals tend to use drugs for excitement. ADHD individuals tend to be characteristic of the stereotypic alcoholic: addicted, excessive users, and out of control. It begins in the early teens and continues until some outside factor forces them to quit. On the other hand, ADD without hyperactivity people use drugs as a relief from the constant flow of anxiety. They tend to utilize more marijuana, which calms the sensory system, thus relieving the ADD symptoms. They tend to avoid cocaine. Marijuana, unfortunately, remains in the brain for a very long period of time and creates a persistent amotivational syndrome resulting in the individual not being interested in anything. ADHD individuals obtain drugs like cocaine because they offer the stimulant properties and excitation they crave.

ADD without hyperactivity people tend to become addicted to marijuana, fearful of ever quitting due to the powers of this substance to relieve them of the overwhelming anxiety they feel on a continual basis. These individuals become panicked at the idea of giving up marijuana because of the release it affords them. New research is targeting short-term memory problems and missing information deficits with long-time use of marijuana. Research reveals cocaine impacting the arterial system, and our documentation of additional impact to the brain has been in the area of frontal, decision-making processes as well as short-term memory problems. Drug use is is no longer an innocent, recreational type of thing. Teens and young adults are attending "rave" parties run by the drug dealers who offer all kinds of drug "cocktails" — a mixture of many kinds of drugs that promises the ultimate high.

Drug variables can include

- Rewarding properties
- Patterns of tolerance
- Cost and availability
- Patterns of withdrawal
- Mode of administration and speed of onset

User variables include metabolism and sensitivity to drugs and an overall mental and emotional well-being or response to stress.

Environmental variables can include peer influence and a conditioned environmental response (allowing the pattern of use to become habitual, conditioned, and repetitious in a cyclical fashion). Substance abuse must be considered a chronic disease.

6.2.26.2 Alcohol

- Penetrates blood brain barrier.
- The sugar in alcohol is toxic to the brain.
- Alcohol drops sugar directly to the brain, which can cause substantial damage to the brain over time.
- Specifically targets the short-term memory and decision-making areas.
- Can often result in hypoglycemia and poor nutritional balance.

Recent research indicates that alcohol impacts a brain messenger called glutamate, which affects the functioning of other messengers — specifically, dopamine and norepinephrine. Therefore, over time, alcohol usage will further disrupt the biochemical balance from which ADD factors emerged, thus creating a cycle that will only become worse. When "blackouts" occur, it is an indication that this neurotransmitter balance has been disrupted because glutamate supplies the memory processes. Blackouts represent the memory processes being affected to such a degree that the person recalls nothing of what took place the night or day before. ADHD individuals again tend to not know when to stop and continue drinking beyond what is safe for them to consume. ADD without hyperactivity individuals tend to use alcohol to get along socially, to self-medicate their anxiety, and to fit in with their peers. Alcohol use begins with teenage years and the onset of social activities while with ADHD the age of onset is much earlier.

In the last 10 years of our research we have found that those individuals with long-term usage of alcohol, especially with binge drinking, are highly susceptible to the effects of excitotoxicity and seizure activity. As a result, it appears to specifically target the memory areas. Thus, the phenomenon of "dry drunk" — an individual who remains as nasty and upset and as inconsistent in mood when sober as when drunk — may actually be showing signs of seizure activity with the emotional outbursts as well as long-term personality changes associated with seizures. The short-term memory is notable in addition to increased deficits of decision making and diminished frontal processes. Alcoholism impacts the two compensatory mechanisms previously used or employed to cope with the symptoms of ADD. Eventually this can create an increase of symptoms of the very disorder from which the person was trying to escape.

6.2.26.3 What to Do

Diagnosis is critical. To accurately diagnose the attentional disorder as well as the nature of the substance-abuse problem it is imperative to understand how the two interact and feed off each other. This will play a crucial role in helping the person to quit drug or alcohol usage. Both disorders must be addressed at the same time using individual psychotherapy, treatment, and 12-step programs. Finally, nutritional supplements, exercise, and diet become very important additions as they work toward sobriety.

6.2.27 Sleep Disorders

There are sleep problems inherent in the ADD population, with anxiety playing a major role. Sleep problems are increased or exacerbated with anxiety. They are often associated with ADD without hyperactivity due to the continual racing thoughts. The amount of anxiety they have results in late-night or early-morning insomnia, difficulty falling asleep, or waking before it is time. This results in

- Restlessness
- Irritability
- More anxiety
- Being on edge
- Unable to concentrate and attend due to sleep deprivation

A number of individuals may also be suffering from sleep apnea. With sleep apnea, the inflow of air is blocked. As a result, the individual stops breathing and awakens with a gasp every few minutes throughout the night. Sleep apnea can be caused by a number of factors and can result in emotional exhaustion with poor concentration and memory. The loss of oxygen can result in damage to the brain that can become substantial over time.

EXAMPLE

We administered a neuropsychological evaluation on a man who had all of the characteristics of Alzheimer's Disease and yet, in all probability, the substantial damage to the brain was due to severe sleep apnea, which, over a period of time, had caused pervasive memory deficits and highly impaired the decision-making frontal processes.

6.2.27.1 What to Do

First identify the nature of the sleep disorder. Is it insomnia, sleep apnea, or anxiety? The attention-disordered population has substantial sleep problems. The ADD without hyperactivity and the Overfocused subtype have particular difficulty due to the degree of anxiety they experience. The contributing attention disorder needs to be ruled in or out. Sleep studies should be completed if there are serious results seen on the evaluation, as well as neuropsychological measures that indicate short-term memory loss. Finally, nutritional supplements can help tremendously. Also, a number of new medications are available that do not have substantial side effects — consult a physician. The only problem with using medication for sleep is that the majority of these drugs are meant for short-term use only (such as Ambien®). There are some medications available for sleeping problems that can be used on a longer-term basis (such as Trazadone®). Consult a psychiatrist for medications such as anti-anxiety and antidepressant agents.

7

Comorbid and Associated Emotional Disorders

7.1 Related Disorders

Emotional disorders often associated with ADD without hyperactivity are the following

- Schizophrenia
- Shizo affective Disorder
- Anxiety and panic disorders
- Post Traumatic Stress Disorder
- Depression
- Social phobias
- Obsessive Compulsive Disorder
- Dissociative Identity Disorder

Symptoms may include

- Alcohol and drug abuse — marijuana is usually the drug of choice
- Stress
- Problems functioning in work, home, and school relationships
- Irritability and nervousness
- Inability to sustain attention
- Mental and physical restlessness
- Easily distracted
- Losing and forgetting things
- Interrupts conversations
- Does not appear to listen to others
- Difficulty waiting for their turn

Emotional disorders often associated with ADHD are the following

- Manic depression, Bipolar Disorder
- Conduct disorder
- Antisocial personality
- Alcoholism and other addictions
- Oppositional Defiant Disorder
- Child abuse

Symptoms may include

- Craves Physically challenging activities
- Craves crisis
- Hot temper
- Impulsive
- Impatient
- General restlessness

The overfocused subtype of ADD without hyperactivity can have some or all of the following characteristics

- Very worried
- Very sensitive
- Very dramatic
- Adolescence elongated over the life span
- Overfocused
- Overreactive

Symptoms include

- Avoidance, procrastination
- Easily stressed and frightened
- Cannot stop thinking
- Always worrying and thinking
- Heavy anxiety

They do not relax. They do not like change or transition of any kind. Research has clearly shown that the impact of psychopathology (meaning that other problematic disorders are present) results in further impact on symptoms of the attentional disorders. Research generally has addressed the comorbidity or co-relationship (meaning that one disorder tends to go hand in hand with another) in children diagnosed with an attentional disorder. Findings are similar as to what would be expected given the nature of the disorders.

The general trends are as follows. Depressed children with comorbid conduct disorder had worse short-term outcomes and higher risk for adult criminality than depressed children without conduct disorder. In other words, those children diagnosed with conduct disorder had greater tendencies to develop adult criminality when the combination was conduct disorder with depression.

Children with ADD and comorbid conduct disorder or Oppositional Defiant Disorder had worse outcomes than children with ADD alone. This means that those children with ADD and conduct and/or Oppositional Defiant disorders had more difficulty than those diagnosed with just the attentional disorder alone.

Overanxious disorder was found with similarity for both boys and girls. Separation anxiety was also comparable for both boys and girls.

Major depressive disorder patterns indicated that rates are low and comparable until adolescence, when girls indicated a very sharp increase. This is a critical issue as girls will be more at risk for depression and possible suicide with the onset of adolescence. ADHD prevalence was still found to be nearly twice as high for boys than girls. However, this may still be a diagnosis issue.

There is more research indicating that girls are being diagnosed with ADD more often. However, girls tend to escape diagnosis as they are less apt to cause problems in the classroom. Girls tend to be referred later than boys for evaluations because they do not cause enough problems to result in being noticed. Additionally, there is a diagnostic issue because much of the diagnosis is based on self-report symptoms and not clinical testing and evaluation. Consequently, there could be misdiagnosis as well the tendency to not diagnose unless there is evidence of behavioral problems or blatant poor performance in school.

Conduct disorder was twice as prevalent in boys as in girls. Oppositional Defiant Disorder, however, had the same prevalence pattern for both boys and girls. Oppositional Defiant Disorder appears to have a life of its own, meaning that this disorder stands alone as a separate diagnostic category and due to its level of severity is not more predominant for either gender over the other. Conduct disorder tends to follow what would normally be expected from boys showing more symptoms of acting-out behavior than girls. It appears to be a gender issue, possibly due to our society and the value system we hold for boys vs. girls.

Alcohol abuse was observed over the age span and was especially high in post high-school years, confirming that it is very important that we observe and address the attentional disorder in a timely fashion. If adolescents are not provided with encouragement or hope they easily lapse into abuse whether that be of alcohol or drugs.

For the 17- to 20-year-old, the prevalence rate was twice as high for boys as for girls. Again, boys tend to more openly display abusive behavior. This leads to their being recognized as ADD more readily than their female counterparts. For example, boys or men will drink openly, while girls or women become what we refer to as "closet drinkers."

Marijuana abuse increased with age and again rates for boys were higher than girls. In looking at the comorbidity, most of the cases that were originally diagnosed at ages 9 to 18 still had the diagnosis at an equivalent level more than 2 years later. This addresses the idea that the attentional disorder does not go away in adulthood and, in fact, only serves to create more problems for the individual.

7.2   Manic Depression or Bipolar Disorders

Bipolar disorders are defined on the basis of extremes that take place with the person shifting from mania to depression. This disorder is seen as genetic and can be traced through the family history. Although present at birth, it may or may not surface, depending on the degree of stress in the individual's life. Therefore, the disorder tends to surface during adolescence and/or young adulthood when environmental stressors are at their peak. Thus, there is the possibility that even with a propensity for this disorder, it may never surface during one's lifetime. The key issue is the extreme and that the individual is out of balance. Symptoms can range from mild to severe, and when severe, particularly with mania, the person can have psychotic features. Over the course of one's lifetime, some or all of the symptoms of the disorder may surface. The disorder tends to wax and wane in its symptoms depending on the outside stresses in the person's life. There is a manic phase and a depressive phase, both of which can range from mild to extreme in nature.

Overall characteristics of the disorder may include

- Binge/purge cycle
- Frequent job changes
- Dynamic sense of personality to deep lows and emptiness
- Dynamism as a whole
- Mood swings can appear in a short period of time
- Cycling varies from hours to days and months

For example, ranks of college kids begin a semester with a full load and only manage to complete three or four credits out of a possible 12 credits by the end of the term.

7.2.1 Defining the Manic Phase

The person appears quite extreme in nature. The phase's mild form may be exemplified in such behavior as buying two items instead of one. In its extreme form, the person can actually appear psychotic or go on buying sprees. One individual, for example, by the time he had finished with a buying spree, had purchased $50,000 worth of cars with money he would never have at one time. During this phase, the person appears unreasonable and communication is all but impossible.

7.2.1.1 Symptoms

- Psychomotor agitation
- Pressured speech
- Hypersexuality or a lot of sexual language
- Lack of or hypersensitivity to feelings
- Grandiose sense of self
- Impossible goals
- Animation
- Impulsivity
- Anger
- Confusing speech — Sometimes they do not make sense and their words are confusing. They may speak in short sentences and shift from topic to topic.
- Inability to sustain one's conversation for any length of time — When in the manic phase, individuals have problems with sustaining thought or conversation due to an extremely high degree of distractibility.
- Over-exercising
- Eating disorders

There is prepubertal mania that tends to be found often with ADHD. Those diagnosed with mania will more often show symptoms of an attentional disorder. Those diagnosed with ADHD may evidence a true diagnosis of mania. In other words, the diagnosis of mania will more often mean ADHD as well, whereas the diagnosis of ADHD will not as often mean the diagnosis of mania. The clinical picture of prepubertal mania is irritability of a continual nature.

7.2.2   Defining the Depression Phase

The depression that occurs is an extreme low. Even if the person does not attempt suicide they can come very close to it. The lows of this disorder are almost a shock to the highs. Individuals will appreciate the medication to avoid the impact of the lows even though they miss the good times of the manic highs.

7.2.2.1   *Symptoms*

- Listlessness
- Loss of formerly pleasurable activities
- Sleeping and eating problems
- Cannot control and regulate food or sleep
- May not be ADHD but looks like it

Behavior in the manic phase will appear like hyperactivity. Bipolar Disorders are highly related to the diagnosis of ADHD. They can contribute to the lack of control of the ADHD individual. Manic symptoms only serve to enhance the lack of controls found with the ADHD individual.

7.2.3   What to Do

Medication is necessary due to the tendency to relapse once the disorder has presented itself in the person's life. This usually occurs with a breakdown of functioning spearheaded by a manic episode. Once this occurs, the cycle has begun and even though there will be periods of remission, the chance of relapse is always expected if some level of medication is not maintained. Watch for symptoms of depression that will not be specifically addressed by the medication for this disorder. Antidepressants are necessary at different times in these individuals' lives to augment the medication they are already taking. Medications used in addition to or instead of lithium are antiseizure medications (Depakote®, Lamictal®, Neurontin®, and Tegretol®), antipsychotic medications (Clozaril) and some of the newer antidepressants (Paxil, Zoloft, or Serzone®). Thyroid function needs to be continually addressed. Issues of toxicity exist with additional over-the-counter medications. Once maintained on an even dosage of medication correct for the individual, the stimulant medication necessary for the attentional disorder will not have a negative impact on symptoms of this disorder. Nutrition, structuring one's life with balance, and working to establish positive relationships are important goals. Psychotherapeutic treatment, especially family therapy, is critical to cope with issues relating to the disorder as well as medical management.

7.3 Adult Child of an Alcoholic

The definition of the adult child of an alcoholic (ACOA) is an individual who has grown up in an alcoholic home. Alcoholic homes may be any home in which one of the primary caretakers practiced something to excess, whether that something was alcohol, work, drugs, food, gambling, religion or simply an excessive manner. There are ACOA children who, as parents, are what we call alcohol phobic. An alcoholic personality is one who looks at things and thinks in extremes. Children raised in an environment with alcoholic personalities have certain common characteristics to describe themselves and to help those significant to them understand their behavior. A group formed many years ago coined the term ACOA, and defined themselves by these common characteristics. ACOA members support each other by working to understand their special station in life.

Overall, the ACOA individual may or may not be alcoholic and may have one of the following addictions:

- Drinking
- Drugging
- Smoking
- Eating
- Working
- Shopping
- Gambling
- Religion

ACOA individuals may become alcoholics to self-medicate or they may become a "true" alcoholic whereby the alcohol is no longer a defense but a way of life. Pressure on the self leads to stress on a continual basis. Physically, there is evidence of chronic fatigue, headaches, and so on.

7.3.1 Symptoms

- Frightened by strong feelings
- Limited by fear of failure
- Stuck in denial
- Focused on others and not on themselves
- Caretaker of others and not able to have their own feelings
- Intolerant of anything that is not how they think it should be

- Limited in their ability to give to others or show their feelings
- In constant need to protect and defend
- Ready to be attacked
- Easily hurt by criticism and interpret it as a sign of not being loved
- Constantly defending and will not face problems to try to correct them
- Always believe that they are bad and they are the problem
- Uncomfortable as part of a family and find it easier to withdraw
- Over-invested in the "me" or the "mine"

Specific symptoms play havoc in the personal lives of the ACOA. They are preoccupied with the "me" due to lack of attention or presence of an alcoholic personality. Due to receiving so little and being so neglected in childhood, children of alcoholics tend to be demanding to make up for what they have lost. Further, at young ages they were conscripted into service or care of the adult and thus never had the opportunity to develop or take care of themselves so they need others to take care of them. This can be seen in the woman-child or the person who is physically overdeveloped and responsible yet at the same time emotionally underdeveloped, childlike, and irresponsible. Outwardly, they take care of others, but in their personal relationships they need to be taken care of. They willingly give to the rest of the world and the rest of the world thinks they are absolutely wonderful. However, in their families, playing the role of parents or spouses, they give very little and expect to be taken care of. In general, they present an overall attitude of "what about me"?

They cannot stand chaos. They grew up in such a chaotic household that they have difficulty when things become chaotic in their adult life. There is fear associated with chaos because in their history this was usually the time when something went wrong or someone was hurt.

They like to anticipate the future and tend to like to control as much of their lives as they can. They want to anticipate and predict as much as possible so they do not have to suffer from the painful unpredictability that was so prevalent throughout their childhood.

They have substantial communication problems. They have no idea how to talk to others. The family in which they were raised did not talk, they reacted. Therefore the tendency is to keep feelings inside and operate alone instead of explaining feelings to others and seeking help.

There is a consistent fear of intimacy. Getting close to someone ensures being hurt. It is very frightening for an ACOA to trust and leave themselves open to the same old hurt and disappointments. They experienced the adult who promised not to drink but did, and who promised to be there but wasn't and so on.

They tend to wear a mask and not expose feelings. They learn not to let their guard down due to the threat of being hurt emotionally or physically. They learn to be tough and make it on their own. How often do you hear of a child who is beaten and then threatened with more harm if they cry? It can become a matter of honor in an abusive household not to show one's feelings.

ADD makes it worse. The presence of an attentional disorder makes it difficult to communicate, therefore there is no desire to communicate. It is harder to communicate as ADD people because they are not truly aware of their feelings due to the disorder. Either they cannot have feelings, are merely trying to cope with the ADD, or their emotions are sleeping, like everything else. If they don't know their feelings, how can they communicate them? ADD without hyperactivity individuals tend to have more conversations with themselves and to keep their feelings hidden.

They tend to be overachievers, are never satisfied with themselves, and have high expectations of others. ADD makes these expectations too hard to attain. With ADD they cannot be the perfect individuals they want to be and are bitterly disappointed by their inability to achieve the goals they desire. So begins the downward spiraling cycle of feeling bad, accomplishing less, feeling bad, doing less, more avoidance, more procrastination, and so on.

The fear of emotions and being overwhelmed by them is increased by the presence of ADD and the inability to compartmentalize emotions due to the attention disorder. Emotions are frightening. Given the basic fear of feelings from growing up in an alcoholic home, it is easier to attempt to compartmentalize feelings. But with ADD and its distractibility, it is difficult to achieve this compartmentalization. Subsequently, the person is overwhelmed by feelings and emotions and finds it easier to withdraw and forget the whole thing.

7.3.2   What to Do

Relapse and sobriety are major issues when some form of alcoholism is involved. The issues of cravings must be addressed in some fashion. Nutritional substances, exercise, and changes in eating habits should be prescribed. With alcohol problems, there are many issues related to hypoglycemia that need to be specifically addressed with both diet and nutritional control. These individuals need to learn how to play to balance themselves, and enjoy life. Issues relating to both the alcoholic home and what was learned as an ACOA need to be addressed in conjunction with the attentional disorder using individual, marital, and family therapy. ADD lowers self-esteem and only serves to increase all of the ACOA symptoms to the degree that the person is emotionally withdrawn. Some professionals are having success with more-rigorous treatment methods involving body work or targeting specific symptomology via resolution therapy techniques. Symptoms relating to ACOA are probably the most problematic when in combination with ADD and, if not addressed, can create the downfall of the person's personal and professional life.

EXAMPLE

One wonderful man with whom we worked for several years was married to a very sup-
portive and, in fact, educated woman who created tremendous changes in the school
system. She moved to provide accomodation for ADD symptoms in the academic set-
ting. She truly understood both ACOA and ADD issues. However, he was unable to
move through the old learned patterns and expectations relating to the household (fam-
ily of origin) in which he grew up. Sadly enough, he never could allow himself to be
loved by his new family — his wife and child. Eventually, his wife had had enough and
the couple divorced. Even at the bitter end, he could not let go of those old wounds from
childhood to allow him to trust and love again. This was probably one the most devas-
tating moments for us as therapists who cared about both of these people and respected
them personally and professionally.

Overall, research indicates that ACOA have

- Reportedly higher levels of depression
- Lower levels of self esteem
- Higher levels of marital conflict
- Lower levels of perceived social support, family cohesion, and
  marital satisfaction

Children of alcoholics have more depression and less self-esteem. They experience difficulty getting along with others, marital conflicts, and see themselves alone and unhappy within their family structure. This seems to be a
negative self-fulfilling prophesy — since they emerged from pain, they will
continue to live their lives in pain.

Coping mechanisms are undeveloped and they see themselves as powerless. When people see themselves as powerless they do not develop adequate
coping mechanisms and find it is easier to give up. They tend to stop trying
at the first sign of trouble, predict the worst, and that is that. This is a vicious
system that needs to be assaulted from all fronts. Family members and professionals need to be prepared to be versatile and ready to try a number of
techniques to break through the wall of the past.

7.4   The Addictive Personality (Addictive Persona)

There is a strong association between parental alcoholism and substance
abuse in the child. It is hypothesized that this occurs as a result of poor
parenting in general, the example that is set, and a lack of monitoring of the
child's activities. Finally, there is a high degree of negativity that tends to promote a self-fulfilling prophesy. Alcoholic parents shift the blame onto the
children, the children become responsible but bad, and then live up to that
expectation.

Research indicates that there is a high correlation between substance abuse and growing up in an alcoholic family, where consistent lack of follow-through is common. Again, the negative outcome occurs; if things do not go well it is easier to give up, escape, use drugs, and forget about it. The lack of structure and perhaps value system provides the idea that substance abuse is acceptable.

Finally, there may be a genetic issue presenting clear tendencies toward alcohol or drug use due to the brain being different in the true alcoholic or drug abuser. To date, a single gene has yet to be identified, but recently there has been evidence to support clear genetic involvement in the presence of addictive persona. What is being identified is that the brains of the alcoholic or rigid, addictive personality are structurally different, with fewer connections in the frontal area to allow appropriate inhibition to occur. Some evidence is being presented identifying the median forebrain bundle as involved in this addictive personality. The median forebrain bundle is a structure with considerable connections to both the limbic system (emotional center) and the frontal area (executive decision-maker — president) of the brain and has been considered the motivational center. The lack of inhibition promotes the rigid, inflexible and out-of-control extreme that characterizes this disorder.

The presence of the addictive personality appears to be due to a number of factors. There is no single personality disorder that could be identified that is consistently associated with this addictive persona. The closest is Antisocial Personality Disorder, which represents that lack of flexibility or rigidity that is observed with the addict. What makes the picture so confusing is that environment may play a factor here in providing the acceptance of escape as a form of resolving problems. In addition, someone may be addicted to some form of escape (gambling, drinking, using drugs, shopping, eating, etc.) and yet they are not this addictive persona. Their addiction is based on a feeling of helplessness, the co-dependent who joins in with the addicted spouse, or a means of self-medication of the overwhelming anxiety that permeates their daily existence. Much of the marijuana use seen in our private practice is in highly anxious individuals who unfortunately find relief from their everyday feelings of anxiety and panic only in the use of this drug. However, after using marijuana, they often search for other types of drugs and/or their personality changes subsequent to marijuana use and they become more irritable, argumentative, demanding, expansive and self-centered, traits that were never observed prior to substance abuse.

7.4.1 Symptoms

- Expansive
- Belittling
- Never taking into account someone else's feelings

More connected to ADHD and to cocaine abuse, substance abuse does not occur for purposes of self-medication. Substance abuse has a life of its own and is internally rewarding. The person likes to drink just to drink, to smoke just to smoke, and to eat just to eat. They do not care who gets affected. They do not care who gets hurt. And they do not care if there are consequences that may be life or death.

They do not stop until they are forced.

7.4.2 What to Do

- Set borders and boundaries.
- Set limits, limits, limits.
- Make them quit because they have to by assigning consequences that will affect them beyond their control.
- Avoid their manipulation.
- Don't take them personally.

7.5 Antisocial Personality

This is a personality disorder that is the adult version of conduct disorder and usually those so classified and seen as juvenile delinquents in childhood will have the symptoms of this disorder in adulthood. Generally, the presence of this disorder means an overall disregard for societal values as well as the values of individuals with whom they come in contact. Antisocial Personality is related to ADHD. The president of the brain is sleeping. The stop sign is down and therefore it is all systems go. They do whatever. Anything goes. There is no way to reach them because they don't experience remorse. Thus, you can't make them feel guilty because they are not anxious. They may lie one day and tell the truth the next, depending on how they feel. They really don't care what you think.

There is low frustration tolerance, they want things *now*. Again, the stop sign is down and there is no inhibition. Interestingly, overall research is showing that Antisocial Personality involves the frontal area of the brain and an overall lack of inhibition. This is similar to ADHD and accounts for behaviors that are common to both disorders. However, Antisocial Personality and ADHD can be seen separately or together. What we are finding is that not only does the brain work differently for both ADHD and this type of personality disorder, but the brain is different structurally, which tends to reveal that the frontal processes do not operate as they should. This type of behavior is similar to some types of head injury, again because the frontal area or frontal processes do not provide inhibition (and/or presidential activity) to pull everything together in regular appropriate behavior.

7.5.1 Symptoms

- There are ADHD characteristics.
- Frontal supervisory system is down.
- There is a lack of caring and there is no way to reach them.
- Control system is down so anything goes.
- There is no way to change them.
- There is no hook such as guilt because they do not care.
- There is a tendency to be critical and judgmental of others.
- There is a lack in motivation and self discipline.
- They are easily frustrated and angered.
- Overall they have emotional ambivalence (love vs. hate) toward others.
- They are impatient and impulsive.
- They are irritable.
- They are unpredictable.
- They vacillate between being cooperative and defiantly resistant depending on what they feel like at the time.

The antisocial personality can be charming, and have a sense of humor provided you don't get in their way. They have the same dynamics as those seen with Conduct Disorder, which progresses from early childhood into serious delinquency in adolescence to Antisocial Personality and criminal behavior in adults. Conduct Disorder and ADHD are two separate disorders. ADHD does not predict Conduct Disorder and Conduct Disorder does not predict ADHD.

Research confirms the hypothesis that those individuals diagnosed with either Conduct Disorder or Antisocial Personality emerge from a similar family background. Thus, these people are genetically at risk to develop this disorder due to the environment in which they grow up. They seem to establish habits from the powerful impact of modeling. Factors of criminal behavior and substance abuse present in one or both of the parents are likely predictors of this disorder.

These individuals tend to be deficient in problem-solving skills and cognitive flexibility, particularly in generating multiple solutions to problems. These individuals are limited in their solution generation resulting in a narrow perspective for responding to conflict situations.

7.5.2   What to Do

Intervention is needed to help assess the learning problems of not being able to think flexibly or to form solutions to the difficulties in life. It is absolutely critical to address and rule out the possibility of an attentional disorder. In dealing with this population from a behavioral perspective, borders and boundaries and specific rules and guidelines are critical. This group does not do well with deals, the point needs to be made and then enforced.

7.6   Oppositional Defiant Disorder

Individuals with Oppositional Defiant Disorder are difficult to diagnosis. The disorder can be seen as early as 2 years of age. What differentiates Oppositional Defiant Disorder from Conduct Disorder is that there is a more-severe degree of acting out behavior such as fire-starting, deliberately harming someone or something. These people tend to be the animal killers, or the hired guns who can kill someone for money or just because they felt like it. They would have been the mercenary soldiers. This disorder has been found to exist over time and the developmental cycle. Like ADD, the disorder can be seen in childhood and persists throughout the life span. Another important issue that further separates and differentiates this disorder from Conduct Disorder and Antisocial Personality Disorder is that there is no difference for boys vs. girls or males vs. females. This disorder cuts across age and gender, it can be seen with both sexes and at any point in the person's age span. Unfortunately, this disorder tends to be overdiagnosed. The description is being used for the child or adolescent who is defiant in order not to fail. What they are saying is that they would rather be seen as oppositional and defiant than as failures. Further, despite the fact that they present the appearance of not caring, the truth is that they care too much.

7.6.1   What to Do

Oppositional Defiant Disorder is seen as a more serious disorder with a life of its own and needs to be treated as such. Very clear borders and boundaries are structured, and a structured, rule-oriented environment is critical when dealing with these individuals. Nothing should be left to chance. They are not trustworthy. One's guard should never be relaxed as problematic situations tend to occur when the pressure is released and the rules are less stringent. Finally, due to the seriousness of this disorder, it is critical to be very clear about the diagnosis and to not misdiagnose especially in the case of very bright children who successfully mask their symptoms because they would rather appear to be behavior problems than failures or stupid. Oftentimes we will clinically see children have violent outbursts that are related to seizure activity and not this diagnosis. Do not take their behavior personally — see it as part of the disorder.

7.7   Child Abuse

Research indicates a connection to a family history of violence and alcoholism. Always look for a history of violence. Abuse is not accepted or condoned by society as a whole. Therefore, for it to occur, it was more than likely accepted in a mini-society or family system. When working with abuse — whether physical, emotional, or sexual (even the covert incest we are now seeing) — there will probably be someone somewhere in the family history who presented similar symptoms. Abuse can generally be traced back to the grandparents or great grandparents. No matter who, there will usually be someone in the family tree who was abusive. Being raised in an environment where abuse was condoned instills the notion that abuse is okay. In fact, it may be so strongly ingrained that the person believes it's more than just okay or acceptable — it's outright correct and proper behavior.

The long-term consequences of childhood abuse result in varied findings such as:

- Poor academic performance
- Vocational problems
- Substance abuse
- Aggressive or violent behavior

Abuse can lead to all kinds of problems, including poor performance in school, job problems, drug and alcohol abuse, and violent behavior toward children. Those raised in a violent setting will model and repeat the behavior as they attempt to cope with and respond to others. Under stress, there is a tendency to fall back on how they were parented and to respond to situations the way their parents did. If a parent was abusive, the child may become abusive or phobic of abuse. With abuse phobia, people go out of their way to the opposite extreme to ensure they do not abuse. This can lead to parenting that is far too lenient and perhaps setting no rules at all. Only by resolving the abuse issue can the reactive state of responding with the extremes of abuse and leniency be corrected.

Sexually abused children have a greater incidence of

- Post Traumatic Stress Disorder
- Borderline Personality Disorder or traits
- Fear and/or anxiety

- Behavior problems
- Sexualized behaviors (over or under sexuality to extreme degrees)
- Poor self esteem

There are different and separate issues for emotional and physical abuse. Children who are emotionally abused tend to feel terrible about themselves. They firmly believe what they have been told no matter what new information they receive as adults. Unlike physical abuse, emotional abuse is subtle and often goes undetected, leaving the child to suffer the serious consequences of its impact. Children, due to a tendency toward egocentrism, are apt to blame themselves and not their parents. Children are impressionable and if told that their actions somehow warranted the parent to abuse them, they believe it. Emotional abuse causes children to believe they are worthless, stupid, unlovable, and deserving of the abuse that is inflicted. No one can convince them of anything else. Furthermore, as the abuse is hidden, there is often no opportunity for an outside source to challenge this belief system. As a result, these beliefs persist through time. For example, we saw a woman for about 5 or 6 years who continued to believe that her parents were right and that she was "bad." Neither we nor her adoring husband could convince her of anything else. The message of emotional abuse is strong and unsinkable.

Physical abuse tends to be easier to cope with. Interestingly, those who suffer the abuse often fare better than those subjected to watching it occur, as it often appears to be worse than it is. In violent homes, it is common to find different effects on those who are abused and those who watch. Those who are abused tend to develop a strength mechanism to handle anything, while those who watch simply develop fear and guilt that they were not the one abused. Physical abuse, as opposed to emotional abuse, is easier to define and understand and therefore can be dealt with and resolved more successfully. Even so, those who have been abused may continue with issues of trust, trauma, and feelings of hopelessness and often end up repeating the cycle and abusing their own children.

7.7.5 Symptoms

Abusive parents

- Are often depressed and hopeless
- Lack warmth, humor, and sensitivity to the needs of children
- Talk to children mainly to give orders
- Ask questions and hurl nasty statements
- Treat children's behavior as though it were intended to annoy them
- Regard abused children as bad, slow, or hard to discipline

Children tend to be more at risk for abuse if they are

- Epileptic
- ADD
- ADHD
- Autistic
- Retarded or dyslexic
- Stepchildren

There is a need to separate the results of abuse from ADHD symptoms they tend to overlap. The impulsivity of the ADHD individual may lead them to become overly angry and to hurt someone without thinking of the consequences. Usually this will not occur unless there is some sort of history. Abused ADHD individuals are more likely to lose control, have little tolerance, and lapse into abuse rather than thinking first about their actions. We had a case involving a child where self-reports from the school indicated that the child was extremely hyperactive, impulsive, and inattentive. Self-report measures from the home indicated exactly the same things. When we administered our clinical testing we found no evidence of ADD at all. It was the child's response to abuse. Abused children come to school preoccupied with how they'll avoid the abuse when they get home. They are angry, overreactive, jumpy, anxious, impulsive and cannot pay attention due to this preoccupation.

7.7.2 What to Do

It is important to address the family-of-origin issues when working through the issues of either physical or emotional abuse. Addressing them in a holistic manner with family, marital, and individual treatment is more successful than working alone with the person. It is crucial that individuals realize the problems are not only with themselves. Separate these issues from the attentional disorder but always remember that the impact of the symptoms of the attentional disorder may well have triggered the abuse. Finally, nutritional plans as well as planning fun time are crucial interventions to bring health and joy to what probably has been a rather dismal existence.

Rule out or address issues of Post Traumatic Stress Disorder and its impact in terms of making the individual more vulnerable to other stressors in everyday life. We have found that individuals who experienced trauma such as child abuse are at greater risk and tend to react and over-react to subsequent happenings in their lives. Having been traumatized, these individuals do not adequately handle further stress in their lives. As their lives become more complicated with children, job, and money issues, they do not cope as well. Finally, due to trauma, research has shown that there are physical changes and changes within the brain that also do not allow the person to cope with everyday life as well as they would otherwise. Some of these symptoms can look like an attention disorder. Addressing the trauma, if it is there, involves different treatment such as using behavioral methods and working through the trauma suggested for PTSD.

7.8   Depression

Depression is a pervasive disorder that tends to predict the negative. It is prompted by grief and loss that is turned inward. When grief is turned outward it becomes anger toward others. When turned inward, the anger can eventually erode the person to the degree that suicide is possible. There are two types of depression, biochemical or endogenous depression from birth or reactive/situational depression that is usually transitory. The type of depression determines whether there is a need for medication. Reactive depression in response to an overwhelming loss may persist for a lifetime and result in a condition that is no longer situational and instead becomes more characteristic of endogenous depression. The idea here is that depression has a genetic quality that can be passed down from generation to generation. Further, growing up in a depressed household may create distorted patterns of coping with and viewing the world. If ingrained in the individual it can lead to lifelong depression. General research indicates that the best predictor of adult depression is childhood depression because the condition and its symptoms are incorporated into the person's psyche.

Those with higher levels of depression have a more pessimistic explanatory style for events that occurred in their lives and this attributional style places the person at higher risk for multiple episodes of depression. Those with depression see things negatively, thus they are pessimistic and continually use pessimism to confirm their belief system, which becomes a habitual way of relating to the world. "I knew it wouldn't work out" to justify when things fail is a perfect example of how individuals continue to feel depressed no matter what happens in their lives.

7.8.1   Symptoms

- Tend to be a victim of the disorder
- Always predict the worst
- Limited by fear of failure and lots of avoidance
- No interest in anything
- A tiredness or total loss of energy (Fatigue is a result of the effort it takes to repress feelings of sadness and maintain everything

inside. The consequence is a loss of energy and thus interest in anything.)

- True negativity and prediction of disaster
- See the worst
- Often hear only the counsel of their own words
- Don't hear anyone else
- Have a notion they are not likely to move out of the depression. The true depressive is stuck — really stuck in a world of negative, have not, cannot have, will not have, and so on. They believe they cannot get what they want and therefore predict the worst so when it happens, it won't be so bad because they knew it was coming.
- Isolation and insulation from others and situations
- Very fearful of hope (if they hope or have expectations they will lose and then be even more disappointed — so it is better not to hope. They do not allow others to come close to them and tend to treat them as objects — outsiders who cannot come close. Viewing others as objects helps to insulate the person and prevent further risk of loss.)

Depression has to do with a feeling of loss or change.

Characteristic physical symptoms

- Overall fatigue
- Sleep disturbance (usually too much sleep)
- Weight loss or gain
- No energy or no interest
- Feelings of worthlessness
- Insomnia or hypersomnia
- Agitation and restlessness
- Psychomotor retardation
- Anxiety
- Hypoglycemia
- Hypothyroid
- Sadness turned inside
- General malaise
- Others feel tired when with them

The presence of ADD helps to continue the depression. There is a grief reaction to ADD that can become anger turned inward. Discovery of an attentional disorder can cause depression as loss and grief are turned inward.

There is a grief reaction on discovering that one has ADD, particularly in older children, adolescents, and, primarily, adults. Often during the evaluation session when they see the scores of their performance on such simple measures, it dawns on them that they have been suffering from something real and that their problems were not imagined. However, when diagnosed (to severe degrees in some areas), the act of attaching a name to their symptoms can cause an extensive grief reaction. When adults learn that their marital or job problems are due to a disorder and that indeed they are very smart, should have been able to go to college and be more successful, and so on, they experience a tremendous feeling of loss. Loss for what could have been had the disorder been diagnosed and treated earlier. Loss for the past. There is grief for the future as well, as they realize that life will always be a struggle for them.

Finally, there are feelings of relief. Relief that it is over and tears of joy for the peace they now may be able to attain. After leaving a testing session, one woman cried on realizing what she had been up against. This same woman cried throughout the whole interview as we reviewed the results because they explained so many of her life patterns and why she had allowed others in her life to abuse her. We are very clear when presenting this data to individuals simply because they need to understand the struggles they have been through and how the severity of the disorder can cause them to be unable to complete the same task a 5-year-old child can do with ease.

Depression tends to be found more often with ADD without hyperactivity because ADHD individuals would not be upset enough to become depressed. Depression really tends to go hand in hand with ADD without hyperactivity and would not be seen in ADHD because that individual does not care enough to become depressed.

With ADD the person stays in depression longer than most because they are so impacted by the presence of the disorder. ADD individuals are already isolated and insulated so depression rocks them even more. If they are depressed and have an attentional disorder it is critical to determine which came first. Are we dealing with true depression or depression as a result of trying to cope with ADD? Generally, operating on the biochemical theory, there can be a biochemical, genetic depression that goes hand in hand with ADD, each tending to exacerbate the other. Or there is depression that is a direct result of the struggle with ADD. Generally, the two can be separated. True depression is more severe and can be traced through the family history as opposed to the less severely symptomatic depressed sadness of a continual struggle with ADD

ADD individuals tend to give up and withdraw and do not try to make changes. Depressives — true depressives — see themselves as victims. They are hopeless and helpless to make changes in their life. They see the worst and see themselves as unable to fix things and make them right. There is no problem solving, only problems. Combined with ADD they tend to give up and not work to compensate for symptoms of the disorder. They give up seeking proper medication. They don't fight for help at work or in school. If things don't work out — well, they tried and that's that. They look for others to save them, rescue them, or fix all of their problems. They tend to exhaust the very people they are trying to get to take care of them and they have little intention of or interest in taking care of themselves. Women are little girls and men are dependent. The spouse tends to be in control and a caretaker.

7.8.2 What to Do

When the disorder is biochemical — frequently severe and longer lasting — medication can be extremely helpful. There are new medications for depression that have minimal side effects and work well with the stimulant medication used for ADD. Encouraging them to participate in social and group activities helps people overcome their natural tendency to withdraw. Use of music is a wonderful way to wake up in the morning and get the day started in an upbeat fashion. A spiritual connection or some religious affiliation also helps people to feel less alone and uncared for. Finally, diet, nutrition, and regular exercise are key components not only to regulate their emotional state and prevent deep lows but to prevent them from becoming ill (as is the tendency among this group).

More often than not, depression does not stand alone. Look for a mixed disorder of anxiety and depression. Rule out other disorders, such as neurological disease, that commonly show symptoms of depression. Generalized anxiety disorder as an intervening factor that continually interplays with depression may need to be addressed as well, especially in terms of medication. There are very effective antidepressant medications, though a combination of several may be necessary to address all the factors of this multifaceted disorder. Finally, note that sporadic depression may be seen as part of the cyclical pattern of manic depression, or Bipolar Disorder. A rule of thumb is to be open to treating depression with both medication and therapy.

7.9 Anxiety

Anxiety tends to be found at its most severe in ADD without hyperactivity, though the motor symptoms of anxiety tend to lead to over-diagnoses of ADHD. These individuals generally tend to constantly shake one foot but sometimes a hand shakes as well. Anxiety and fear is what makes ADD without hyperactivity individuals lie with a perfect poker face and avoid and procrastinate because they would rather be seen as behavioral problems than admit to their failures. They don't want anyone to be mad or upset with them.

7.9.1 Symptoms

- Ranges from generalized anxiety state to panic disorder
- Pervades the person before they even know it
- Creates a constant fear and anticipation of disaster without the knowledge that it can be handled
- Involves the autonomic nervous system or automatic system, therefore once anxiety has occurred it must be handled
- Panic leads to more panic
- Includes feeling a loss of control
- There is procrastinating and forgetting to do things due to fear of failure
- May also be a subtle form of anger, the passive-aggressive type
- Uses avoidance due to a constant fear state
- Whines when angry and apologizes for being angry
- Avoids conflict
- Fears abandonment
- Undecided because afraid to be wrong
- Can be manipulative and secretive
- Experiences moodiness
- Involves identity confusion due to fear of identifying needs and taking a stand

These individuals do not want anyone to be mad at them. They can be angry, but they cannot tolerate anger from others. They will lie to avoid others getting angry at them. They will be secretive with their feelings so as not to upset anyone. They will manipulate and use passive-aggressive behavior to elicit a desired response because they are fearful of a direct, head-on collision. This is the person who doesn't get mad but gets even. For example, in the movie *Prince of Tides*, the mother, in a very passive-aggressive manner, cooks dog food as a meal to punish and get even with her husband for his raging temper.

Those with anxiety are unresolved as to what they want, who they are, and what they need both from themselves and from others. The moodiness is the result of the constant confusion and frustration that is due to the inability to make a decision and stick with it. Anxious individuals hate their fear and *hate* being wimpy.

Generalized anxiety is present all of the time, waxing and waning depending on what is going on with the individual. This tends to be a genetic biochemical anxiety that is present in the family history. Anxiety, once past a certain point, has a life all its own. It enervates or impacts the automatic system in the brain, causing the person to go on automatic pilot. Anxiety hits the internal organs, which is why there can be responses such as feeling sick, fluttery feelings, and so on. Individuals with anxiety may think that if they stay in bed they can keep the anxiety at bay, but it remains. These people get so scared that they cannot pull themselves out of the anxiety and it can then move them into a full-scale panic attack.

General research findings support the idea that anxious children experience a broad range of somatic (physical) complaints when compared with the "normal" population. Anxious children tend to have somatic complaints, such as, tired, don't feel well, constant colds, headaches, backaches, stomach aches, and so on. Adults tend to follow the same pattern.

Physical symptoms of generalized anxiety

- Trembling
- Shaky
- Muscle tension or soreness
- Restlessness
- Easily fatigued

Physical symptoms of panic disorder include the above symptoms to a mild degree as well as

- Frequent urination or trouble swallowing
- Feeling keyed up and on edge
- Exaggerated startle response
- Difficulty concentrating — mind going blank
- Trouble falling or staying asleep
- Irritability

Physical characteristics of panic attacks

- Shortness of breath
- Tachycardia
- Chest pain
- Sweating
- Dizziness, unsteady feelings
- Abdominal distress or nausea
- Trembling or shaking
- Choking
- Feelings of detachment
- Flushes or chills
- Fear of dying

- Fear of going crazy

ADD perpetuates anxiety and panic disorders and people cannot trust themselves to handle it. With the symptoms of ADD, these individuals are unable to trust themselves enough to know if they should punt, pass, or run. Symptoms may be present that contribute to the anxiety because they can't rely on themselves to take care of things. Finally, there is so much failure related to this disorder that self-esteem is too diminished to allow them to count on their own abilities.

Low self-esteem associated with ADD leads to a more continuous cycle of anxiety. More anxiety means less ability to compensate for the ADD. This is the cyclical relationship of anxiety with ADD without hyperactivity. All of this eventually leads to depression and feeling victimized. This is the essence of the self-fulfilling prophesy that so plagues the ADD population. They sabotage themselves by not compensating for symptoms of the disorder and the ADD remains larger than life. They are stuck with no options. ADD individuals who are anxious and feel futile would rather not try than try and fail. They avoid because they are unsure of how to do things. It is easier to withdraw, procrastinate, or put things off, than to risk the shame and embarrassment of poor performance related to the attentional disorder.

7.9.2   What to Do

It is important to understand anxiety as a very serious disorder that has farreaching consequences and not to underestimate the impact of its presence. If genetic, it is always there and comes and goes depending on the environment and how the person feels at the time. This can be a crippling disease, preventing people from attaining their life accomplishments, goals, and so on. Fear can run people's lives and keep them from close relationships. This can result in their dying before they ever lived. Having presented all of this, the first step is a clear diagnosis a definition of the nature of anxiety assessement of a genetic history in the family, and a determination of how the anxiety impacts the person's life. Establish where the anxiety is an issue. In dealing with generalized anxiety, use techniques of hypnosis, general relaxation training, and cognitive self-control therapy. Teach them to use motivational statements such as, "I can do it." Refer to the great amount of literature on coping with anxiety that talks about all the people who have *beaten* this disorder. Inform them that when anxious or worried about something that they know they must do anyway, it is best not to think about it. The anticipatory anxiety for a feared event can become highly overwhelming. Obsessing about something does not help lessen the anxiety.

With panic disorder, it is important to understand that once the automatic symptoms appear, it is a done deal. Best to go with the flow, get up, walk around, take breaths and do whatever needs to be done to get through the physical discomfort of the event. Those who describe panic attacks talk about being awakened in the middle of the night. For example, they may say, "I woke up the other night with a panic attack, my heart pounded, I could not catch my breath and I had a tightness in my chest that felt terrible. I tried to lie there and go back to sleep, which did not work. After a few minutes I got up, went into another room, put on some music and concentrated on a project on which I had been working. After a few hours, I had calmed down enough to go back to sleep." A common mistake people make is trying to move out of the panic attack once it has started or they just sit there with it instead of doing something. Anyone who has ever experienced a panic attack knows how awful it can feel.

Finally, nutritional supplements have proved extremely beneficial in coping with this disorder by alleviating both the immediate symptoms and protecting the brain from future illness such as hypertension and increased risk sensitivity to environmental toxins, viruses, and illness. Using specially tailored nutritional supplements helps to calm the system. Our tendency is to try nutrition first, and then turn to the excellent new medications that are now available, whether the antianxiety agents or the new SSRI antidepressants. (Luvox® is a recent medication being heralded as treatment for panic disorder. Inderal® is used for panic symptoms that are more temporary, such as public speaking). Addressing the impact of depression on anxiety and how closely these two conditions are interwoven is very important. Often, generalized anxiety will lead to depression and vice versa.

7.10 Borderline Personality

Borderline Personality Disorder is a watershed diagnosis that appeared in the last 15 years or so and since that time has emerged as a very important diagnostic category to help individuals understand their frightening and inexplicable behavior. The movie *Fatal Attraction* characterized the extreme borderline personality and revealed the peculiarities and idiosyncrasies of the disorder. There is a considerable pathology to this group, meaning they have very severe psychological issues that are not always amenable or able to be resolved with individual psychotherapy treatment. Overall research has documented that this diagnosis carries with it higher rates of depression, substance abuse, and antisocial disorders. It is associated with a history of significant family pathology or disorders and maternal inconsistency. The onset of this disorder tends to occur with the presence of highly inconsistent maternal involvement — with mother being there either too much or not at all. The mothers of people who suffer with Borderline Personality Disorder inconsistently exacted discipline and often broke promises, which confused the children. This left them unable to decide whether their mothers cared about them. It also instilled the question of whether their mothers could be trusted to do as they said they were going to do.

7.10.1   Symptoms

- Their world is clearly split with good and bad people and/or things.
- There is a rigid separation of positive and negative thoughts about the self and others.
- Stormy relationships are common because they believe they are always being victimized by others.
- They move from clinging dependency to angry manipulation with those close to them.
- There are job problems and extreme difficulties managing their lives.
- They range from wonderful to awful.
- Temper outbursts are common and come unexpectedly — when least expected they explode about something insignificant or trivial.
- They are very fragile individuals who are highly sensitive and can break easily.
- They project onto others what belongs to or represents them.
- They assume that others have the same feelings, thoughts, and beliefs.
- Their facial features change through the years — they can change their appearance to look so very different that they are not easily recognized.
- They switch quickly in temperament and disposition.
- They can be depressed, enraged, delinquent, lawless, antisocial, anxious, fragile, crazy, psychotic, manic, childlike, wonderfully sweet, and considerate but the end always justifies the means.
- They appear to lack moral consciousness as they trade their value system for what they believe is right.
- They can move quickly from the rational to the irrational and anything can set them off.

The mark of the Borderline Personality is that out of nowhere they come up with something that makes absolutely no sense at all and once they arrive at this totally irrational place, you can't talk them out of it. That is that. If you try to tell them something else they believe you are trying to rationalize your own guilt or fault. They need to be right. They are always right and they will prove it no matter what, no matter how absurd or irrational the situation becomes. Because they are fragile, their world needs to be structured. They demand comfort and safety and, therefore, cannot tolerate opposing thoughts. Borderlines twist and turn things into what they want to believe.

People are objects to be used. They attach to no one for fear of being hurt. They are extremely rigid individuals.

With ADD they don't get it and this leads to increased irrational thinking.

They tend to miscue, misassume, miscommunicate, and miss the point, which sets off an emotional reaction. With the Borderline Personality in combination with ADD they will miss information, arrive at erroneous conclusions, and will not be convinced of anything else. Borderline Personalities can easily move into a *lock* whether that is a lock on an idea, belief, notion, or plan for what they want to do or how they want to handle a situation. Symptoms of the ADD disorder contribute to the irrational thinking as they continually miss information and are more likely to be upset and move into the lock. The lock may also be used as a means of structure to cope with low self-esteem symptoms of ADD and establish structure and safety in an ever-changing world. The ADD Borderline Personality needs to be right and does so by locking into the idea to maintain stability in their thoughts, how they view the world and feel things should be.

7.10.2 What to Do

These individuals need to be handled carefully. They tend to overreact and to not back down. In speaking with them, you should be as clear as possible verbally and then ask the person to feed the information back to ensure that the correct message has been heard. Medication is difficult with this group due to the everchanging diagnosis: when they are anxious, they benefit from anti-anxiety agents, when depressed, antidepressants are in order; when there is loss of reality and irrational thinking, an antipsychotic is needed. The problem is that each of these medications needs to be in the system for a period of time to work effectively and, so, just about the time one begins to work another disorder can appear. Emotions shift and secondary diagnoses of depression, anxiety, and psychosis change. Recently, we have seen some positive results with use of Zoloft®, Effexor®, and Serzone® to address the fragility. By addressing fragility, the person tends to be less argumentative and emotionally reactive. Depending on the behavior at the time, targeted coping mechanisms for the anxiety, depression, rage, mania, and so on would benefit from exercise and nutrition.

Finally, do not take their behavior personally or see it as connected to you as a significant person in the Borderline's life. Diagnosing the ADD and treating it may help some of the miscommunication problems and thinking problems. Use of stimulant medication may trigger more reactiveness, so in deciding whether to medicate the ADD one needs to weigh the possible negative effects it may have on the borderline disorder in relation to the positive effects it will have on the ADD.

7.11   Posttraumatic Stress Disorder

Posttraumatic Stress Disorder (PTSD) was originally identified in victims of war, flood, or some other unusual disaster. Trauma is defined as an event that threatens or causes death, undue harm, or serious injury to an individual or someone significant to them. Often the event is so severe that they were unable to do anything to stop it. Observation of these individuals showed symptoms impacting their emotional skills, physical health, and thinking ability. We now realize that this disorder can occur as a consequence of all kinds of stressful situations including emotional, physical and sexual abuse, death of someone significant, and any situation not within the context of "normal" that is totally unexpected and shocks the person. What we have found in research is that the severity of PTSD or related problems is dependent on the age at which the trauma occurs, people's gender, the support available from their families, and the general atmosphere of the home environment. Having experienced trauma of some sort, these people become more at risk for the inability to cope with further trauma in their lives or even everyday events that become slightly overwhelming. PTSD individuals may overreact to an event that does not pose a high degree of threat. Coping with everyday life and stressors becomes increasingly difficult as they age and have more responsibility in terms of children, job, family, and so on. The alarm is always in set position.

If someone has been abused, there are many trust issues, much defensiveness, and a tendency to not communicate feelings. When trauma occurs, whether it is in the form of significant loss (i.e., special people in their lives), abuse, or some environmental disaster, how the person reacts determines the degree of the trauma's long-term effects. When a traumatic event occurs and surprises someone, it may leave the person untrusting because he was caught "off guard" in such a violent manner. These individuals tend to remain "ready" so not to get caught again. This eternal vigilance creates a defensive, careful, suspicious reaction to everyone and everything. Symptoms of PTSD are further exacerbated by the fact that the adrenaline system remains in a constant "ON" position in response to long-term stress.

7.11.1   Symptoms

The strongest predictors of PTSD symptoms are

- Exaggerated startle response
- Illness due to stress-related chemical imbalance
- An irritable family atmosphere followed by a depressed family atmosphere

- The overall disfunction of the parents, particularly the primary caregiver

Individuals who find themselves stuck in trauma either did not have a supportive, encouraging atmosphere that allowed them to talk about what had happened or they were too young to cope with the issue, which led to a general feeling of powerlessness.

EXAMPLE
We once participated in a legal proceeding where a child was the center of the battle and, as such, was subjected to a constant battery of questions and evaluations. Indeed, at his fragile young age, this child had been evaluated more than an adult. Consequently, after 4 years of this activity, the boy began to show signs of PTSD.

When age, fragility of nature, or an unsupportive family create feelings of helplessness during a traumatic event, the individual turns to withdrawal and denial as a means to cope. Unfortunately, repression and denial allow the trauma to live on and continue to impact their lives, kind of like a low-grade fever. Consequently, they are unable to be completely productive, share emotions or live with spontaneity (they are overly rigid).

The presence of an attentional disorder compounds this pattern as it further impacts the ability to cope with trauma and resolve it. The combination of symptoms from trauma and attentional disorder, especially ADD without hyperactivity, produce a system where each feeds the other, which can generate severe problems.

Trauma continues with diagnosis of ADD, and the communication problems as seen with the attentional disorder make it easy for these people to withdraw and not be close to those significant in their lives. Factor in an attentional disorder with trauma and fear increases as the individual has less well developed coping mechanisms. Thus, all of the symptoms relating to trauma such as withdrawal, flatness of feelings and poor communication are heightened.

EXAMPLE
One woman diagnosed with ADD without hyperactivity talked about her childhood being so traumatic due to the symptoms of ADD (in addition to other emotional and family-life issues) that she had to mentally and emotionally enclose herself. She developed a "friend" to operate for her. While she was aware of this split, she realized at the time that it allowed her to cope with the situation. Once on medication she was no longer able to maintain this separation and her life began to happen directly to her instead of to her "friend." She no longer had a shield to protect the child within her; the small person was flooded with feelings of fear, anger, rejection, and so on.

General symptoms

- Fear of life
- Avoidance and procrastination
- Associated with ADD without hyperactivity
- Shyness and fearfulness can lead to withdrawal from people
- The person continues to be traumatized and never moves out of it

Due to trauma, there is a pervasive fear of life, avoidance, procrastination, and the tendency to maintain the status quo for stability. In ADD without hyperactivity there is the tendency toward shyness and withdrawal, which, again, is heightened by trauma. With this combination, the individual is not able to resolve the trauma and move out of it if having to battle two factors at the same time.

Thinking abilities are affected. PTSD is subtle and can be confused with the fogginess and spaciness of ADD without hyperactivity. Trauma is diffuse and nondistinct. It is hard to get to the trauma and deal with the emotions of it. There is a fogginess associated with trauma that needs to be separated from the fogginess associated with the ADD without hyperactivity. Sometimes the symptoms will overlap. Things get confusing, particularly when considering the research that shows that there are biochemical changes with PTSD that affect the same systems as ADD. Finally, the trauma itself may be related to a number of factors rather than just one issue or event. This requires continual prodding to get these individuals to release, experience the emotions, move out of the "lock" of the trauma and move forward.

7.11.2   What to Do

The two disorders, ADD and PTSD, need to be differentiated and separated as distinct entities and then examined for their overlap of symptoms. How one relates to the other, where they are separate, and where the symptoms overlap in the person's life is critical information to begin to cope with the presence of PTSD. Further, one must understand the far-reaching consequences of PTSD and the degree to which they impact individuals' ability to function in their everyday lives; how they affect goal achievement, task performance and personal relationships. Trust issues and continual fear are considerable barriers toward developing long-lasting relationships, leaving the person feeling quite alone, which further increases the effects of this disorder.

Referring the person to support groups, conducting individual and family therapy aimed at resolving old issues and building a new future that is not reliant on the pain of the past is crucial. Old traumas may create phobias and require guided desensitization whereby the person is gently asked to face the thing that triggers fear and work through it to understand that the old situation and the old helplessness can be resolved in the present, although it could not in the past.

EXAMPLE

We worked with an individual who reported that his job was on the line because he could not climb a high tower that was part of his daily job requirement. In the past, this man had been a member of a motorcycle gang. He could do anything and viewed everything as a challenge. In fact, he prided himself on being able to do everything and anything. This man came from a pretty tough family background — an abusive and alcoholic household. His method for surviving was to meet and conquer every challenge. He expected he would die by 40, and if he died earlier, he didn't care. When he turned 40 and looked at his family, he suddenly decided he cared about life and wanted to live. Practically overnight he became afraid of everything from riding elevators to climbing this high tower at work. He had not dealt with the trauma of his difficult childhood. Instead, he had lived dangerously with the notion that early death would be fine with him. We hypnotized him and he turned out to be a pretty good subject. It was surprising that he was able to trust us that much. During one of the hypnotic sessions we took him through his fear by guiding him up the tower while fellow employees watched him. He started to sweat and his breathing became heavy. However, by using self-talk statements like "you can do it," he moved triumphantly through the anxiety reaction and climbed the tower, setting himself free from the crippling fear. One more session solidified the progress and he has been fine since.

This type of treatment does not always result in success so easily (in this case the man had also been in therapy for several years). Sometimes, traumas are multiple and one fear response is replaced by another.

Finally, address the thinking problems and provide a means to generate alternative solutions to problem-solve everyday issues in their lives. Teach them how to identify workable solutions and rule out nonviable ones to increase flexibility and creativity of thinking. Medication can be helpful in addition to diet and nutritional supplements, which are central to the treatment of this disorder. This disorder commonly overlaps with symptoms of an attentional disorder (without hyperactivity specifically). It is important to realize that this disorder has a great impact on the person hormonally with regard to anxiety and stress reactions and places them at greater risk for future health problems.

7.12 Dissociative Identity Disorder (Previously Multiple Personality Disorder)

The cause of Dissociative Identity Disorder (DID) seems to be related to childhood trauma, sexual trauma or abuse that is so horrible that it must be split off and dissociated from the host consciousness and lodged in the alters. DID is defined as the existence in the person of two or more distinct personalities or personality states. With DID, the individual experiences trauma that cannot be tolerated because of a lack of defense and coping strategies. Those affected tend to be fragile and vulnerable and simply cannot cope with the trauma. To survive, they adopt a means of coping by which they split themselves into parts and assign the trauma to one of the "others" they've created. Much like denial, creating another personality to deal with extreme trauma allows the person to cope as the event is seen as disassociated from themselves and happening to someone else. The problem becomes more serious if traumatic events continue and more personalities are formed to assume responsibility for them. How fragile these people are determines how much they will integrate their personalities into their own existence or separate them into clearly distinct entities with different voices, appearances, and so on.

7.12.1   What to Do

Identify the presence of this disorder and understand the individuals' behavior within the context of their past experiences. Identify the trauma and treat these individuals similarly to those with PTSD. It is important not to miss the traumas in their lives and know whether they can be resolved in a therapeutic situation. Nutritional supplements can be helpful in addressing the consequences trauma exerts on thinking ability and brain functioning.

7.13   Schizoaffective Disorder

This is a term used generally to describe individuals who have high degrees of fragility and the tendency to develop symptoms characteristic of full-blown psychosis or schizophrenia. There tends to be a genetic base with a clear presence of family history of schizophrenia or overall fragility.

7.13.1   Symptoms

- Shy and keep to themselves
- Fearful of others
- Very mistrustful in general
- Fragile individuals with ability to have a psychotic break
- They miscue and can miss information, similar to symptoms of ADD without hyperactivity — they do not "get it"
- Can be present with both ADHD (to a considerably lesser degree) and ADD without hyperactivity
- Aggressive behavior of ADHD creates an aggressive type of schizophrenia rather than the withdrawn behavior that is so often seen with this population

- Poor social convection — inability to read social cues and express self in an appropriate social manner
- When irrational, words do not make sense
- Unfinished sentences and thoughts — use of fragments rather than whole sentences and rarely complete ideas
- Lack of rule-governed behavior, or very compulsive
- Low profile — for not upsetting anyone
- Schizophrenia — a range from withdrawn to full-blown psychosis with lack of reality, delusions, and hallucinations
- Lack initiative
- Feelings are not known
- Unable to sense other people's feelings
- Unintentionally aloof and indifferent to others at times
- Fragile and emotionally bland or devoid of emotions
- Calm, gentle, not easily angered, and peaceful
- Work quietly and independently and are seemingly untroubled

Research indicates that individuals are at greater risk for development of schizophrenia if there are symptoms of:

- Attentional problems
- Psychosis (loss of reality)
- Social isolation

The greater the stress on the individuals the more likely they are to develop the symptoms of this genetic disorder. ADD without hyperactivity is more commonly related to this disorder because there is withdrawn and fragile behavior and they have more conversations in their heads than anywhere else. The highest-functioning form of schizophrenia (which is really a term meaning loss of reality) is seen in the Paranoid Schizophrenic, who is very mistrustful. Schizophrenia is a genetic disorder. The tendency is always there for it to develop. However, signs of the disorder are not seen until there is a high degree of stress in the person's life. The first breakdown (loss of reality) typically occurs in adolescence and by early adulthood is pronounced as things become more complex and problematic.

Some individuals can have the genetic tendency for schizophrenia yet never see it develop as their lives remain without complications and stress. For example, a bright young man diagnosed with ADD and a genetic predisposition for schizophrenia was having trouble with his college courses. It was determined that Ritalin would help control his situation but could possibly initiate a schizophrenic reaction. He chose to try the medication anyway and schizophrenic events did occur. He was taken off the medication, provided with an antipsychotic medication and then resumed Ritalin. Since then, he has been fine and is doing so well in school that he is applying for his doctorate.

7.13.2   What to Do

Understand that these are very fragile individuals who are highly sensitive as a result. Teasing and joking with them can easily turn into an upsetting event in their lives from which they will have difficulty recovering. These individuals tend to be immature and childlike and need very clear and gentle guidance about how to handle themselves in social situations, work settings, and so on. They will miss information as a result of the attentional disorder and be too shy to ask for help. Instead, they are more comfortable struggling along in confusion. Identify if there is an attentional disorder due to the overlap and masking that can occur with this disorder.

Finally, there are new medications such as Clozaril®, Risperdal® and the antiseizure medication Depakote®, that have fewer side effects than medicines of the past. Medication is critical for treating outbreaks, loss of reality, and breakdowns and must be administered on a very strict schedule. Setting limits on environmental variables to create a stress-free environment is very integral to their care. Diet and nutrition are also important factors in the treatment of this disorder.

7.14   Impulsivity

Serotonin is the neurotransmitter indicated by impulsivity. It is important to differentiate true impulsivity due to a biochemical imbalance in the serotonin system from impulsivity that occurs with ADD (when the person becomes frustrated and suddenly gives up). You can see true impulsivity in the ADHD child or adult who thinks of something and just does it, while others would consider consequences before acting. When you ask an ADHD, "Why did you do that?" they often respond with, "I don't know."

7.14.1   What to Do

Separate impulsive behavior observed with an attentional disorder or other diagnosis from true impulsivity. Impulsivity can occur as a result of pent-up frustration or feelings of hopelessness and helplessness. Borders and boundaries as well as structure and consequences serve to curb true impulsivity as much as is possible.

7.15 Obsessive Compulsive Disorder

Is it a disorder or a defense mechanism to cope with the world? When examining Obsessive Compulsive Disorder (OCD) it is important to determine whether the obsessive compulsive behavior is a defense mechanism used to provide stability and control to one's environment or if it is a syndrome of and by itself. OCD can range from mild (defense mechanism) to severe (presence of the disorder with all of its characteristics and symptoms). The disorder of OCD has a genetic biochemical basis that can be traced to family history with the existence of high anxiety, fragility, or both. What I call the "true" OCD involves symptoms such as continual hand wringing, door checking, hand washing, and so on. Often this disorder can be a precursor to the development of Tourette's Syndrome.

The term defense mechanism is used to define those who develop a need to defend themselves from their environment and cope with its difficulties. By defending, they alleviate anxiety and instability in their lives. They always do things the same way, do things perfectly, withdraw into work, and so on. Traits of the obsessive compulsive are perfectionism, a drive to attain goals, and overachievement. Some OCD people are great collectors, as if surrounding themselves with possessions provides stability. Accompanying this personality type is a high degree of anxiety and obsessive compulsive behavior that helps to provide stability in these peoples' lives.

7.15.1 Symptoms

- Compulsive preoccupation with details
- Compulsive preoccupation with routine
- Compulsive preoccupation with stability
- Difficulty discarding unnecessary objects
- Difficulty expressing tender feelings
- Work, work, work — workaholic
- Empathy with others' feelings is inhibited by compulsive behavior
- Getting the job done is most important
- Anxiety is masked with compulsiveness
- Perfectionists
- Poor self image
- Rigid insistence on doing things as they have done in the past or in their own way
- Skeptical

- Accurate
- Dependable
- Pay attention to detail
- Productive
- Always get the job done
- Punctual
- Persevering

These are the traits of the obsessive compulsive. You will find that many (if not most) doctors, dentists, and lawyers are somewhat obsessive compulsive and perfectionistic in nature to have earned that degree and made it in their profession. Obsessive compulsive behavior tends to be associated with ADD without hyperactivity and often is a defense mechanism to cope with the symptoms of ADD. Perfectionism is a way of controlling the fear of ADD symptoms by only doing what you can do well and doing it so well that no one sees the symptoms of the disorder. When perfectionism is part of OCD it is difficult with ADD due to the symptoms of the disorder. The "not getting it" contributes to the feeling of lack of control. Feeling a lack of control promotes the need for more control. More control leads to increased tension, increased tension leads to more compulsive behaviors and rituals to provide stability. Bright individuals with severe ADD tend to work harder than others to mask the symptoms of the disorder. They try to be perfect, and to avoid and procrastinate what they cannot do. They concentrate their efforts on presenting a picture that everything is fine. Thus, the need to be perfect increases with more-severe symptoms of ADD.

7.15.2   What to Do

For the OCD disorder there is medication to relieve the drive and compulsivity. Medication is important, as the nature of this disorder causes these individuals to lose control over their behavior. With regard to personality traits, self-talk and setting limits on work and perfectionism can be very positive. New and old medications such as Luvox®, BuSpar®, Lithium, Prozac®, Risperdal®, Tryptophane, Clonidine®, Klonopin®, and Anafranil® are being tried with this group. When working with the OCD personality, suggest setting limits. Regulate the time and effort they exert on tasks and help them to set reasonable and rational goals. Because there is so much stress, the person will definitely benefit from nutritional supplements, diet, and exercise. Finally, it is critical to separate and treat symptoms of the attentional disorder since the effort spent masking them increases their struggle and could lead to serious physical results. Planning fun time is almost unheard of yet it is a necessity for these individuals. These are the personalities who by their 40s and 50s are in serious physical condition and can no longer compensate for symptoms of the attentional disorder.

8

Assessment and Why It Is So Important In Diagnosing ADD

8.1 Current Problems of Testing for ADD

It is said there is no test to measure ADD, no single method of measurement for ADD. In fact, there is a considerable degree of controversy over how we currently evaluate for this disorder. At our clinic we have implemented a battery of tests measuring all aspects of ADD. Over a period of 10 years, this battery has proven clinically effective in evaluating an attentional disorder for ages as young as 5 years and as old as 79 years. We always begin with the actual testing that forms the clinical picture and determines if the disorder is present in terms of performance on neuropsychological tests.

Neuropsychological tests are very simple paper-and-pencil tests that specifically measure different aspects of the brain and are called brain-behavior measures. Performance on each of these tests is compared with the predicted intellectual potential of an individual. For each of the tests we have scores that we would expect the average person to obtain, based on the exact age of the people being evaluated. Their performance on each test is then compared with what we would expect them to score based on the averages obtained when the test was administered to other people.

Norms are what we identify as the average score obtained based on an evaluation of a group of individuals taking the same test. When a test or measure is normed, the researchers go out and administer that test to all kinds of people who supposedly make up the *normal* population. The idea is to screen out anyone who is not the average, so those individuals who have some type of outward emotional or mental impairment are not included in this normative sample (e.g., mental retardation, autism, Tourette's Syndrome, and other disorders are screened out). The test is then adminstered to this normative population and scores are obtained for the age range the test is supposed to measure. So if the test measures ages 5 through 50, then you have scores that are what we would expect the average 5-year-old, 6-year-old, and so on up to 50-year-old to obtain on this particular measure.

The picture gets a little more complicated when we bring in standard deviations. The *standard deviation* is the number that represents the degree by which the score is different from the mean, the distance from the mean. So if someone had a score of 5 and the standard deviation was 1, and the average normed score was 4, the score of 5 is one unit or one standard deviation above the mean. If the score people obtained was 4, then their score would be average. If the score people obtained was 3, their score would be one unit below the mean or below average. In this manner, we can determine the degree to which the score differs for the people being tested from what we would expect average people to do for their age levels and how much their scores differ from that.

Evaluation is based on the people's identified intellectual potential and comparing their score obtained on each measure. What if individuals have the intellectual potential for being average? Then, we would expect average scoring on each of the attentional measures in our battery. If they have an above-average potential, we would expect above-average scoring and if they have a below-average potential, we would expect below-average scoring. This is how we can determine to what degree the disorder is mild, moderate, or severe. We can take each variable, distractibility, slow thinking speed, information processing, and spatial factors and compare results to determine if the disorder is present and to what degree. Then we factor in self-report measures to confirm or contradict our diagnosis.

There may be a problem in determining someone's intellectual potential. More often, we find that the intelligence tests that are the gold standard for intellectual assessment are not accurate. They are impacted by attentional symptoms, the greatest effect being speed and spatial variables. Half of the intellectual assessment is timed. Therefore, you can imagine just how inaccurate such testing would be.

To determine intellectual potential for the adult and adolescent (above 15 years) we use a measure that is based on word recognition, known to associate or correlate highly with the IQ assessment. However, often this measure is affected by people's poor vocabularly and worse yet, their inability to recognize a word and sound it out correctly. (Those spatial variables hit again.) We also have another measure. It is a measure of the whole brain potential. In other words, this measures the power or potential of the brain and often provides an accurate reading of one's potential. This measure can be affected by slow speed because it is based on time and spatial issues. So then what? Often, if the above two measures do not provide what appears to be an accurate reading, we can find another measure within the battery that will reveal what seems to be an accurate reading. When we say "what seems to be an accurate reading" we refer to a measure that is not so obviously impacted by speed, spatial issues and distractibility. Usually we are able to find some measure to determine someone's potential in an accurate manner. However, there are the isolated cases (approximately one in ten) where the symptoms are so pervasive that some attentional symptom (whether information processing, speed, spatial issues, or distractibility) manages to impact every single measure. It is then that we must estimate or hypothesize what their potential might have been. These are the cases that we will often re-test once these individuals are on stimulant medication.

An example of this would be individuals who achieve all average scores. They have average scores across the board for the intellectual evaluation, the IQ test. They have average scores for all of the neuropsychological measures. However, it can be seen as we go through the tests that these people could have been doing really well and then all of a sudden they lost it and began to do poorly, resulting in an average score. But it can be clearly seen that if they had continued to perform at the same rate with which they started, they would have come out with a superior score. And it can be seen that the problem they encountered was due to one of the symptoms of the attention disorder. So what does this mean? We believe that this provides evidence that their performance would be significantly altered if the attentional symptoms did not interfere. The idea being that if attentional symptoms impacted every measure and every measure is scored as average, then imagine what they might have done had there not been this interference. We hypothesize that they have a much higher potential based on qualitatively seeing very different ranges of performance within the same measure and that the scores are globally repressed to the average range.

Results of evaluating two different children point to the necessity of using clinical measures and neuropsychological evaluation in addition to examining the whole picture. We evaluated a child whose self-report measures from the school system indicated the presence of ADHD, as the child was acting out in school and displaying aggressive behavior and lack of attention. The self-report measures from his parents yielded the same picture. Results of clinical testing however, presented no evidence of an attentional disorder. Why? Because the child's behavioral problems were the result of child abuse, not ADD. Child abuse can cause a child to become angry and aggressive as well as inattentive, impulsive, and overactive — the same symptoms as ADD. At school, such children can be worried about going home or what is going to happen that night or the next. They may worry whether their mother is okay. They may be preoccupied with how to avoid making the abusive parent angry. The result would be distractibility and appearing inattentive. They would be anxious, due to worrying about what was going to take place at home and anticipating the worst. Anxiety can easily result in fidgeting behavior, the continuous moving and shifting in their seats. They may appear impulsive, saying to themselves, "oh what the heck, I don't care anymore," just to stop worrying. And they may be angry, taking out their aggression on their peers or talking back to the teacher or being defiant or oppositional in some manner. It is well known that symptoms of PTSD will present the same symptoms as we may see with ADD. PTSD can be the result of growing up in a dysfunctional, alcoholic, and/or abusive family.

Another clinical evaluation of a different child indicated the presence of ADD without hyperactivity. The self-report measures from both the parents and the school, however, indicated no evidence of an attentional disorder. But the neuropsychological testing clearly revealed the presence of an attentional disorder with all the characteristics of slow speed, distractibility, spatial issues, and information-processing deficits. There was no genetic history of ADD so what was it? This child suffered from early birth trauma to the brain. A lack of oxygen or anoxia can easily create minor or mild brain dysfunctioning that would result in attentional symptoms. The reason that attentional symptoms would be seen is that this is one of the first areas of the brain to be affected by anything because it is so vulnerable to insult.

These two examples clearly illustrate the importance of considering both clinical and self-report measures when seeking to diagnose ADD. This is why we do not rely on self-report measures, or on parent or teacher reports, to determine the presence or absence of ADD. This is the reason there is so much over-diagnosis and misdiagnosis. We cannot stress enough the need to use testing, evaluation, and, we believe, neuropsychological measures to test for ADD and to rule in or out other issues such as brain damage, emotional issues, home environment, and so on.

8.2   A Different way to Test for ADD

Neuropsychological measures or brain-behavior measures (tasks that tell us how the brain is working) tend not to be impacted by anxiety, depression, and/or other emotional factors. These tests are based on very simple tasks that everyone can do. Mostly, these are paper-and-pencil tasks, matching tasks, card sorting, etc. Often, these tasks become fun because they do not stretch the person beyond their abilities and thus do not produce anxiety. These tasks are not boring and do not tend to be subject to or impacted by the reduced psychomotor speed characteristic of depression. We have tested approximately 3000 individuals and no one has yet complained of the battery as a whole, just a few specific tests that were extremely difficult for them. Conversely, timed measures will tend to reveal more of the slow cognitive (or thinking) speed related to ADD as opposed to depression. Due to the variety of tests used to measure the same patterns, timed measures can assess slow thinking speed.

We have checks and balances for every symptom of ADD. We have different types of measures to assess distractibility, speed, information processing, and spatial problems. We have different measures to rule out interfering variables of motivation, fear of math, poor vocabulary, and so on. People don't know what we are looking for so we get a very accurate reading. In other words, they can't throw the test. They may give up on one measure but we have another way of measuring the same symptom. Medications that have an effect on the testing are antidepressants because they impact distractibility. When we know that someone is taking an antidepressant, we know to factor this into the evaluation of their score. The only other type of medication that would affect these measures is a stimulant medication such as Ritalin®. There is an effect if the person's blood sugar is low, so we can account for that.

There is an effect if there is anxiety but only on one specific measure and we are able to factor that in as well. By the time we finish, we are sure whether we have ADD or not. There are the times we think there is some additional diagnosis and then we will pursue further testing, whether that is neuropsychological or psychological.

EXAMPLE
Mario was a 45-year-old man who had come in for his test results. Before the evaluation meeting began, he indicated that the assessment was the easiest type of test that he had ever taken. He said it was lots of fun but he had no idea how we were going to identify ADD from those tests. We thanked him, indicating that this was the intention of the battery, simple tests that anyone should be able to do. However, he was very surprised when we started to score his results and found that his scores were well below the average.

The testing is scored with either the parents present, the adult individual who took the test, or the adolescent and his or her parents. This allows tested individuals to be part of the evaluation and, more importantly, to see for themselves the results and the specific meaning those results have.

We request that parents be present when their child is tested so they can understand the nature of the child's disorder. By observing the specific tests administered, parents can see the problems firsthand. Surprisingly, we have found no test bias for the neuropsychological measures that would prevent our including parents in the testing process. These measures are so intrinsically interesting that children are only minimally aware of the parents sitting in the back of the testing room. They are completely engrossed in the tasks at hand.

The only section that might be affected by parents being in the room is the intellectual assessment, primarily the verbal measures. When the examiner is asking for answers to specific questions that the child cannot readily answer, the child will look over to the parents for help. If they are doing well they will remain focused and continue to interact solely with the examiner. Usually on the performance tasks of this intellectual assessment, the child will remain engrossed in the task. We do not worry about these results however, because usually the intellectual assessment is already problematic and biased, being so highly subject to other academic/learning issues. Finally, the responsibility of the examiner is to record all of the responses of the person being tested, and, in this manner, it can be documented when motivation or anxiety or some other variable, such as the parents being in the room, has had an impact and this is then noted in the evaluation. By going over the evaluation specifically with the parents before completing the report, we are able to document and determine exactly what did occur with their child and agree on any external variables or effects that may have impacted the testing. If there has been an impact by the parents' presence that is significant we will readminister portions of the evaluation that are not subject to practice effects, or we will wait the required 6 months to re-evaluate without practice effects. However, to date, this has not occurred to an extensive degree. If we feel that we have a bright child and have not obtained a good intellectual assessment, we might re-administer portions and average out the two scorings.

At the time of assessment, parents (and adults being tested) are presented with the results in the form of means (averages) and standard deviations. From a very clinical perspective, this allows the parent or individuals to see the difference in their skill level or functioning over a wide variety of situations and how far their scores vary from their hypothesized potential. As a result, we never have to convince anyone to take medication. They see the need for it because they have watched or taken the tests and received the results.

8.3   Why is Specific Testing so Critical?

Specific assessment allows us to clinically see ADD, what it is and how it occurs and affects the ability to think. As psychologists, we experienced problems in the past as we attempted to measure an attentional disorder as a "concentration" problem rather than measure it as ADD, which consists of a number of factors. We attempted to target the attentional problems as the only measurement of ADD and, as such, have often misdiagnosed on the side of false positives and sometimes false negatives. Most importantly, as psychologists, we tended to just pronounce diagnoses. We now recognize that this is one diagnosis that needs to be "proven" to individuals, especially if we are going to ask them to be on medication for the rest of their lives. Consequently, we have to conduct multiple measurements to prove that the disorder exists, to what degree, and for what specific problematic issue. In the end, we tend to see no evidence of medication compliance problems when the person totally understands the nature of this disorder and the degree to which it impacts them.

Intellectual assessment used to be the only measure we utilized for ADD, in particular a factor called Freedom from Distractibility. Now we find that this does not accurately rule in or out ADD. In addition to the intellectual assessment, psychologists now utilize specific tests that attempt to measure continuous performance. There are controversial issues regarding these measures since the brain is still mysterious, thus rendering testing difficult with regard to determining the assets and liabilities of its functioning. Finally, there is the issue of using statistical vs. clinical evaluation. We have found that there are specific patterns of response characteristic for both ADD with and without hyperactivity. It is critically important not to base diagnosis on a single score because this tends to give us skewed data that could paint a false picture. Statistical analysis vs. clinical analysis is highly controversial, as each presents continually different results.

We test specifically for ADD. If we can see it, we can fix it. Hence, we arrived at our present battery of tests by initially attempting to target the specific deficits associated with ADD. Then we measure deficits associated with frontal and parietal functioning, look at self-report and clinical measures and finally form the whole picture of the disorder and determine whether it is ADD with or without hyperactivity. This particular compilation of measures has proven very successful in discovering specific patterns helpful in allowing us to rule in or out an attentional disorder as well as to discriminate between ADD with and without hyperactivity. The specific patterns observed with these measures in addition to the actual scores, and how scores obtained differ from scores that would be predicted based on the person's intellectual potential, result in a very systematic manner of testing and evaluating ADD.

By determining the specific assets and liabilities and categorizing them as mild, moderate, and severe, remediation programs and suggestions for learning can be proposed. In addition, coping mechanisms based on individual strengths and weaknesses can be suggested. We have found that it is not enough to diagnose ADD and simply treat it with medication. This is a very powerful, subtle, and pervasive disorder that requires a combination of medication (to get the person off to a running start) as well as coping strategies based on their strengths and weaknesses. Because a child, adolescent, or adult is diagnosed does not mean that they can just medicate the problem and change the course of this disorder. Too often, what we see is individuals who were diagnosed in childhood continue to experience numerous problems and unfulfilled potential in adulthood. This occurs because, although they have taken the medication, often they were taking an incorrect dose (not having adjusted for age increases). They have not made the necessary changes to employ the use of coping mechanisms that become part of their daily living. The little things such as the planner, being aware of being distracted in certain environments or settings, not allowing interruptions, using feedback to confirm appointments, directions, and instructions, and so on.

The purpose of an ADD evaluation that is specific and designed to identify exactly where the problem areas are is to provide very definite information about the way the brain operates specific to the individual and how it compensates for the deficits associated with ADD. What is the price paid by this compensation? Everyone is different, some have more of one symptom, less of another. Being able to analyze the symptoms exactly provides people with the knowledge of what to fix first, on what to focus, and upon what they can rely. The knowledge is staggering and provides control ADD people thought they would never have over this often confusing and sometimes unseen, but deadly, disorder.

Many individuals are already compensating for symptoms of this disorder by the time they seek evaluation. This is especially common with the adolescent and adult population. Often an adult will already be compensating for symptoms and the evaluation merely provides confirmation of what they have been doing on an unconscious basis just to allow them to function in their environment. The more logical and the brighter the individuals, the more the assessment provides confirmation of deficits for which they are already compensating. We advise them to continue doing the same things they were doing. In this case, the evaluation clears up the confusion, provides explanation of their lives to date and gives them the choice of what they want to do next. People have been so busy compensating for symptoms, they never thought to choose what symptoms for which to compensate, of what symptoms to let go, and, basically, the most efficient way to use their energy.

EXAMPLE

Recently, we evaluated an extremely bright young man who had been given all of the advantages of education. He had graduated from college and had been working for several years. His family was professional. He was, therefore, expected to achieve. Because everyone was aware of his intelligence, whatever he did had to be great and had to be the best. At the time of evaluation he was working in a nondescript job barely making ends meet financially. He did not know what to do. He could do so many different things and he could do them well. It wasn't an issue of picking a career because it was what he was good at. He was good at everything. However, there was a pressure to be great, and of that he was unsure. He knew he could do something well but the question of great remained unanswered. So he never picked a focus. He did all right in his job but he never emerged from the masses to shine and allow his brilliance to be seen. He never felt good about himself or valued his intelligence because to him, it just held him back and made him so confused he could not focus on one particular career tract. He was so fearful of failure. Someone so bright was not allowed to fail. He had to do it right on the first bounce. The thought was so overwhelming and frightening that he never tried that first bounce. Here is an example of someone who looked like they had it all — but what good is it if you can't use it? The guy who plods along, who is good in one area and, through trial and error, including lots of failures, eventually becomes great in that area, ends up being further ahead.

Another individual stated that she felt a whole load of anxiety fall from her when she was evaluated, just to know that she was not "crazy," and that the things she had been handling in her life were due to some specific issues, could be explained, and it was not her imagination that the simplest tasks could be so incredibly difficult.

Adults often cry during the evaluation session when we go over their results because someone is describing exactly the way they have lived; someone is understanding their struggle without even knowing them. The patterns are so clear that there are many commonalities that exist and can then be predicted due to the presence of some symptom or cluster of symptoms of this disorder. The tears represent the struggle they have been through, the times they have been called lazy and the people who have concluded that they just don't care and are nothing but a washout.

8.4   A Good-Quality Evaluation Convinces Accountants, Lawyers, Doctors, Teenagers, and Disbelievers

The evaluation is very critical for the individual who would not believe the presence of this disorder. They wouldn't believe it unless it was shown in a concrete fashion, with averages (means) and standard deviations, and using math and clear black-and-white evidence. Individuals who are extremely bright have pocket areas of symptoms and/or mild evidence of symptoms that possibly show up on self-report measures. It is only with this type of specific clinical evaluation, this battery of different tests, that their actual problems can be identified. Their spouses say that they don't listen, they miss the information, they deny it, until they score low on the information-processing measures. It can be an insult for a psychologist to pronounce these people ADD without first proving it to them, because it is as if someone knows them better than they know themselves. The idea that someone they just met, even if they are a professional, can be so arrogant as to give them a diagnosis is insulting. Unless we prepare to spend years with these individuals, they don't have to trust us just because we have a degree and experience in a field; they have the experience and degree in themselves.

EXAMPLE
We recently saw one young man who was beginning to experience some problems in college after attaining excellent high-school grades in what appeared to be a very easy, effortless manner. Testing indicated that he had some very clear and severe problems, but he had managed to compensate and they would never have come to light on an assessment that did not include a number of checks and balances and different ways of looking at brain functioning. If we had not used a battery of tests, specifically measuring aspects of ADD, he would not have been diagnosed with ADD and would have continued to ask, "what is wrong with me?" to understand why he could not perform to the degree that he rightly expected.

What this battery is able to do measure symptoms of the disorder in both a specific (and what we call "discrete") as well as a more generalized manner, whereby other issues can enter into the equation as variables. Very bright individuals may compensate for the disorder on a specific measure where they can utilize processes of logic to strategize a single symptom of ADD. Yet, when given a very simple measure that is more general and more vulnerable to interference from several ADD symptoms, they cannot compensate and, therefore, difficulties are observed. The problem is more the interaction of ADD variables than the specific individual ADD symptoms of distractibility, information-processing deficits, and so on.

Sometimes it is the spatial issues that are actually the worst. The person has been so busy successfully compensating for ADD symptoms that the price has been the lack of development of spatial functioning. Then, it is solely the spatial problem that is taking them down academically and affecting reading skills and language acquisition. We even see major spatial problems with 7-year-old children. This suggests that these children have been working so hard to do well and using so much of their energy that their brains are showing a lopsided development even at this young age. Usually this group is made up of the worriers, the ruminators, and the ones who need recognition and perfection to be okay.

Finally, it is very important to note that there are many very bright individuals who establish excellent careers, but by their 40s are worn out. The stress of having to continually compensate and expend energy to a considerable degree just to maintain their status quo, has been an exhausting experience. These individuals are not able to participate in a business meeting or enjoy a new learning situation, because of having to spend so much time simply trying to make sure they have all the information. There is no room left over to become creative and to interact within the situation. The same is true of learning.

One individual remarked that he had gone through college just trying to maintain his grades. He does not recall any of the information he supposedly learned, and never had the opportunity to just enjoy learning and allow his mind to be creative with ideas and conclusions. All he was able to do was just try to obtain the basic information. Information does not register over a long-term period if not attached to something relevant. His learning simply focused on taking in and understanding the information presented. There was no opportunity to attach significance to the information for recall at a later date. There was no opportunity to generalize learning and apply newly learned concepts to form some new and novel idea, which is what makes learning exciting and fun.

8.5   For the Adult, Being Diagnosed is a Very Emotional Experience

Being diagnosed in this manner, by having one's life laid before them through a series of measures that appear so simple a child could perform them, is initially embarrassing and shameful and later emotionally devastating. As one score after another is produced and is widely divergent from the "normal" population, people begin to understand why life has been such a struggle for them. The spouse has tears as all of the past miscommunication, misunderstandings, and continual arguments finally make sense. There is empathy and understanding to replace the anger and frustration.

EXAMPLE

A mother of five children described the aftermath of her diagnosis as an intense onslaught of emotions that arrived unexpectedly and with full force. She caught scenes in her head of childhood experiences that could now be explained and understood. There were now reasons for the difficulties occurring in her past and present life and she had a specific name and measurement of them.

The common question from both parents of children, spouses, and the adults themselves is, why didn't we find this before? The hidden disorder of ADD without hyperactivity is difficult to diagnose because these individuals do not cause problems, do not call attention to themselves, and are very adequate with coping mechanisms through intact logic processes to strategize and compensate. Thus they appear as if "all is fine." Unless the child, adolescent, or adult creates or suffers from emotional issues that would somehow call attention to themselves, or they are not performing in some capacity at work or in school, how could a problem be recognized? We wish we could tell you that, as psychologists specializing with the attention-disordered population, we are always able to spot this disorder. But unfortunately, that is not the case. Often the disorder is spotted by an astute family member or teacher who notices that something is not quite right; the cue is usually a high degree of anxiety that does not make sense. If the child always does well on a test, then why would he or she be so anxious before the test begins? If someone continues to perform well on a consistent basis, why do they continually worry about the day that they can't perform?

Parents are very hurt after evaluation and often ask themselves why they didn't find this. They feel like bad parents or blame someone else, e.g., therapist, teacher, or physician. Parents, on learning that their child has an attentional disorder, react in a variety of ways. They may blame themselves for not finding it earlier and after they are done blaming themselves, they are then in pursuit of someone else on whom to place the blame. If they did manage to catch the disorder at an early age, the question is then, "Will this thing be fixed and, if so, how soon?" This thing needs to be fixed overnight, as correcting the wrong quickly would erase any guilt that it exists or was not caught earlier. Parents will say, "Well, I guess that he or she got it from me; I am the one responsible for this." There is a universal principle, that whenever there is a problem, someone or something must be to blame. Parents need time to process the understanding that they give their children their genetic heritage unknowingly, the good with the bad, whatever that is.

One parent will nudge another and say "I told you so," or, "that sounds a lot like you" and we end up testing the parents. Often the evaluation process begins with the child and proceeds throughout the family to other children and parents and siblings of parents and grandparents and so on. This becomes quite helpful to children. If they identify with one of the parents, then having this disorder doesn't mean they are bad or stupid. The idea of Mom or Dad having ADD too makes it okay. Parents and children work together to develop their brains through the different brain-training programs and they work together to use the coping strategies. They understand each other.

Parents are initially relieved to finally understand their child. However, this initial relief subsides and turns to concern for the welfare of their child, and to feeling overwhelmed over what to do next. We attempt to stress to the parent that the task is to begin to adopt specific training programs, methods of intervention related to the deficit area of their child, means of using the child's strengths, and ways to address all of the consequences of the disorders such as social training and problem-solving skills. Medication is only the means by which to arrive at a level of capability to begin to cope with the disorder. It is not the *only* treatment for it.

8.6   Overview of the Measures Used in the ADD Testing Battery

The battery is made of a number of measures designed to gauge and assess each of the areas identified as making up an attentional disorder.

8.6.1   Is the Information Getting In?

This refers back to the model of how information gets into the brain. The information needs to get into the brain simply from an input standpoint. Basic attention and concentration are necessary to get the information into the brain. There are measures that allow for the measurement of input and for the determination of whether information is getting into the brain just based on basic attention and concentration abilities.

Certain patterns are observed in these measures that can be related to differential diagnosis. Using these patterns, it can be seen if the task was found to be boring and, as a result the information was not received, this is symptomatic of ADD and would indicate an input problem. Another pattern would be as the information became more complex and fast paced it did not get in. Seeing this, it could be predicted that the person would experience difficulty in real life as things became more complex or complicated and as the pace increased. If there is a severe score, hearing might need to be checked and/or there could be a severe disorder of ADD. Finally, there is a means to determine if there is some type of progressive condition in the brain beyond ADD, generating this input problem. If there is a history of input problems as well as other indications of dysfunctioning within the brain, then further investigation using neuropsychological measures would be in order.

Thus, if there is a problem with input, we know that the person would experience difficulty getting information into the brain, and as a result, may miss bits of conversation, directions, instructions, and communication in general.

8.6.2 Is the Information Getting Processed?

The next level is information processing. There is a measure to determine the ability to take in information, process it, and then utilize that information within the higher levels of the brain. This measure requires the person to add two numbers, call out the answer, remember the last number, and add it to the next number. There are four trials that increase in time and provide a measure of what will occur as we ask more of the brain, and life issues or learning becomes more intense or difficult. What this measure provides is the knowledge of whether the information is being processed. Research supports that this measure is very powerful in its ability to detect any issues of brain injury as well as information-processing skills. To some degree, math skills are needed, but primarily the measure does what is expected. It measures information processing. We know this because we conducted our own research by testing children on and off Ritalin who had already been diagnosed with ADD and found to have this problem. They performed significantly better with the medication than without. This suggests that information processing was being measured rather than math skills. Furthermore, we have tested accountants and mathematicians who perform poorly on this measure, despite their already proven excellent math skills.

We have found this to be one of the most powerful measures in the battery: it is the most difficult for ADD individuals to complete while non-ADD individuals do not evidence a problem. Sometimes the distraction of one's own thoughts interferes with the ability to complete. People with ADD find this task very frustrating and this is the one measure that stimulates low frustration tolerance for both ADD with and without hyperactivity. This is the measure on which the ADD peson says "I quit," "I give up," "I can't do this anymore."

We see a pattern with children where sometimes they will keep going and will not give up no matter what, no matter how many answers they get wrong or cannot do. This identifies the child who will keep trying over and over. We call them tenacious because, like the bulldog, they hang on. Then there are the children who try but when it becomes too hard they whine, complain, give up, and feel defeated and frustrated. We say about them that *when the going gets tough, they're gone*. Then there are the children who know how to do the task, take one look at it, decide that they can't do it, and without even attempting or trying the task, they decide on another, easier course. These are the avoiders, the procrastinators, the ones who will try if they think they can do it and work forever, and, to the same degree, give up the minute they smell or sense failure. These are the ones who fear failure to such a degree *that they will not try*. They take no risks, everything has to be a sure thing and they limit themselves by what they will or will not do.

Again, there are different patterns that can be observed. Usually those with ADD without hyperactivity will experience a problem on this measure because they are "not getting it" and they become confused. This is characteristic of the population. If these people start out relatively within their intellectual potential, they quickly begin to experience problems, and difficulties emerge as things progress from the simple to the complex. Initially, they look good, appearing to understand what is going on around them. But as things become more intense or time becomes a factor, their systems become overloaded and they begin to miss information. This is particularly problematic for the highly intelligent individual who is acutely aware of the rapid decrease in their abilities as tensions mount. Their difficulties are exacerbated as they try to look good by attempting to compensate for their deficits and as obsessive-compulsive personality traits begin to emerge.

Sometimes, the pattern shows problems from the beginning, often to a severe degree. If the disorder is severe enough in nature, a great deal of information is missed and the individual may appear to be very spacey or confused. The other pattern that is observed is one in which they will perform fine (or within their expected limits) for three of the trials and on the last one their performance drops off. This individual is practiced in compensation and only falters as things become increasingly intense. There are many patterns on this measure to explain how a person operates.

This measure is highly critical in separating or ferreting out an attentional disorder especially in a very bright individual, where other measures would not reveal any difficulties. There could be additional reasons that a person would score worse on this measure than we would normally expect for ADD, such as PTSD, sleep apnea, seizure disorder, hypoglycemia, etc.

8.6.3 The Applied Measure of Information Processing — Looking at Information Processing from a Different Perspective or Point of View

There is confusion that results in problems with information processing and it becomes important to determine how the brain handles this problem. With ADD without hyperactivity the problem-solving skills of the frontal processes tend to be intact. If individuals have a problem with information processing they can modify that confusion with the problem-solving skills of the frontal processes. So what they don't understand they simply try to figure out by using the pieces they do have and attempting to use logic to make up for the missing pieces.

An example of this would be someone who could not understand a set of directions. They would throw the directions away and simply figure it out themselves using logic. This can become a problem, however, if a person goes in the direction that, to them, logically makes sense but, since they are missing a piece of information, they've headed in the wrong direction. These are the individuals who insist that something logically makes sense and cannot understand when you attempt to tell them that it just is not so. We can see this phenomenon on an applied measure of information processing where the individual is asked to perform a new learning task based on an examiner saying "correct" or "incorrect." What the task is asking the individual to do is remain in connection with the examiner, input and process the information of "correct" or "incorrect," and, based on this information, use it for feedback to modify their behavior. This is how we learn a new skill. We keep getting feedback in one form or another and use that feedback to do a better job over and over. What happens with ADD without hyperactivity is that they have difficulty processing the information and remaining in tune with the examiner. We do not score this for perseverance, instead we look at this measure from a clinical analysis. With severe ADD without hyperactivity, there will be a great amount of confusion, followed by finally getting the correct response. Once they get it they can use it. We see evidence of a capacity problem and loss of focus. Sometimes, they will spontaneously recover or they may then become confused and take a long time to get back on track — if they ever do.

Individuals with a severe problem processing information can also produce perfect or near-perfect performance on this measure by utilizing their logic and problem-solving skills. If this occurs despite severe information-processing problems, then it becomes obvious that the person is of a high level of intelligence or really relies on logic to compensate for these deficits and has fine-tuned this area of the brain. We have been able to hypothesize higher potential for individuals who obtain very low IQ values when they can perform well on this measure. Understanding brain functioning suggests the brain would not be able to perform at such a high capacity if the individual were truly mentally retarded. Sometimes, though, people make the task more complex and really confuse themselves.

For ADHD individuals, the pattern is observed where they simply are unable to do the task and cannot learn from feedback or their mistakes. Also with ADHD they tend to continually lose their places. They display an inability to figure out what they need to do because they can't learn from feedback. A great deal of frustration is observed because of low tolerance. ADHD will perform poorly overall with numerous mistakes.

8.6.4 Is There a Vulnerability to Distractibility from the Environment and/or a Tendency to be Behaviorally Distractible?

Distractibility is gauged by a divided attention task that is very effective in providing a measure of the gating mechanism. The person has to perform a task where they must use the gating mechanism to gate out and focus on information and not allow the interference that is part of this task to distract them. Someone can do well on this measure using logic but they will not do well on the applied measure of distractibility. If the person is taking an anti-depressant medication this is the only task in which this type of medication will be helpful and they can attain a higher score as a result.

Next is the question of whether these individuals are vulnerable to environmental distractions. Are they distractible in and of themselves? This next measure is the type of task that determines evidence of behavioral distractibility. Mild to severe levels of distractibility can be determined as well as how the individual would be able to compensate. There are specific patterns of response that would differentiate ADD from ADHD. Finally, if there is a high degree of distractibility for both groups, it will be evidenced by a high number of errors when the task is too simple for errors. This points to the need for external structure to a greater or lesser degree.

8.6.5 Is There a True Problem of Planning and Organization with the Frontal Processes Being Involved?

Frontal processes are measured by a task of planning and organization. To begin, directions and the ability to follow them serve to determine if there is an information-processing problem. It is also on this measure that the determination of a spatial problem, characteristic of inattention, occurs. At times, with ADD without hyperactivity there is a spatial problem characteristic of problematic parietal lobe functioning. This problem can result in time-management problems, a general underestimation of time and poor planning of the day that is not equal to or commensurate with the number of tasks the individual has planned. In addition, this measure can be used to detect organicity, motor issues, and emotionality and has been researched in depth to provide information on these issues.

8.6.6 Are the Frontal Processes Down and Are There Cognitive Flexibility, Problem Solving Ability, and Sequencing Skills?

Other measures of frontal processes include tasks employing the use of being cognitively flexible, switching sets and maintaining sets as well as determination of sequencing problems characteristic of ADHD. These measures have been controversial in the research due to problems of measurement, yet we have found very clear patterns consistently differentiating ADHD from ADD.

These patterns are clinically identified and if an attempt is made to statistically analyze results simply based on correct scoring, the conclusions will be incorrect and lead to erroneous determinations. Second, we cannot measure frontal areas of the brain directly because the frontal area is so dependent on the processes below it and has such integrative functioning. Thus, we refer to the frontal area as frontal processes. When measuring, we understand that this measure needs to be evaluated from a clinical perspective to present certain patterns for ADD in general as well as for defining ADHD vs. ADD. The measure is timed and, as is characteristic for ADD without hyperactivity, will be problematic and results will not fall within their expected levels, thus revealing slow cognitive speed. However, if frontal processes are well developed, or the individual is very bright, then this may be the area that is highly intact and a problem may not be seen at all.

It is also important to realize that frontal processes, when being used to compensate for other deficits, may be overbuilt to the demise of other areas.

ADHD patterns indicate use of the same incorrect solution over and over again for the same problem although it didn't work the first time. Errors for ADHD will be present throughout the measure in addition to some impulsivity as they speed through the task to get to the end without really trying because it has become difficult for them.

Typically, the pattern characteristic for ADHD is one of giving up very easily if things become even slightly difficult, which demonstrates very low frustration tolerance. For ADD without hyperactivity, there may be evidence of slow thinking speed and a tendency to lose concentration or focus, which is typical of a capacity problem. With a severe disorder, there may be confusion. The pattern will be that they start off fine and about one third to half way through the measure they will become confused. This is caused by the capacity problem and an inability to sustain attention, focus, and energy. When confusion occurs, it pulls them off task and they may not recover. They may become distracted and unable to recall what they were doing a minute ago or know what to do next. Finally, if someone performs really poorly, beyond that expected for ADD, then there may be additional issues related to the brain and further evaluation may be needed.

8.6.7 Is There an Overall Impact of Slow Cognitive Speed?

There is a measure of pure motor speed that will determine the presence of slow thinking speed. There is the classic problem of slow cognitive speed for ADD that is very characteristic of the disorder without hyperactivity. One does not see a problem with speed for ADHD. This may also be reflected in reading problems and the spatial issue may not be noted. This measure is compared with other measures of thinking speed and more information is determined about when and how the person will experience a problem with speed and may need untimed testing.

8.6.8 Finally, to Rule Out Any Impact to the Brain

The final measure, to screen out anything else going on in the brain, assesses the general integrity and functioning of the brain. This holds up well in research as a screening device for brain dysfunction. This can also be used to measure someone's potential when intellectual assessment is reflective of continued problems with learning and time. What is helpful about this measure is that sometimes we see a higher score than that seen intellectually. If this correlates with the person's history as well, perhaps other measures in the battery can serve to determine that the person's potential is not being fully met.

8.7   IQ and IQ Potential and Relating This to Scoring on ADD Battery Measures

As stated before, for the intellectual assessment of children, the most updated versions of the Weschler Intelligence scales are used. We have found it neither helpful nor productive to perform the Weschler with adults because of the issue of time. Half of the intellectual assessment incorporates time and may thus be more a measure of time than of ability. Second, with ADD, learning is problematic and thus impacts verbal performance as well. So in an effort to determine the person's potential, we use an IQ potential that research shows to correlate or associate very highly with the Weschler and has been proven to provide an accurate measure of intellectual potential. This measure, however, is also verbally loaded and if these individuals have had a problem with reading, spelling, or phonemic skills, they will do more poorly, which will negatively impact scoring and, in this case, their potential. Thus, with a severe disorder, there are times when the examiner becomes aware that true potential cannot be identified using this measure or any of the other measures. However, more often one of the measures in this entire battery will prove to be a pretty accurate measure of the person's potential.

The Weschler Intelligence scales cannot be used to establish the presence of ADD or to rule it out. This measure does provide information on these individuals' learning patterns and what they have learned. Some of the subtests can also be used to provide some information regarding ADD. A note of caution is in order, however, as the scoring of this measure assumes that children increase their skills with age, which does not always occur with the ADD population. Therefore, when scores are compared based on the expectation that these children are improving their skills, the scoring will be off, i.e., not valid and generally incorrect.

9

After the Evaluation: How Tests or Clinical Findings are Used to Develop Coping Mechanisms to Address the Symptoms of ADD

9.1 Coping with ADD: What Do We Do Now that We Know the Problem?

A clear and specific evaluation will help these individuals in developing further mechanisms or ways to adapt and provide strategies to maximize their performance. It is also important to separate ADD without hyperactivity from ADHD for a number of different reasons. First, the general population tends to typecast the ADHD individual as restless, out of control, and behaviorally problematic. For the most part, this is pretty accurate. However, this is not the picture of ADD without hyperactivity. These individuals are very sensitive, they care about what people think of them, and they have difficulty with criticism because they don't like to fail or have anyone unhappy with them. Therefore, if we see someone as ADHD we tend to treat them more roughly, knowing that they really don't care about anyone else's feelings and nothing really upsets them unless they are somehow prevented from getting their way. If there is a misdiagnosis, however, and we treat an ADD without hyperactivity child, adolescent, or adult as ADHD, there could be long-term consequences in terms of the impact to their self-esteem and extreme sensitivity to anything said to them (while they do not appear to be sensitive at all).

9.1.1 What to do if the Problem is Input or Information Processing

If individuals have an input problem and/or an information processing problem then it is clear that they will tend to miss information from their environment and thus will tend to miss bits of conversation, directions, instructions, and communication in general. Those with an input problem, similar to an information-processing problem, will tend to be described as forgetting things because they did not have the information in the first place, and although appearing as a memory problem, the issue is truly the lack of information. Thus, I will often tell parents, spouses, and significant others of the ADD individual, to establish eye contact and then deliver the message. They can also use another modality, such as visual in the form of a sticky note, but do not assume the person has the information if you attempt to tell them as they are racing out the door, or in a rush, or have other things going on at the same time.

Individuals who miss information, either due to input or information-processing problems will often be accused of not listening. This is evidenced in the school setting as an auditory comprehension problem when teachers notice that children frequently miss the assignment and what they are being asked to do. They are seen as having difficulty understanding class material or remembering it the next day. Children and students will avoid and procrastinate homework assignments simply because they do not know what they are supposed to do. Consequently, they will sit and stare at a blank sheet of paper for hours trying to figure it out, or they only know part of the assignment and have to guess at the rest.

A *feedback mechanism* needs to occur where individuals can feed the information they think they have received back to the person to ensure that they have the correct information. While this may sound peculiar, it can often be an excellent social technique and empathetic response to provide the teacher, spouse, parent, speaker and anyone who communicates with them, validation that they are being heard or "listened to." This method of feedback will also clear up the communication problems that occur on a daily basis in the ADD household. It is common to think we said the movie was at 10:00 and our spouse thinks that was 10:30, or we thought we were meeting at the drug store but it turned out to be the video store. The parent could be at the drug store while the child is at the video store and they are both waiting for each other. Then 20 minutes later one goes to find the other only to arrive angry and frustrated and ready to blame. A final example is an appointment that was for Tuesday at 2:00 yet one party thinks that it was for Wednesday.

The feedback mechanism may work like this: the person says "What I hear you saying is…, is this what you said?" or sums up a conversation by saying "OK, what we are agreeing on is this, or is this what you mean?" and so on. This guarantees that when the conversation has ended both the speaker and the listener are clear that the correct information has been transmitted. Using tape recorders for classes will provide the same thing. People are continually surprised by what they hear on the tape as opposed to what they thought they actually had heard in class. If possible, a tape recorder at a business meeting will help individuals know that they are gathering all of the necessary information so they can then relax and begin to participate in the meeting, mobilizing all of their creativity and problem-solving skills. Instead, ADD adults have to be continually fearful they have missed information, or they are constantly finding themselves daydreaming only to return to the conversation and find that the topic has changed and they have no idea what was said or what just occurred.

The same is true for the classroom situation. If students know they have the information on tape, they can then begin to enjoy learning. They are free to use the knowledge and apply it to information they already have that can become the "exciting" part of any learning — that experience of "Oh, I understand now!" The problem of missing information is one of the most frequent complaints and the subject of a great deal of controversy between parents and children, spouses or friends. Often frustrating experiences of missed appointments, missed connections, and late pick-ups are due to this phenomenon. Consequently, ADD partners in a marriage to a non-ADD person (or two ADD people together) will think that they are not being listened to or heard, or are not important in the other person's life. Spouses assume that if their husband or wife truly loved them they would listen to what they had said.

This is why if someone calls for marital therapy and suspects ADD we will discourage them from beginning the therapy until the suspected ADD person has been formally evaluated.

Finally, this issue of information processing is probably the most stressful aspect of ADD, both for the spouse and the ADD individual. A consistent lack of information tends to lead to confusion and can provide a feedback loop. When people find themselves confused, they use it as a signal to go back and gather more information. Confusion for the ADD individual will tend to be moderated by the frontal processes of logical problem-solving. An example of this is individuals who throw directions away and proceed to assemble an item by themselves.

There is a possibility that someone will logically determine something, while missing a very vital piece of information and draw bad conclusions or go off in the totally wrong direction, swearing that logically this should make sense. However, based on the information they have, they believe their conclusions are correct. Thus, they will not understand when you try to explain to them why something is incorrect. If they continue to argue with you, it is time to stop and ask what their conclusions are based on.

When confusion is so overwhelming that the individual is unable to compensate with problem-solving skills and continually remains confused, this may represent severe problems in these areas. We tend to observe this with severe degrees of ADD without hyperactivity and/or with the aging process. (As one grows older brain cells begin to be lost and as a result we cannot compensate for the disorder as well as we did previously). Consequently, there is more confusion through which the brain needs to work. This picture is also observed with individuals who have participated in long-term substance abuse, particularly alcohol. We are now learning that alcohol can result in substantial damage to the brain and failure of the brain to recover or rehabilitate itself if injured further.

9.1.2   What to Do if the Problem is that of Vulnerability to Being Distracted by the Environment

Imagine a gate that allows a little information in while keeping out the rest of the information. When there is a vulnerability to being distracted, that gating mechanism is not working to allow the individual to weed out extraneous information and focus on relevant information. This vulnerability to distractibility can mean that people are distracted not only by what is happening around them but also by what is occurring inside their heads. For example, we all have been caught in a situation where we are thinking of something, only to totally miss what someone just said to us. By the time we recover, we find that we have missed part of the conversation and now must pick up the pieces and attempt (with as much social grace as possible) to understand where they are in the conversation and what they are trying to tell us. An ADD person with a vulnerability to distractibility has this happen to them frequently. Thus, they may appear as if they are not listening when, actually, they have difficulty sustaining attention to task because they are so easily distracted by the least little thing.

In addition, these individuals have difficulty maintaining eye contact. They seem to be unable to think and look at the person at the same time and are distracted by the visual stimuli of the face. They have difficulty completing tasks or remaining focused and, as a result, tend to shift from one task to another. These individuals, fearful of their own distractibility, will interrupt others or blurt out the answer before the question is completed because they are afraid they will forget what they were going to say if they quietly wait until an opening in the conversation is available.

If there is a vulnerability to distractibility from the environment then coping mechanisms should be practiced. White noise, such as the snow on the TV set when the station has gone off the air for the night, is particularly helpful. Introducing a noise that does not require attention or concentration blocks all of the other noises and sounds that would otherwise be disturbing. We have found that music at night, e.g., instrumental in nature or a song the person has heard so often that they are no longer listening to the words, helps the person to sleep by blocking out the common sounds of a door creaking, dog barking, and so on. However, individuals often cannot sleep because they are still thinking and those racing thoughts continue on into the night. Headphones with music help to additionally block out not only the external sounds but the internal thoughts as well. Similarly, the use of a portable CD player offers more-intense sounds and when used with headphones may allow for focus and the blocking of distractions.

EXAMPLE

One individual described her work environment as too quiet. What she meant was that she could hear all of the noises and sounds that never bothered anyone else, such as the copy machine, the coffee machine, the fan system and so on. The distractibility increased her anxiety and she had difficulty concentrating on her work.

9.1.3 What to Do About Planning and Organization Problems: How to Cope with Being Distractible in a Behavioral Sense

It is important to separate the high-speed motor activity of ADHD from the meandering, wandering distractibility of ADD. Sometimes they can look the same if there is the addition of anxiety. Anxiety and distractibility will make these people look as if they are on a high-speed chase going nowhere. Distractibility that is behavioral in nature will differ for ADD with and without hyperactivity. Both groups can appear to always be on the go, moving from one unfinished task to another and evidencing either mental or physical restlessness or both. It is important to distinguish anxiety as the differentiating factor, i.e., whether the restlessness is due to anxiety or the motor hyperactivity of the ADHD individual. These are ADHD children and later adults who are seen as running, not walking. Both groups can evidence impulsivity, but for different reasons. The ADHD person is impulsive due to low frustration tolerance and for the ADD without hyperactivity person it is due to exhaustion and being tired of trying. The distractibility can result in difficulty completing tasks alone (without a monitoring system) and can impact follow through as well. Planning and organization problems may occur as a result of the distractibility and confusion of the ADD without hyperactivity or it could be due to a true planning and organization problem from the frontal processes being problematic, which relates to ADHD.

One coping mechanism for the behavioral tendency to become distracted as well as for the problem of planning and organization, is the use of a planner. Setting goals with times and dates can will oneself to complete tasks in a timely fashion. All of the tasks the individual needs to complete, e.g., dates, appointments and so on, are placed in this planner for the person to reference on a continual basis. Ironically, another problem common for ADD individuals is to misplace things — including the planners.

Ritualizing the habit of consulting the planner daily helps people not only by reminding them of what they need to do but also by instilling the importance of the book so they are less likely to lose it. In lieu of a planner, ADD individuals may have some sort of a backup method for task completion, such as encouragement and/or assistance from a parent, spouse, or office manager. However, they may tend to become overly dependent on that person for planning and task completion. For example, I have had individuals who called me daily to report on what they are going to do for that day as a means to plan and organize.

A daily assignment sheet that goes from school to home helps ADD children with task completion, ensures that they know what they are supposed to do, and fosters good communication between home and school. Tasks can be broken down into smaller units and these people can teach themselves to develop task completion skills. It is critical to lay out all of the materials needed for task completion and to clear away materials not needed. ADD without hyperactivity can self talk themselves through a task until it is done by using internal statements, such as "just keep going until you finish,"

"Don't go off to that, just stay on task." ADHD individuals do not tend to have the availability for this internal control system and benefit more from external controls to provide the means to stay on task and not become distracted. External methods to ensure that the individual remains on task include writing checklists, reinforcement and feedback at different points of task completion, time cues, and close monitoring in general.

Bright individuals with ADD without hyperactivity tend to develop obsessive-compulsive traits in an attempt to compensate for the deficits or pocket areas of problems and to combat failure by trying to do things perfectly to look wonderful. These same individuals will tend to procrastinate and avoid any situation in which they do not think they excel. Obsessive-compulsive behavior can become so paralyzing for these individuals that they will clearly and manipulatively avoid situations that they believe will result in negative outcomes. What happens with the obsessive compulsive is that they take too long to get things done and everything becomes a major project. Thus, it is important to set time limits on task efforts.

Or what often happens is the complexity of a task appears so overwhelming to people before they start that they may not start at all. Goal setting is very critical to accomplishing tasks. ADD individuals either do not set goals at all or tend to set lofty goals that are impossible to accomplish. It is important to address the reality of the goal, both in terms of whether it can be accomplished at all or whether it can be completed in a realistic time frame. Additionally, it is necessary to implement an external feedback system, particularly for ADHD individuals, so they know when the goal has been attained.

Structure and *use of routine* are critical for the ADD individual. Routines are performed to accomplish daily tasks. There is a routine to prepare for school or work in the morning, a routine when one arrives home from school or work, and a routine prior to going to sleep at night. The child has certain tasks each morning, begins homework at a certain time in the evening, and prepares for the next day before going to bed. The use of routines provides a structure to accomplish tasks, not become distracted, and complete everyday things that could otherwise prove problematic in daily functioning. The routine allows for daily chores, household tasks, work preparation, homework, and the other small details of daily life.

9.1.3.1   More Suggestions

- If you are vulnerable to distractibility don't try to do paperwork in an office crowded with people or interrupted by phone calls.
- Distractability can derail ADD people and create confusion. It is all they can do to get back on track.
- Know that these individuals can become easily overwhelmed in a chaotic situation.

- Don't try to talk to them as you are leaving or they are leaving, especially if there are information-processing problems.
- Don't attempt important conversations at parties, in crowded rooms, or in a restaurant.
- The more distracting the external noises, the more problematic the environment, so attempt to keep these conversations light rather than about things the person would be expected to remember at a later date.
- Take frequent breaks but do not allow interruptions.

9.1.4 What to Do about the Slow Cognitive or Thinking Speed Characteristic of the ADD Without Hyperactivity Individual

Primarily to combat the slow cognitive thinking and/or slow time that is so prevalent in this population one may need what is called *untimed evaluation*. The idea is to measure the ability without using time constraints. We have consistently found that time constraints severely limit the individual's performance. Often all that is being measured is time, not someone's ability. This becomes particularly problematic for evaluation, e.g., achievement and intellectual testing. Evaluation that is not timed has made a great difference for the individual who is unable to complete tasks and finish tests quickly. Often in analyzing students' performance from a qualitative perspective, it can be identified that they answered the question correctly or were able to complete the problem, but their time was not quick enough. If the score is based on both time and the correct response, what will ultimately be measured is only the effect of time. The result is that generally ADD individuals do not perform well on intellectual or achievement testing primarily due to this issue of speed. Time constraints need to be removed for both in-class and standardized evaluations.

It is exciting to note that colleges are now helping these individuals by allowing untimed evaluation as well as providing notetakers to help combat the information-processing problem. It is becoming more and more common for colleges to be aware of these difficulties and to offer students provisions whereby their tests are read to them, tests are untimed, and rooms are free of distractions. If specific provisions are not available, such as a learning center, then professors have been asked to increase their time available to spend with students to discuss their needs regarding a specific class in which they may be struggling. Recently, there has been some controversy around this issue and lawsuits regarding requests for accommodation that were not honored. When people won such court cases, usually they were able to document a consistent slow thinking speed that impacted timed measures as well as a consistent reading problem. In those cases, accommodations were granted by the court for a separate testing room as well as additional time to complete the test. Those cases where the court did not grant additional time were in the absence of a documented historical problem with timed test taking, and the individual when taking timed tests scored in the above-average range. Generally, the court concluded that a person was entitled to accommodations when the impairment they were documenting had substantially limited their performance, which could be proven by evaluation by an expert or psychologist.

It is common in the public school setting for accommodations to be made for untimed evaluation. This becomes more of an issue at the level of junior-high and high-school. It is at that time that testing becomes more critical and examinations are less frequent and, thus, carry greater weight. Resource rooms or learning centers at the junior-high and high-school level provide a method of testing that can be untimed or in a room free from distraction.

Schools are also offering untimed entrance exams, and nationwide examinations such as the ACT or SAT have provisions to be given untimed. Exams for further study and extended degrees at the master's or doctoral level, such as psychology, business, law, or medicine — the GRE, MAT, LSAT, MCAT, respectively — can also be taken untimed. Even some of the licensing exams, such as the exam for real estate, for a builder's license and so on, can be administered in the untimed condition. Many testing situations these days offer untimed evaluation as well as a room that is free from distraction. This indicates that it is becoming more widely recognized that ADD individuals have specialized needs and there is increased cooperation to provide methods or specific provisions that have been successful in isolating their true potential and ability.

There are, however, some isolated problems that emerge by taking these entrance exams or achievement testing with special accommodations, as some groups will be discriminatory as a result. Under a great deal of controversy the military has adamantly refused to admit anyone taking medication or identified as ADD, nor do they allow accommodations in their evaluation procedures. We saw one man who was discriminated against once he took his MCATs with untimed evaluation and admitted ADD on his entrance exam. The pattern was initial interest followed by consistent disinterest. Medical schools that were formerly interested never returned his calls and this occurred with such regularity that it became painfully obvious that he was being discriminated against.

This slow processing of information or slow thinking in general needs to be taken into consideration when goal setting and planning. People tend to bite off more than they can chew; they tend to overwhelm themselves thinking that they can accomplish more than they can. This problem is increased by the time-management problems occurring with spatial issues. It is a fairly common ADD issue to underestimate how long something will take to complete. One of the things that is helpful is to estimate the amount of time a task will take based on previous completion of a similar task. These individuals can admit to themselves that previously something took a lot longer than they expected therefore they will allow more time to complete the task. For example, if you know that it takes a specific amount of time to complete writing a paper, or making a specific phone call, or an appointment of some type, use the past to predict and anticipate the present. If it takes longer, then that realization allows the person to plan better the next time.

9.1.5 Misunderstanding Time

Children can easily lose track of time. The ADD without hyperactivity individual may lose track of time due to distractibility and confusion that results in a general lack of awareness. The ADHD individual, however, does not have the ability to be aware of time. With the frontal processes being down, they are truly not aware of time frames. They can be gone for 4 hours yet see their absences as a matter of minutes. Thus, the ADHD will continually argue about time due to the true absence of a sense of time.

It is helpful to use watches with alarms that can be set for a variety of times throughout the day to remind them of deadlines, appointments, and scheduled medications. Such monitoring is helpful to make the person more clearly aware of time and to exercise that area of the brain for rehabilitation.

9.1.5.1 More Suggestions

- Issues of a lack of time sense can be helped by first being aware of the time problems and using cognitive retraining to be more aware of time.
- Set the alarms on watches or on the computer.
- Constantly ask the ADD individual what time it is to instill in him or her the idea and concept of time.

9.1.6 Sequencing and Flexibility of the ADHD Individual

ADHD individuals are unable to sequence activities and goals. Thus, one cannot expect them to set a goal, figure out the steps to attain it, and then proceed. These individuals are in need of specific support in the delineation of the structured steps to reach the goal in question. The ADHD individual needs to work with others to break down the specific steps leading to a goal. It is not reasonable to expect that these individuals can arrive at the steps in a sequential fashion to attain their desired goals. When left to their own devices, they rarely follow through.

9.1.7 How to Improve Problem-Solving Skills for the ADHD Individual

Problem-solving skills need to be taught in a very specific step-by-step procedure. The feedback mechanism is not working and the tendency is to repeatedly use the same solution that does not work. To make sure that the same ineffective solutions are not continually applied, a step-by-step procedure is instituted.

9.1.7   *Problem-Solving Four-Step Process*

1. Identify the problem and then restate it. The idea is to clarify that this is the problem that the person specifically wants to fix.
2. Generate multiple solutions and encourage flexibility. Teach the child, adolescent, or adult to be creative and just think of anything. This means battling the tendency toward rigidity and the tendency to look at things from a black-and-white perspective.
3. Examine each and every one of the possible solutions generated to solve the problem. Weigh the pros and cons in an effort to thoughtfully select the best possible solutions available.
4. Arrange the list of best solutions in a hierarchical fashion based on which ones are expected to work best. Administer each possibility one by one. If the solution does not work, provide feedback as to why and attempt the next solution. Continue this process until the right solution is applied and the problem is solved. In this way, these individuals are taught to use feedback both to recognize success and learn from their mistakes.

This concrete program teaches the ability to be flexible and to problem solve. The inability to do this is the reason that ADHD individuals frequently depend on others to avoid making poor decisions and finding themselves in some sort of terrible predicament.

9.1.8   Test-Taking Behavior

Many of these individuals experience difficulty taking tests. Teaching them in a specific manner how to take tests can be highly beneficial. Teaching how to recognize "trick" questions, key words, and double negatives, as well as how to group similar items, can prevent any test from becoming an overwhelming endeavor.

9.1.8.1   *Suggestions*

- Skip the questions of which you are unsure and finish those you know you can answer. It's better to complete what you can than to get stuck on one question for a long period of time and not have enough time left to complete the test.

- Study skills are critical issues — learn how to outline the chapter, read the beginning sentences and ending sentences, use the areas that are emphasized in bold or italics in the chapter.
- Read silently the multiple-choice questions. This helps to avoid making the mistake of dropping words or adding words and reading the question wrong. Watch yourself for the tendency to skip words.
- When studying for multiple-choice tests it is best to read and reread the text and notes to make sure to study all of the little pieces of information, the factoids.
- For essay tests the information has to be memorized. The best way to do that is to rewrite the information so you can memorize it. For instance, take 20 pages of notes and rewrite them, pare them down to 10 pages and then rewrite to 5 pages and finally to 2 pages. Memorizing automatically takes place with the rewriting that occurs.
- When it comes time to take the test, first go through all the essay questions and, in the margin, write down all the facts that you have memorized, all the dates, the names of people, events, and so on. After this step, go through each of the questions. You can now think about each answer and fashion your answer in a coherent, orderly manner without having to remember what you have memorized at the same time.

9.1.9 How to Improve Social Skills for Both ADHD and ADD without Hyperactivity

Socially, ADD individuals often do not fit in with their peers and spend their time on the periphery of the group. They tend to associate with the less popular children and, in general, feel more awkward than their peers or contemporaries. They have no idea of how to relate, fit, or blend with others. Unfortunately, no one gives us a handbook that tells us how to act socially. ADHD individuals tend to act more inappropriately and, as a result, are rejected. ADD without hyperactivity individuals tend to be isolated and neglected. They are shy and can just fade out of the situation. Before attempting any of the following suggestions or remedies, first determine if the social issues are related to some type of an underlying psychological or physical disorder. Any underlying issues that would result in difficulties with social skills should be specifically identified through additional evaluation. This may be either some type of a physical evaluation or a psychological evaluation.

The two ADD groups each have specific issues related to their particular diagnosis. The ADD without hyperactivity individual tends to withdraw and find himself or herself easily neglected. When people are quiet, it can become very easy to ignore them and forget that they are part of the group. ADD individuals tend to act inappropriately and are highly unaware of the borders and boundaries of others. They are continually agitating people around them in what appears to be a very inconsiderate manner with little regard to the feelings of others. This assumption may be false considering the high degree of sensitivity ADD individuals experience as a whole. They appear to be able to dish it out but cannot take it back. The problem is that often they have no idea that they are dishing it out in the first place.

The picture can become rather confusing when considering the reason that someone behaves socially in the manner that they do. If people are truly ADHD they may be so disconnected from anyone but themselves that they don't care what others think and intend to do as they please at any given moment. If there is a co-related disorder, such as Oppositional Defiant Disorder, in a similar manner they remain so uninvolved with those around them that they do not concern themselves with whether their behavior is socially appropriate. With ADHD, due to the lack of inhibition, they tend to do as they please without regard to the consequences. As a result, when the above or similar conditions are in operation generally they are not upset with their behavior and have little desire to make the necessary changes. Individuals falling into the above categories would not be likely candidates for a treatment program emphasizing social training because they would not be agreeable to doing things differently. They tend not to hear others who try to tell them when they are inappropriate unless it is clearly stated in a very blunt and concrete manner. Fortunately, these individuals actually make up a very small percentage of the total population.

Symptoms characteristic of ADHD and related disorders, however, are seen quite often but usually not due to the above-listed disorders or conditions. These symptoms emerge for a variety of reasons and the knowledge of such reasons can be important to rule out any hindrance to social skills training. Any psychiatric disorder resulting in a fear of intimacy and closeness will also create a definite deterrent to the learning of social skills. Fortunately, the majority of the population presenting the above symptoms will be good candidates for social skills training. It is important to enroll your child, adolescent, or the adult in specific social activities or social training programs to begin to cope with these social problems.

First, there needs to be a framework to understand, from a more global perspective, why things are done one way and not another. This provides the reasoning for the suggestions to follow. It allows ADD individuals (usually ADD without hyperactivity) to utilize logical reasoning processes and, once they have the framework, they can be highly creative in generalizing and creating different alternatives. The problem is a lack of understanding of social behavior, the whys and wherefores.

Social skills are taught by indicating specifically how to act and what to say. There is a considerable lack of information about appropriate social behavior, practical knowledge, and common sense. There is difficulty with many common situations such as what to do in a movie theater when one sees smoke and fire or what to do if someone starts to fight. Providing real-world examples or just simply talking with them is helpful in improving their skills. Taking children to movies and using movie plots as a means to relate how people act in certain situations works well also. Children who have older siblings without ADD benefit from watching them and learning from their social skills, e.g., how to dress and present themselves, simply choosing the perfect dress for an event, etc. Lots of information and examples can be helpful.

You are in a grocery store and you watch a child do something and the parent responds inappropriately — a simple situation yet socially incorrect. You imagine that your child saw the same situation, understood it the same as you did, and drew the same conclusions. This is not the case. ADD children do not pick up all of the information and it becomes necessary to tell them in a very specific manner exactly what has occurred and what it means.

ADD without hyperactivity individuals are not able to view the whole of things and miss the big picture. As a result, they may do the wrong thing at the wrong time, say the wrong thing and not realize it. They miss the big picture when it comes to understanding abstract ideas and concepts. Thinking tends to be layered, e.g., this affects that and means that, and then this will happen and that will happen and lead to that and so on. Often attempts are made to have a person grasp the seriousness of a situation by layering one thought on top of another to understand the consequences only to have that person, e.g., spouse, child, or student show *absolutely* no understanding of what is being explained to them. Sometimes people are not very empathetic due to their inability to realize the full consequence of things — seeing the big picture — or a solution might be developed without thinking of another solution — missing the whole picture. Anticipating the results of one's actions is problematic due to an inattention to the whole. The parent says to the child, "Why did you do that?" The child responds, "I don't know. The parent does not believe the child. These children truly do not know, they *miss the whole picture* to understand that their action would result in the consequence that it did. They don't always see the big picture or how things relate to one another. Socially, this can create all kinds of problems and all kinds of messy situations.

Finally, targeting improvement in communication skills, in general, is critical. ADD persons are not terribly skilled at communication. They may miss stating part of the information mostly because it is still in their heads in a conversation that they had within themselves. They also talk without the use of proper nouns, "Can we do *this* tomorrow?" What is *this*? "Remember when we were *there* and *this thing* happened?" The receiver has no idea what these people are referring to in their speech. They also tend to talk in half-sentences because they have finished their sentence in their heads already and moved on to something else.

ADD people need to learn how to share thoughts and feelings, rather than keeping everything inside. They need to understand that body language, gestures, and tone and inflection in the voice are all methods of good communication. In the same manner, there is not always the understanding that they have used an inappropriate tone and have communicated an emotion they did not intend. They don't see that they are coming across angry. It is common for them to say, *I am* not *angry,* in a very angry tone. Sometimes voices become loud without people realizing it. They don't realize the impact of the loudness of their voices on others.

ADD individuals tend to have private conversations; they talk to themselves rather than to others. Sometimes they may say something internally without realizing that they never said it out loud. In conversations others may wait while they think about all the things that they want to say and rule in and rule out what they can and cannot say. All this occurs during a noticeable pause. The other may wait for them to respond and think, *boy, are they slow.* The other does not realize all the thinking that is taking place behind the scenes. Although their outward appearance may be a bland face, devoid of expression, this is actually covering up the activity taking place internally. The other may, meantime, assume that they have been ignored. There is a lot of work and energy that takes place for the ADD individual to have social conversations due to the fear of saying or doing the wrong thing — which creates the need to censor everything.

The thinking patterns of ADD without hyperactivity are more characteristic of the above-described tendencies: to think internally, to worry about what is said and rehearse conversations, and to miss the whole picture, thus making mistakes and feeling inept socially.

ADHD is very different. Their tendency is toward black-and-white thinking (there is no gray, things are either this or that). Rigid thinking results in their dismissing the thoughts of others and only listening to themselves. It means that their opinion is the only right one and only their opinion matters. This can lead to assumptions that are incorrect, both about the individual and the significant others in their lives. Improved communication will help them to see more gray areas.

9.1.10 The ADD Population in General is in Need of Information. Now What Do We Do?

Finally, because both of the ADD groups are desperately in need of information, the new interactive CD ROM computer is expected to fill this void by being so interesting. It is so fascinating that the brain is externally stimulated. Therefore, the ADD person may not need medication because the degree of stimulation bypasses the effects of the disorder.

We think that the computer will be an excellent way to teach ADD children and ADD adults to rehabilitate the brain. We tell children that this is their weight-training program for the brain. The computer provides information that is so stimulating they are able to take it in and use it. It goes directly into the brain without encountering the effects of this attentional disorder. Now the information that was too boring to learn in the classroom is learned from the computer. The computer is multimodal, meaning that information is presented using sound, pictures, color, movement, and a number of modalities to communicate the information to the brain. Remember the movie *Fantasia*? What was so novel about this movie was the combination of sound, movement, and color to communicate the information, or the story line, of the movie.

There are wonderful games that can teach children and adults math, spelling, reading, and vocabulary. One of the things we find frequently is that ADD individuals are not a particularly expressive group. For many, reading can be difficult due to the spatial issues, so they stop reading, learning new words, and increasing their vocabulary. Due to the lack of words, they tend to keep their thoughts inside, which results in both depression and repressed or hostile, explosive anger. Lacking the words, ADD individuals do not know how to adequately express themselves. Conversation remains vague, therefore, they do not communicate their needs so their needs remain unmet and they remain unhappy.

Computers are a nonreactive, unemotional method to help ADD individuals learn and become more efficient in their learning in a variety of ways.

- *The material is stimulating enough to hold their attention and help sustain focus.* The excitement it generates supersedes the symptoms of ADD. Computer programs resemble self-instructional training and allow individuals to proceed at their own pace as well as develop internal speech.

- *Self-monitoring* is another plus as individuals are taught to monitor their own behavior and learning curve using these programs. There are concrete instructional packages that are well sequenced and help the individual to develop reading, comprehension, writing, and spelling skills by using feedback and error monitoring.

- Individuals receive *immediate feedback* and can use that to *modify their behavior.* For instance, social skills and anger management can be taught on the computer.

- The computer can provide *routine and repetitious practice* at whatever level is needed by individuals and the programs can be easily tailored to their style of living. This creates a positive learning experience and motivates people to increase learning.

- By presenting *limited information* at one time, *distractibility decreases* as does the tendency to shift from one project or topic to another.

It also provides the ADD individual with a framework for finishing a project, learning experience, and so on. (Although we see avoidance and procrastination, this is not the natural tendency of the ADD individual).

- Another way of getting information to the ADD person is through movies or television like the Discovery Channel. Again, this emphasizes the multimodal approach and the use of a story to make history interesting. Seeing a movie about a war, or a specific event such as the *Titanic*, or a period of time, increases knowledge as well as interest in a subject that would not have been thought about previously. Adding a story to something increases its meaning and places the event in a perspective or framework for greater understanding. Sources like the Discovery Channel allow the opportunity to learn interesting, new things about a topic, which again increases both our awareness and interest. The whole idea is to make learning interesting, fun and special.

9.1.11   Spatial Problems

There is no pill to fix the spatial problem, which is the result of a lack of use of that area of the brain. To correct a spatial deficit it must be used. The problem is that this can actually be harder than anticipated. ADD persons (without hyperactivity) tend to use logic much of the time and attempt to avoid these spatial areas. Therefore, if they can solve a problem using logic, they will. A method must be developed to force these people to specifically use this area. If they say that they are good at something and that they really like it, they may have already figured out a way to do the task using logic. If they say they are not good at something, or they don't like it, it may be the type of task that will benefit the brain with re-training.

What we now know about the brain is that if you don't use it, you lose it. In other words, the brain develops through constant use. The more certain parts of the brain are used, the more connections between the neurons are developed. These pathways can become so developed that they operate without requiring any direct thinking and with little or no energy.

An example would be driving or any type of developed skill. In the beginning, specific steps are learned. There is a specific procedure that is memorized and learned. It gets better and better with each trial. Within the brain, the pathways are becoming more developed. Finally, these pathways become so well developed that when driving, the exact steps that were learned so long ago are automatically performed, i.e., the driver may be thinking of something else and may even be doing something else. This is how the brain becomes more efficient: A skill is learned and it remains learned. The same thing happens if people learn how to play tennis or roller skate and then don't do it for years. When they return to the activity, although a bit rusty, they still remember what to do.

What is particularly exciting about the computer is that younger children benefit greatly from its targeted approach, which can help form a permanent improvement in areas of the brain since it is used during the time when the brain is still developing (before 13 years of age). The computer is the method best utilized to address spatial issues and has been found to be highly successful in treating this issue.

EXAMPLE

One 5-year-old boy was tested and found to have very serious spatial issues that affected his evaluation. His scores were lower as a result. This child participated in spatial training for a period of 2 years and was re-tested. This time we found that his drawings had improved to a considerable degree and as a result he tested at the level of his true potential, which happened to be in the gifted range. It is not that the training created intelligence, the training released the potential that was already present.

9.1.11.1 Specific Suggestions

- Computer games address spatial problems. "Sim City" is a program that requires the individual to build a city. This task is fun, interesting and targets spatial abilities. Usually ADD individuals tend to buzz around, building parts of the city and then joining the whole thing together rather than building the city by the instructions. *It is important to make sure that the person is doing the step-by-step process. Otherwise, they are simply using logical skills again.*

- In building something by using either a computer program or something like Constructs™ or Legos™, the parent constructs a design and asks the child to form the same design. This requires the child to use parts to form the whole, rather than tbreaking down the whole into its component parts.

- Three-D puzzles, darts, ballroom dancing, and country line dancing are also useful. Dancing with various steps, twists, and turns can be highly spatial in nature. Have you seen the one person who is going the wrong way when everybody turns? That is the one with a possible spatial problem.

- Generally, anything the ADD individual tends to avoid doing for fear of failure will probably have a strong spatial component to it. ADD people are already aware of what they can and cannot do. Therefore; they are our best teachers as to what is more *spatially loaded* and what type of task they cannot use logic to solve. This is true for kids as young as 5 years of age who already know what types of tasks to avoid.

This spatial issue has far-reaching consequences in terms of the impact on the development of basic academic skills of reading, handwriting, math, and spelling. The greater the spatial problem, the more out of balance things become in terms of brain functioning. The more logical the spatial problem, the worse it becomes due to the lack of use and the more difficulty they have with the basic skills. The brightest people can have the worst spatial problems due to their over-development of logic skills and, to the same degree, the under-development of spatial areas.

9.1.12   The Constant Homework Problem

- Homework needs to be done in a proper study area, where things are tidy and the area is not chaotic or crowded. Choosing a good location that is comfortable for the ADD person and provides adequate lighting and comfortable seating is critical.

- Use planning and organization to set up a schedule to make sure homework is completed on time. More often than not, homework is avoided or not completed. These individuals tend to wait until the last minute to finish the task, which only increases their anxiety, frustration, and anger at themselves. ADD persons will always say that they work best under pressure. They do finally get the job done under pressure because they can no longer afford to worry about it and so they just do it. However, the anxiety that goes along with this situation is not a positive experience. What they remember when all is said and done is the anxiety and how they had to rush around like crazy to complete the paper or the task or whatever. They still don't feel good about themselves nor have the confidence to complete the task, so the process just repeats the next time. If the homework or task is scheduled at a certain time each day, then it is just done at that time, without all of the above thinking, worrying, predicting, and so on.

- A research project should be scheduled. A little bit is worked on at the same time each day until it is completed. The task is taken in small steps and does not create the overwhelming fear of completing the large project. By having the time allotted each day to work on a project, or any task, it will get done.

- Homework time is best when scheduled directly after school, as it continues the school day. If the homework is put off and not done as soon as the child arrives home from school, attention may get focused on other things and then it becomes harder to return to the homework. Often this allows more time for avoidance, worry about the task to be completed, or upset that it has to be done at all. Often homework is saved until late at night, completed in too hasty a manner or only partially completed. This means that children or adolescents can take a break when they arrive home — have a snack, maybe exercise for a half hour — and then the homework is started. The homework is always started *before* dinner.

- Use chunking of time: studying for a maximum of 2 hours (depending on the age) and allowing for 15-minute breaks. People come back refreshed after a break. If the person gets stuck on something — some problem, some part of a paper, writer's cramp, etc. — leave the task for 15 minutes and return. The break can be a short walk, stretch, exercise, or sitting down to eat something, but not the TV because it is too addictive and it is easy to never return to work.

- Sometimes children need to be externally motivated toward their homework since it is not part of their value system. Thus, until learning becomes internally exciting, children need external motivators. Constant praise and value of their performance will eventually result in internalized motivation. Other motivating tactics are: working out a behavioral program where they earn points to get something they want or to do something they want to do; using charts to record those times they have completed the homework and then giving them both an immediate reward at the time of completion of homework and a reward later in time once they accumulate the points they need. This can even be done using a calendar on the refrigerator. Each day homework is completed on time is checked off and a certain number of days earn some reward. There are many books on this subject (see References).

- By adolescence, there should not be an external reward system used or needed. By this time, the reward should be internal or simply part of their routine. If it is not, generally it does not work to try to place adolescents on a behavioral program. The idea would be to have the time scheduled so that they get used to doing the homework at that time, no questions asked.

9.1.13 Addressing the Emotional Issues of the ADD Adult, Child, or Adolescent

In treating the ADD adult, it is important to address the issues of grief and loss. These individuals see the impact of the disorder on their lives after being diagnosed and are filled with grief and remorse that they did not address these issues sooner. They are upset that they allowed their lives to be run by this unknown disorder and feel very guilty about not seeing it in their childhood, when they just dismissed the symptoms that now are so obvious to them. In a blaming process, they are angry at the parent who did not get them diagnosed early or who did not see the problems and do something about it when they were younger.

In a step-by-step mourning process, such adults must work through the issues of grief and loss. They may experience the stages of loss, anger, guilt, remorse, anger revisited, and then sadness, acceptance, and resolution before they can truly move forward and begin to address the problem. After mourning, they can work to change the way they see things or view situations. In general, they may change the way they approach life and how they deal with situations and people in their lives. This can result in job changes, lifestyle changes, and sometimes marital changes.

Marital changes occur when the ADD adult resides with a co-dependent spouse who takes care of them. Codependent spouses may be too angry and no longer want to be involved with ADD people, despite their changes. The ADD people may no longer want to be taken care of and spouses cannot change or give up the control they had when taking care of them. For whatever reason, the marriage cannot accommodate these changes and will be unable to continue. We really try to avoid this. If two people have established a good base and a good connection with one another, they can shift, change, and weather this storm together.

Sometimes these adults are *unable to resolve the anger and hurt*. They are enraged at the professionals who let them down or the school officials who did not notice their learning problems. They cannot escape the constant plague of not being good enough. The low self-esteem is a never-ending spiral from which they cannot escape. There is a fear of failure that chokes any new ideas or goals that they may entertain. At the first sign of trouble, they are ready to abandon any goal they have undertaken and to return to their ambivalence and avoidance. Fear is their enemy and their constant companion. Failure to achieve their goals keeps them angry, frustrated, and unable to achieve their potential. They remain stuck and hopeless.

Similarly, parents with ADD children need to address their grief and loss at discovering that they have a child who is *not perfect*. They need to understand the difficult path that lies ahead. Furthermore, they may feel guilty they did not see the disorder sooner or may have reprimanded their child for symptoms caused by the presence of the disorder rather than a true punishable event — they got angry when they should have understood. Parents, too, need to go through the grief and mourning process to successfully begin addressing the issues of their ADD children.

It becomes important that this disorder is not seen as a disability, but rather as a part of life and something that can be overcome with coping mechanisms and not giving up, *always* keep trying.

If ADD adults, spouses, children or parents of ADD do not formally resolve the issues of grief and loss, they will be unable to work full force at developing new ways of existing. They will tend to feel sorry for themselves, give up and not try to address the symptoms of the disorder. Thus, people may refuse medication, or may not take the medication properly, they may try only some of the ways to cope with the disorder or give up and simply hope it will go away.

A common interaction with the person diagnosed is "You mean I am going to have this for the rest of my life?" "Yes, and either it runs you or you run it." When issues are not addressed, this often leads to problems between spouses or parent and child.

9.1.14   The Tendency to Give Up Is Common

It is common for the ADD individual to initially be excited — buy all the books, gather all the information, attend support groups, buy the planner — and then, after a month or so, discard the materials, especially if they don't see immediate results.

Because this population is sensitive, they tend to give up rather easily, rather than seeing it through and working it out. This can often lead to blaming others and not taking responsibility for one's actions. It is someone else's fault, not theirs. They do not see themselves as able to change or that they have any abilities with which to change; it is easier to give up and continue to avoid things.

They are not lazy, but depressed and anxious. They have little belief in themselves and their ability. Rather than risk failure, they remain stuck. Those close to them, however, need to remember that this is due to their fears and their inability to believe that they can actually make changes occur.

9.1.15   The Anxiety of the ADD without Hyperactivity Individual: What Can Be Done?

People with ADD without hyperactivity make up a group of individuals who are highly anxious. The anxiety tends to run through them. There may be a genetic history of anxiety in the family. The individuals may tend to have a generalized anxiety substrate that waxes and wanes depending on the external stressors. Due to this constant generalized anxiety state, as these persons grow older they become increasingly vulnerable to their external environment, particularly the toxins that we are now finding can result in cancer and strokes. These same individuals are seen as high risks for digestive-related disorders, such as irritable bowel syndrome, colitis, and so on. Also seen are sleep disorders with either early or late insomnia or continual waking throughout the night.

Such individuals are always thinking, their thoughts race and they become mentally restless. As a result, they do not get a full REM sleep or restful sleep. They end up suffering from sleep deprivation that results in increased levels of irritability and cognitive deficits that serve to amplify and increase the symptoms of ADD.

Stimulant medication can magnify anxiety levels. Therefore, people cannot tolerate a high enough dose of the medication to get positive results. They see the medication as not working and tend to quit after a brief trial period, never realizing that they were not taking enough to make a difference and never had a sufficient trial of medication to determine whether it would work. This happens often. Therefore, the anxiety needs to be addressed in some manner to allow the ADD person to take enough medication to see if it makes a difference.

We have found that taking calcium at the same time as the medication allows them to tolerate a high-enough dose to see a difference with the medication. The calcium tends to calm the system down and decreases the anxiety. This allows for the stimulant medication to be tolerated without the heart beating too fast and without nervous feeling and unable to breathe. They are then able to take sufficient stimulant to elicit a positive response. A thorough vitamin regimen also becomes extremely important for these individuals because they are so vulnerable to both their internal and external environment. It can help to decrease the effects of stress that are so much a part of their lives.

It is also important to take the stimulant medication with food. Low-blood-sugar reactions can trigger anxiety-like symptoms in people. They may feel anxious, nauseated and not hungry without realizing that this is due to low blood sugar. They actually need to eat even if they don't feel like it.

In ending this chapter on suggestions of what to do about the symptoms related to this disorder, we cannot stress enough the issue of the emotional response to ADD and how important it is to understand this before treatment occurs.

- The emotional responses to ADD create additional problems that, in turn, increase the severity of symptoms of this disorder.

- Due to the downward spiral of the continuous emotional reaction to ADD, emotional symptoms can often become worse than the ADD.

- We often tell both parents and ADD individuals that their emotional reactions of not trying, avoiding failure at all costs, limiting themselves in school or on the job, not being creative, and not taking a chance on things often costs them more than the ADD itself. We need failure to learn. It becomes impossible to learn without failing because we cannot always know everything. The most successful people have failed numerous times and learned from their mistakes.

- ADD people begin with problems associated with ADD and they compound the symptoms with problems that are worse due to their emotional reaction.
- This must be understood to treat this disorder and truly help the individual with these problems. Usually the brighter the individual and the more serious the deficits, the greater the degree of difficulty.

10

How To Tell Your Child About ADD: What It
Is and Isn't and Why Take Medication

10.1 Discussing ADD With Your Child: The Facts,
Just the Facts

This phase is extremely important if for no other reason than to stop the endless folklore about ADD. If you have read this far in this book, you are aware
that far more is unknown than known about ADD and that this cumulative
field (psychology, neuropsychology, medicine, education) is changing so
quickly that "current" information does not stay current for long. Thanks to
recent development in research methods involving QEEG-, PET-, and CAT-
scan studies, MRIs, and breakthroughs in pharmacology, important information is constantly discovered. Unfortunately, your local library is probably
one of the last places to start learning about ADD. By the time a "current"
publication (yes, this one included) makes its way to the library shelf, the
information is often outdated. Therefore, start your own ADD research
project at the bookstore and choose publications with a current (relatively
speaking) copyright date. Another good source of information is the nearest
university library, department head, or media specialist. The local C.H.ADD
(Children and Adults with Attention Deficit Disorders, headquartered in
Plantation FL) chapter or support group generally has a keen eye for note-
worthy, credible information.

Deliver the facts to your child. Report what you know, not necessarily
what you think. There is a vast difference between when we were trained
and worked as schoolteachers in both general and special education, We
were "taught" our professors' biases and folktales about ADD. Clear, specific, direct information was at a premium and too often just not available.
We then passed those biases on to other professionals and nonprofessionals
and contributed to the growing amount of folklore, certain that we spoke
only the humble truth dispensed to us from one of the assistant gods. When
discussing ADD with your child, use your knowledge and understanding

— be ready to apply what you have learned. Otherwise, you are not yet ready to have this important conversation.

10.2   Where's This Kid Coming From, Anyway?

Dr. Beckley's many years spent as a schoolteacher, consultant, psychologist, and dad has taught him that, as a general rule, kids do not listen to what grownups have to say regarding the vast culture of children. We can tell children that "x" will happen if and when occurs. Many children may record that message into their memory banks, be able to repeat it on command, and reassure the adult that the parental edict has influenced their behavior. You are well versed in seeking your child's compliance when completing tasks, running errands, and studying for tests. It is often the most well-intended parent who gives the least understanding message to the child.

Words to avoid with an ADD person

- "Relax." (I know that I always relax when my trusted physician snaps on those rubber gloves and says the very same thing to me.)

- "Honey, this blood test is for your own good and it won't hurt, you've had this test before." Actually the necessary but evil blood test is for the physician's own good. Most kids I know hate blood draws.

  Dr. Beckley has been an insulin-dependent diabetic since the age of 14 years; he undergoes blood draws on a regular basis and still we catch him whining.

- "This medicine will make you smarter and help you get better grades." (which only confirms children's assumption that they are stupid in the first place and need to get smarter).

- "Get organized, it's easy." (again confirming the child's self-diagnosis of terminal stupidity and being a total loser). The child says to himself, "If it's so easy either why can't I understand it or I struggle to understand that which everyone else believes is easy. I told you Dr. Ross, I am pretty stupid, eh?"

  Many children of all ages appear in our office awaiting confirmation of a diagnosis of "stupidity" a.k.a. ADD and as living proof they are sentenced to taking medication ("smart pills for stupid children"). They tearfully report to us that the absolute worst kid in the class takes those pills and now of course there seem to be two worst-kids-in-the-class-award winners. Children traditionally feel powerless, and worst of all, hopeless, when handled by well-intended but poorly informed parents and teachers. The overwhelming majority of kids do not have words to communicate those feelings of woe. However, even if they did have the necessary language skills, they would never tell you or me. Kids tell us in many ways that they would much rather be seen as "crazy" than "stupid." Crazy has rebellious overtones while stupid is shameful and thus incurable. Despite the best intentions, kids feel shameful and hopeless. Not feeling capable and not being truly valued increases the emotions of shame and self-doubt.

A child's self-esteem and worth quotient results in part from how they see themselves when compared with other children. We cannot dictate to our children how they are to feel when bullied by another child or intimidated by an adult. They often feel how the collective mind of their classmates dictates they should feel. To sermonize, moralize, or lecture a child only serves to further confuse and polarize between how one feels and how one is supposed to feel. How school was when you were a kid is pointless. Today's kid will benefit by viable information and an empathetic parent.

10.3 What We Say and How We Say It Can Validate Their Experiences

It is very important that ADD is discussed at children's developmental level and is applied to events in their everyday lives. This helps children to understand why some tasks are completed with ease, while others are overwhelming. The parent functions as the child's translator of the world but not always as his/her evaluator. Parents can think of themselves as consultants and can use examples of issues that have been a struggle and then relate the examples to the attentional disorder. The idea can be presented that ADD is an answer to what has (not) been going on academically and before that the diagnosis was not fully understood. The idea should be stressed that the problem is now known and understood. It is, therefore, far easier to remedy it.

EXAMPLE

Our son really understands what problems belong to ADD and what don't. He was talking about his ski lesson and told me that he decided to take his medication for the lesson because his cousins had noticed that he appeared "kinda drifty" and he noticed that he really wasn't getting what the ski instructor was saying to him. He will also go down to the office and track down his medication on days when he feels out of it and knows he has forgotten his pill. We have managed to point out the changes to him when he is on medication and when he isn't and as a result he has been able to recognize this for himself and now uses the medication when he feels he needs it. This is usually in school and when studying. However, he also takes medication for his sports activities.

10.3.1   The Issue of Bedwetting

It is important to understand the impact of this disorder when there is the issue of bedwetting. Kids need to understand that they may wet the bed because their brain just continues to sleep and therefore does not wake them up to go to the bathroom. At the same time, this is why when ADD kids say they have to go to the bathroom they mean *now*, not later. There is no warning and "accidents" can happen because they simply don't have enough time to get to the bathroom. There is no warning because the brain continues "sleeping."

10.3.2   The Brain Is Partially Sleeping

An explanation that seems to generally work well with kids is that their brains are sleeping: sometimes they are sleeping more and sometimes less. There is nothing *wrong* with their brains, just sleeping. As a result, they cannot work to their potential or to the best of their ability. It can become very frustrating to *know* they can do something but yet not be *able* to do it.

10.3.3   The Brain Talks To Itself

The brain is constantly talking to itself. That is how it works. The brain continually interrupts interactions. It talks to itself chemically and electrically. With ADD, it talks to itself through the chemical system. Sometimes there is more of the chemical and sometimes there is less, it just depends. Therefore, sometimes there will be more signs of ADD, especially during boring activities, and sometimes less, when life is a bit more exciting.

10.3.4   If Something Is Exciting We Don't See ADD

If something is really exciting and neat it will bypass this whole system. There won't be signs of ADD. ADD is not seen in crisis but is seen in boring activities. It is not seen at the beginning of the task but in the middle and at the end; it is not seen with something that is really likable because of the interest in it.

10.3.5   What Is Boredom, Really?

Kids often say they are bored and they can be bored about just about everything. But that boredom really means the brain is not aroused, stimulated, or turned on to do its job so they say they are "bored." Consequently, they *are* bored but, because they are, the brain doesn't get turned on. So it is not just an issue of being bored, there is a cycle that continues for boredom to beget boredom. The idea is stressed that we need to do something about ADD. It is not just about boredom. We need medication to wake up the brain because the person is going to be bored with some classes and that is just how it is. The student still needs to work hard and learn in those classes.

10.3.6 When the Going Gets Tough, They're Gone. Don't Give-Up!

Medication is necessary to make the brain work because ADD people cannot be stimulated or excited all of the time. Things will not always interest people but their brains still need to memorize, attend, and concentrate at least as well as anyone else's brain. Kids need to understand that the medication works because it stimulates their brains and helps to promote functions of memory, attention, and concentration. Stimulant medication promotes these same features in all brains. If any medication does what it is designed to do, the patient should merely be getting an even break just like anyone else. Interestingly, stimulant medication can also stimulate emotions that kids (especially boys) never knew they felt. The idea is that now the patient knows what the problem is and can fix it. Things can be much different from what they have been in the past. The outlook can be very positive and exciting now that the patient knows how to deal with things and how to make them better. Now patients can achieve and attain skills more in line with their capabilities.

10.3.7 Just Like Diabetes

Taking medication for ADD is like taking insulin for diabetes. It does not mean that these children are bad or a problem. It is necessary to help them operate to the best of their potential. Just like diabetics need insulin to live their lives to the fullest, the ADD person needs medication. Medication allows them to make the first step toward management. It is not, however, the whole journey. The ADD individual has to use additional coping mechanisms to develop weak skills. The use of coping mechanisms and compensatory strategies to deal with problem areas or symptoms due to the attentional disorder are methods they will use daily. As proper eyeglasses allow a child's vision to operate at 20/20, medication allows the brain to operate at its best.

10.4 Why Does the Medication Work?

Kids need to understand that the medication works because it stimulates the neurotransmitters in the brain and charges the area that is sleeping. If medication does what it is supposed to do, children should merely be getting an even break and be just like everybody else. Sometimes it can also stimulate their emotions so they may have more feelings than usual.

10.4.1 When Do They Need Medication?

Whenever they need to think clearly they need medication. Ritalin is not a happy pill. It is a thinking pill. They do not need to take it all of the time. They take it when they need to think for school and doing homework and may need to think while playing sports, taking lessons, participating in a social activity, etc. It just depends on what they are doing. It also depends on the degree of outside stimulation. For instance, they don't need it at an amusement park, the movies, or Disney World.

11

Adolescence and ADD: A Class by Itself

11.1 Introduction

One needs to remember, when dealing with adolescents, that they are in a continual state of turmoil. Emotional, social, hormonal, cognitive, and growth issues are all coming together at once. The brain is peaking in its ability to perform abstract thought and the body is growing in spurts. While this is an exciting time, it can also bring with it some negatives. Blood-sugar levels bounce, which can lead to symptoms of hypoglycemia and irritability, followed by exhaustion after eating. Teen eating habits are notoriously poor. When they don't eat, the body reacts by signaling its lack of proper nourishment with a low-blood-sugar reaction. When they do eat, they eat everything that is not nailed down and the body responds with exhaustion.

If the adolescent is ADD and taking medication, the required dosage will vary frequently in this period of constant change. We have found that Ritalin does not work as well in times of stress, which often impacts the way medication is metabolized in the body. Adolescence is also a time that high stress and changes in medication levels can add to the emotional instability. Teenagers react to everything and see everything as a big deal. They are often confused and dizzy, not knowing which end is up. Stimulant medications and low blood sugar can enhance this effect. Therefore, at times, they can scarcely think ahead because their heads are clouded. For ADD people, all of their issues are heightened. There is anger, questioning, and depression due to the emotional changes that are occurring. They question who they are, where they are going, and what they have done so far. In short, a life review occurs. Teens attempt to seek their own degree of truth — what is truth for them. They really don't want to give away secrets or show any kind of emotion, as this would provide clues as to what they have been doing or where they have been while they are still rehearsing. It is like looking at the artist's painting before the artist is ready to show it. They don't want anyone to see them before they are "done." Thus they show a "deadpan" of emotions, and rarely show excitement about anything. There is a fear regarding their ability to perform. They are unsure that they can do something and unsure that things will happen the way they want. They would rather not talk about it. It is one of those times when they don't talk, they just move through it. Often life feels like a war zone and the adolescent just gets up and does it again, day after day.

11.2 Findings of Longitudinal Studies

- Substance abuse was found to be independent of ADD. ADD is not a causal factor for substance abuse.
- ADD symptoms seen in childhood were present in adolescence.
- More disorders were seen in ADD adolescents of anxiety, mood disorders, conduct disorders.
- Adolescents, whether diagnosed with ADD or not, had greater family conflict.
- Patterns were identical for children and adolescents with ADD of psychiatric comorbidity involving cognitive, interpersonal, academic, and family functioning. This confirms that ADD is not just a childhood disorder but one that remains constant from childhood to adolescence.
- ADD children or adolescents had higher rates of Conduct Disorder, Oppositional Defiant Disorder, mood disorders, and anxiety disorders.
- Adolescents had higher rates of bipolar disorders and substance abuse but the age differences were the same for children vs. adolescents regardless of ADD. ADD is not a causal factor for bipolar disorders or substance abuse in the adolescent.
- Psychiatric comorbidity (such as depression, anxiety, bipolar, schizophrenia) in the adolescent can lead to the under-diagnosis of ADD. Therapists can become so preoccupied with the crisis situation of the adolescent that the underlying ADD disorder goes unnoticed.

11.3 Specific Issues and Concerns with Adolescents

11.3.1 Attachment

Recent research findings on attachment and adolescence include

- Early attachment with parental figures determines the degree of positive feelings toward connection with another human being.

- Being connected to another human being later translates into values such as trust, loyalty, and respect for the family unit.
- The respect for one's elders, the value of honoring one's parents, grandparents, authority figures, and so on, emerges from this early attachment and the meaningfulness of people.
- The bond that is formed with the parental figures establishes the value of people and provides the basis for future decisions regarding conflict resolution in relationships. People will give in or compromise if they value people. They don't get stuck in being right.

11.3.2 School Performance

School performance becomes more inconsistent. As classes become more complex and topics more involved, learning requires a greater amount of effort, and performance quickly becomes problematic. Commonly, those bright individuals who were surviving to this point, by high school show anxiety levels that have increased tenfold. They are struggling to continue compensating for deficits of this disorder that may or may not have been diagnosed. As a result, all of their energy is spent maintaining school grades and performance. There is no energy left for socializing. They can, therefore, easily become isolated and withdrawn. At this point, learning becomes a chore and it is all the teenager can do to pick up the information, much less enjoy learning or being able to be creative in the classroom. The reading that they had done up to this point was based on development of a sight vocabulary, reading contextually, and figuring out the words they did not know from the other words in the sentence. Although comprehension may have been problematic in the past, they could always manage to figure it out because the sentences were less complex and things were explained over and over. But now it is different. There is a multitude of information. It can be too much to take in and yet still complete these process of figuring out the meanings because they don't know enough words to just simply read the material.

Distractibility is increased due to the emotionality that is present. There are so many more things to consider, worry, and think about. Often teenagers read down the page only to find that they have no idea what they just read, or their friends interrupt them to talk and they lose their place and can't get back on track. (They don't, however, want to miss anything socially.) They may skip three lines on the page and have no idea this occurred until at a later time when they are wondering where the information for a test question is. Scan-trons are an absolute nightmare. Often exams are failed due to reading the multiple-choice question wrong or losing their places on the scan-tron and filling in the wrong answer. Fear and anxiety can make the learning disappear. Exams are failed for many reasons, which leads to more anger directed internally.

EXAMPLE

We saw a 15-year-old boy who was very angry and argued with everyone. He had an obvious skin problem due to anxiety and never stopped tapping his foot during the therapy session with him. Social skills were highly problematic and he had success-fully alienated everyone by that time. As we explained the seriousness of his attention disorder and he saw his deficits firsthand, his foot shook more. At first appearance, he looked like an ADHD, impulsive, acting-out, inappropriate. However, testing revealed an extremely bright individual, with ADD without hyperactivity. The pri-mary problem was information processing. Due to constantly missing information, he had to work extremely hard in his classes just to pick up information, maintain the excellent grades he had always received, and be able to continue to please his father. There was no energy left to learn how to fit in with his peers, to learn how to be social, or to enjoy learning, and he was, therefore, incredibly angry.

When adolescents do poorly in school and thus cannot do well socially, self-esteem is depleted and they are at risk for depression or acting-out behavior. Depression is anger turned inward or outward and adolescents fre-quently turn their anger outward. This can often be misinterpreted as being oppositional or defiant.

With ADD without hyperactivity, there can be an increase in anxiety, facial blemishes, and depression. They care too much, while saying they do not care at all. They say they are not anxious, while their legs are shaking and they are continually changing positions. The emotions are spilling out of them. However, they have no idea and cannot explain what they do not even understand. This is where evaluation becomes useful.

EXAMPLE

We had a 15-year-old girl in our offices. While we were in the process of explaining the test results, she burst into tears and could not stop crying. We stopped what we were doing and attempted to try to understand what was happening. In the presence of her mother, we discussed the problems between the parents as well as her relation-ship with her father. She continued to cry. We decided to evaluate her psychologically with a personality assessment and projective tests (the ink blots, etc.). It was through the psychological evaluation that we learned that she missed her father and was very wounded by him. He was an alcoholic who had been close to her as a child but now was continuously drinking.

Only when other significant issues are addressed can the adolescent begin to address the ADD symptoms, work on the coping mechanisms, and under-stand the disorder. Until that time their minds are still clouded with other issues, fears, and concerns.

ADHD adolescents are a different group entirely. It is in adolescents that conduct-disorder behavior and/or delinquent, acting-out behavior occurs. They push the limits to see how far they can go and then they push some more. There is no attachment to anyone or anything. They do what they want when they want. They have no rules or restrictions. Others should not get in their way or they will be sorry. Nothing is their fault, they place the blame on everyone else. Others are blamed not as protection to avoid feeling guilty or bad, but because they truly believe that others are at fault.

Because teens hide their emotions they can easily appear to not care or be unmotivated. This is where avoidance and procrastination become so highly evident and the pattern of working under crisis begins. They put things off until finally the deadline forces them to abandon their fears and begin working on the dreaded project. Teenagers may not take care of themselves hygienically either because they forget (ADD) or they actually do not care (ADHD). It is imperative to separate the ADD without hyperactivity from the ADHD at this age. It is important to recognize the teen who truly wants to be successful but does not know how to accomplish this task and is ready to give up and drop out. ADHD teens do not care what you or anyone else thinks and they will do as they please. As problems become worse the stakes get higher and they end up in court having committed a variety of offenses ranging from car theft to breaking and entering to running away from home and school truancy. Outwardly the two subtypes look very much alike. Evaluation is the only way to tell the difference, and with adolescents a psychological evaluation is necessary to truly understand what is going on with them that they cannot tell you.

ADD without hyperactivity teens who avoid and procrastinate can be motivated toward crime just to look cool. They associate with friends who make them feel better about themselves. They end up in the wrong place at the wrong time and suddenly find themselves in big trouble with the legal authorities. They are embarrassed and ashamed. They have now truly fallen down in the eyes of those who are important to them. So they put on a mask and act like they don't care. The angrier and more frustrated parents become, the more adolescents tighten the mask down so no one knows how bad they feel. Inside they become smaller and smaller and less and less significant. They do care and yet they don't want to care. They are afraid of everything and they feel they have to act as if they fear nothing. It is exhausting. These individuals are usually the more fragile and sensitive and, thus, they cover up and hide their problems and difficulties. They must be acknowledged before they begin to feel nothing. They do care and feel, and, therefore, must be understood before they totally give up their goals and make it impossible to ever achieve them. They anticipate failure and in a self-fulfilling prophesy make their worst nightmares and fears a reality.

11.3.3 Junior High School as a Transition Experience Is Frightening

Junior high years are particularly difficult for ADD individuals. In elementary years, environmental stressors are fewer and there is more external structure so they can concentrate on compensating for the disorder. As children, they are told what to do and don't they have to think about it. Their decisions are made for them. By the time they reach junior high, the decrease in structure creates a chaos that is literally overwhelming. Just getting from one class to another on time becomes a task that increases in difficulty in high school. Not only must they adjust for things becoming more complex but there are also new social aspects that have been introduced. The world becomes threatening for ADD children.

The ADD child now must deal with cognitive and physical changes in an ever-changing setting. I cannot say enough about how the social adjustment and the need to fit in become so incredibly difficult during junior-high years as information-processing problems cause them to constantly miscue. The ADD child who reports problems to the teacher, not knowing what else to do, is often labeled as a misfit. The ADD adolescent knows that asking adults for help in how to handle the peer group would be disastrous. There is nowhere to turn. This is the time ADD people withdraw. They can't get help from anywhere and they have no idea what to do.

EXAMPLE

One adult ADD without hyperactivity individual talked about her experiences as an adolescent in school. She found junior high to be an overwhelming experience. Changing rooms several times a day, switching subjects rapidly, and having only 20 minutes for lunch kept her disoriented and tense. The running theory among the students was that if you didn't make at least a "C" in every class, you were either stupid or "bad." "Bad" kids failed on purpose and stupid kids got placed in "Special Ed." She firmly believed these views and, therefore, used all of her time and energy to keep up that "C" average. While doing this, she had difficulty keeping track of other things. She couldn't ask for help lest they find out how stupid she was, so she just continued to struggle. Gym class was another nightmare. There was no privacy at all in the girls' locker room and shower, where jokes about overdevelopment or underdevelopment and general verbal torment were constantly being hurled. All of these made her shrink further inside herself. She found herself angry about how she was, anxious about how she looked and sounded, and fearful about possible failure. It led her to feel totally helpless and hopeless about where she was going and her future.

Another evaluation that we completed with a teenager in high school caused the individual to burst into tears on learning that she truly was very bright and very capable of doing all that she wanted to do. She could not believe after all these years of seeing herself as "stupid" that she actually was capable and had the ability and potential to do what she dreamed of doing.

11.3.4   Task Completion

Task completion is a difficult endeavor for "normal" teens, but with ADD as an added factor, it becomes virtually impossible. Due to the continual distractibility and lack of focus, they appear impulsive and cannot see anything through to its end. As a result, their friends cannot always count on them to be where they say they are going to be, and to do what they say they are going to do. It is not their intent to hurt anyone and they feel very bad when this occurs. However, "I'm sorry" statements last only for so long. ADHD teens will show up when they feel like it, when their interest is piqued, or whenever there is a payoff.

Task completion becomes a problem for both groups because they have so many things to do and cannot organize their time. They feel overwhelmed, they cannot figure out how to do all the things they are supposed to accomplish. The problem with time management due to spatial issues results in planning way too much for the time slots available. When unable to meet all of their goals and unable to figure out the space of time to complete tasks, they feel hopeless and task completion becomes one more battleground for them.

11.3.5 Social Skills and the Peer Group

ADD teens tend to be loners. They only have time for school, and because they lack the necessary social skills, are not socially "tuned in." They can only handle a few relationships at a time. They daydream their life away and become lost in their own thoughts. They complete all of the social milestones later than their peers. If they do not retreat, they associate with a group that they can tag along with and act as they belong. Usually this is not the popular group because that would be too intimidating for them. This group is usually the drop-outs. They have a coolness to them and they receive acceptance based on being different from the rest. By joining a group based on being different, whatever they do is now acceptable and okay because it *is* different. ADD teens cling to these groups, defending their new friends, from whom they are actually very different, because at long last they now have a group of friends. They tend to like whoever likes them. They are so desperate to be accepted that they give up their ability to choose.

EXAMPLE
We saw a 16-year-old girl who, when she first came in, had part of her hair dyed purple and her nails were purple to match. She dressed in clothes straight out of the 1960s, purchasing them from the resale shops and garage sales. She was a beautiful girl and childhood pictures of her revealed someone you would see on a shampoo ad. However, her beauty was hidden beneath the purple hair and dark ringed eyes and pierced nose. She told me that her goal was to be as different as she possibly could because this is how she was known in her school. She had to show up in the most outrageous outfits that she could — one time even in a velvet evening gown because that was what was expected of her and was her established reputation.

11.3.6 Getting Along With Others

Common problems listed by most adolescents are that they don't get along with their parents and/or their parents do not understand what is bothering them. With ADD adolescents these issues are important because their struggles are greater. They feel incompetent, unfulfilled, worried about their futures, unsure of themselves, and they continually question their abilities and assets. This is even more the case with ADD without hyperactivity as they are the ones who care and are fearful about what others think of them. The more sensitive they are, the more overfocused they are and the more emotionally extreme they become. They can be moody due to keeping all of their thoughts and feelings inside. They are children, being forced to operate in a grown-up world about which they know nothing and in which they have no confidence. Because they are so sensitive, they never want anyone to know lest they can be taken advantage of.

EXAMPLE
We saw a 14-year-old male who had a history of arrests as a juvenile for a variety of misdemeanors ranging from stealing to school truancy. He had lived in numerous places by the time we saw him and was being transferred from one facility to another. Outwardly, he looked as tough as nails and the more you thought that he was tough the better he felt. He appeared arrogant, condescending, and removed from people. He seemed to look down on everyone. There was absolutely no warmth or friendliness; he was definitely cold. A psychological evaluation revealed an underlying sensitivity and a preoccupation with the harm that had been done to him in the past. As a child he was thin and frail looking. He had been teased incessantly by the other kids in his class. When he could not do the work, was caught being distracted, or couldn't stay in his seat the teacher would reprimand him. This only added to the teasing. He had formed a tough personality to protect the hurt child inside and his own fragility. The anger that he felt as a child remained inside and became part of his everyday living. His personality had changed and formed around the anger that he continually felt.

ADHD adolescents do not appear to go through these types of struggles. Rather they are busy flexing their muscles, straining the reigns held by their parents, seeing how far they can push things and how far they can get. They are always determined to get what they want. ADHD adolescents will talk sarcastically, have a million excuses for their behavior, refuse to take responsibility for their behavior, and always blame someone or something. They can be defensive, put others down, use name calling, make light of things, and deny any involvement in whatever they are accused of. ADHD adolescents may monopolize discussions, practice obnoxious behaviors that are often inappropriate for the setting, and are likely to ignore others. They may be subject to temper outbursts and *always* need to be right. Their rigid thinking prevents flexible problem solving, and they will attempt to dominate their surroundings.

ADD without hyperactivity adolescents may also practice the exact same behaviors for different reasons. However, their behavior is due to low self-esteem, the fear of someone becoming angry at them, and desperately wanting others to think that they are more acceptable and okay than they truly feel. They need to be important. Whereas ADHD will not back down and rethink things, ADD without hyperactivity adolescents will back down because they really are connected and they really do care.

11.3.7   Sexual Maturity

Recent research indicates that

- Girls who were early in development of sexual maturity were more likely to exhibit later difficulties with depressive eating and delinquent, acting-out symptoms.
- Adolescents saw themselves as different and asked what was wrong with them. This self-perception often led to serious mental health outcomes. Early-maturing girls were more likely to have attempted suicide.
- There was a pressure placed on early-maturing girls to engage in sexual behaviors appropriate to their appearance, thus the early sexual activity.
- For boys, early and late maturation resulted in adjustment problems as well as higher levels of depression, a higher emotional reliance on others, and the development of dependency on others to meet their needs.
- Later-maturing boys reported more self consciousness, more conflict with parents, more trouble in school, and less social competency.
- Later-maturing girls did better in school as if they compensated for less sexual activity by spending more time studying and improving themselves academically.

11.3.8   Clarity

Adolescents are spacey and ADD adolescents are even more so. It takes a very special individual to work with adolescents in treatment because this group really needs to have a sense of who and where they are. The adolescent frequently seems silly. Everything they do is a big deal to them, so it must be to others, therefore they tend to be narcissistic and very self-involved. Sometimes their conversation feels like idle chatter about nothing and they make no sense at all. They tell stories in the greatest of detail, yet cannot recall their homework assignments or the day they are due.

The spaciness occurs with the preoccupation that they have at any particular moment with any given thing, which they will not even recall in a week's time. Sometimes they become vague due to overwhelming emotions. They cannot make decisions, don't know what to do, and are *so* confused.

Teens are very sensitive, flighty, and emotionally at risk. The ADD adolescent is even more at risk. As their emotions overwhelm them and occupy their thoughts and time, they appear more and more spacey. The common question becomes, "Are you there?" This is why we need to worry about the failure of ADD individuals, especially perfectionistic, bright, ADD without hyperactivity adolescents, who feel more terrible and hopeless about themselves and their future. Adolescents become so involved with their emotions that they are unable to figure out where the emotions came from in the first place and to what they are connected. Emotions build out of proportion until they cannot be fixed. Once they feel hopeless it becomes difficult for them to see things differently and they become stuck in their own out-of-control feelings that they don't understand. Therefore, when someone, such as a therapist, comes along and identifies the disorder and the problem, the adolescent who has long since given up remains confused and helpless. He or she is not going to respond with joy and immediately begin to make changes in his or her life by incorporating all of the helpful hints that might be provided. By the time we see teenagers they have gone past the state of feeling badly and are sunk into the confusion of their own depression. They cannot relate to what is being said. Therefore, we must resolve the issues of depression and of emotions that clog their thinking on a daily basis and create the spaciness that we see outwardly. Then we can work on coping with the ADD. Often, by the time of adolescence, it is the emotions and their method of coping with formerly undiagnosed symptoms that create most of the problem, not the actual ADD symptoms themselves. By this time, the emotional consequences can be far more disastrous than the disorder ever was.

11.3.9   Off-Task Behavior

There tends to be a high level of off-task behavior and a great tendency to be quite unorganized. Off-task behavior can be the result of the symptoms of distractibility as well as the consequence of the depression seen so often in this population. Adolescents with ADD tend to develop a very passive attitude toward learning. Symptoms of ADD without hyperactivity often result in feelings of helplessness and hopelessness. The anxiety leads to depression and feeling so overwhelmed that they can no longer cope. This creates suicidal tendencies and eventually the idea that nothing matters.

The true ADHD individual, however, never really experiences depression. He or she simply sees that the going has now become tough and so it is time to go. They move on, do something else, or get someone else to take care of them. Adolescents with ADD without hyperactivity also leave when things become difficult but they don't move ahead. They leave due to avoidance. This leads to the depression and feelings of being worthless. They tend to leave both the problems and the solutions to others and prefer to remain in their own world and continue as they always have. This is partly because they have little energy for anything outside of all that is happening to them internally on a physiological level and partly because symptoms of the disorder have built to the degree that they are ready to quit. They are tired and angry with the struggle. They do not see the possibility of change nor of a future.

Off-task behavior needs to be separated from (1) the emotional consequence of feeling so bad and so helpless or hopeless that nothing matters. (2) the "so-what, I-don't-care attitude" of ADHD, (3) the overwhelmed feelings of incompetence, and (4) the avoidance and procrastination. Off-task behavior can be blamed on numerous emotional or motivational issues as well as simply being distracted or due to poor, sustained attention and the lack of capacity to remain on task for any lengthy period of time.

11.3.10   Substance Abuse

Recent research indicates that

- Alcohol use, teenage pregnancy, and psychiatric disorders in adolescents were related to trauma and adverse life events.
- The trauma for females was sexual abuse; males were victims of other types of violence.
- Alcohol consumption may be perceived by adolescents as providing a means of their own emotional self-control.
- The early use of cigarettes, alcohol, and marijuana was related to later psychiatric/psychological disorders, depression, and antisocial personality disorder.
- Substance abuse is not specific to ADD and occurred to the same degree for both ADD and non-ADD adolescents.

Substance abuse in adolescence varies and depends on the nature of the ADD disorder. Generally, the ADHD individual will have been abusing some substance for years prior even to reaching adolescence. ADHD individuals, at very early ages, tend to become involved in more hard-core drug use, such as cocaine and heroin, for their stimulant properties. They drink to live and live to drink. These patterns may begin as young as 9 years of age.

ADD without hyperactivity individuals may also engage in extensive alcohol use but as a means of self-medication to ease them into the social scene. Drinking tends to begin during adolescence. They will also use marijuana as a means of calming themselves down and attempting to fit into the group. They become addicted to daily use of marijuana as a means of remaining calm and coping with escalating problems in their lives. Marijuana, they find, is helpful in allowing them to think better because it impacts the sensory system. However, problems escalate further with the drug use. There is a lack of motivation that occurs with the use of marijuana that is far reaching and affects every level of their lives. Teens on marijuana do not feel motivated and have little interest in anything. There is also an agitation that occurs and they may argue constantly. Their mode of operation is to defend and attack, defend and attack on a continual, never-ending basis. You say black and they say white just to disagree. We now know that short-term memory is impacted by marijuana use and increases problems with information processing, which leads to missing information, poor communication, and miscommunication.

It can be difficult to determine a diagnosis of ADD in adolescence especially just by using self-report measures. Poor insight, lack of social ability, poor monitoring, and confusion are common with "normal" teens and thus create difficulty in diagnosing ADD. Many of the symptoms they display could be due to the type of substance they are abusing. A common complaint is that the use of Ritalin or stimulant medication will lead to further substance abuse. Actually those who abuse Ritalin are few in numbers. Individuals who abuse the drug tend to be ADHD, highly addicted, not ready for change and still practicing abuse. Otherwise, the use of medication can actually prevent the onset of substance abuse. Many teenagers who abuse drugs were once diagnosed with ADD and placed on medication when young. The medication made a difference and they improved their performance in school. Then they were taken off the medication because everyone thought that the problem had been fixed. Unfortunately, things became worse again in a couple of years. The panic, anxiety, and depression can lead adolescents to substance abuse. Had they remained on the medication and understood the nature of the disorder there is a high likelihood that future substance abuse would not have occurred.

11.4   If Emerging from an Alcoholic or Dysfunctional Home

Adolescents are more at risk if emerging from a traumatic, alcoholic home environment. Recent research findings report that

- Specific types of traumatic events were associated with the occurrence of PTSD symptoms in adolescents. A link was found between the exposure of the adolescent to violence and symptoms of PTSD. There is a victimization that occurs from witnessing violence.
- Adolescents who were continually exposed to violence developed difficulties with concentration, short-term memory loss, attachments to those significant to them were anxious in nature, and they displayed an aggressive or otherwise tough mask to hide their fears.
- Violence exposure led to the development of more-internalized thinking patterns and the increased likelihood of the development

of depressive and anxious symptoms. The development of intrusive or unwanted and uncontrollable mental images plagued their everyday thinking.

- Trauma and other adverse life events were found to be associated with alcohol use in adolescents. Females, more so than males, had a history of sexual abuse; males were victims of other types of violence.

- Alcohol was viewed by the adolescent as providing a means of emotional self-regulation. They were in charge and could exercise their own control.

11.4.1 The Overfocused Subtype in Adolescence

The overfocused subtype of an ADD without hyperactivity is highly vulnerable in adolescence. The drama, the oversensitivity, poor sleep patterns, irritability, sleep deprivation, blood-sugar problems, etc., all come to a head in adolescence. All of the ruminating and overfocused thinking that has been internalized bursts forth and emotions erupt, overwhelming adolescents, and all of those close to them. Suddenly these individuals have turned into raving lunatics, maniacs out of control, and one thinks is this ADHD? Can a child be ADD without hyperactivity until adolescence and then become ADHD? *Our answer is no.*

What happens is that this dramatic, overfocused subtype reaches an emotional peak and there is a considerable degree of acting-out behavior that occurs with temper tantrums and out-of-control emotionality as well as wide mood swings and overall discontentedness. Nothing pleases them and they don't know how to be happy nor how to make themselves happy. They want to be close and then they don't want to be close. They fight with you and tell you to go away and then cry and say that you don't really love them because you are not helping them. They want to be young and to be taken care of yet they want to be grown up to have the freedom. They don't know what they want and neither do their parents.

These emotionally reactive, sensitive beings are the ones who create the airtight mask to keep everyone at bay. They do not want anyone to know how vulnerable they are. They keep everyone away, but their messages are mixed because they really want to be close. They are scared and always anticipate the worst.

Then there is the what if. What if this happens and what if that happens. In this manner, they effectively talk themselves out of taking any type of risk. Change only occurs with risk and these individuals therefore do not change. They become stuck in their own fears and eventually their own hatred of their fearfulness. The anger that they feel inside is projected outward to those around them and they can become quite nasty to live with. They are critical of themselves and of those around them as well. The continual ruminating becomes a recital of how bad they are and how terrible they have become and how nothing will work out — ever. There does not appear to be a future, things become too dark to continue, and death appears as a blessing. These feelings can be the genesis of suicidal thoughts.

The internal ruminating causes an overfocus on any mistake that is made. The smallest mistake is analyzed and re-analyzed to the degree that they don't even want to talk about it anymore, much less fix the problem. As a result, problems are not faced and things continue the way they had in the past. The avoidance and procrastination remain in place as permanent methods of coping and the downward spiral never ends, nor shows promise of ending. It is so important for those working with these adolescents — their parents, teachers, or therapists — to understand what is occurring behind the scenes and to know that what they see outwardly usually is not what is going on internally. It becomes far too easy to infer someone's feelings and to react to what they present to us, rather than to search deeper for reasons to explain their unacceptable behavior or emotions.

11.4.2   What Do We Do for the ADD Adolescent?

Active parenting plays a crucial role. Parents who are continually attempting to find new and creative ways to reach this unreachable child meet with better success than parents who feel helpless and hopeless and tend to give up. The idea is to provide adolescents with as much information as is possible to give them the choice for change and the opportunity to do things differently in their lives. This is a time of providing the information and then letting them go so they can flap their own wings and attempt to soar into the world.

11.4.3   Involve Them in the Diagnostic Process

It is important to involve the adolescent in the diagnostic process. We tend to encourage individuals who were diagnosed in childhood to be reassessed in adolescence just to show them their assets and liabilities and where the ADD hits and where it doesn't. This encourages them to begin to form good strategies to compensate for the presence of the disorder and to develop good study habits. Finally, if adolescents see the presence of the disorder, they recognize the need for medication, which eliminates the usual problem of compliance. Compliance problems tend to occur more often when adolescents do not know why they are taking the medication and no longer wish to go along with a program they didn't sanction.

We have found in our experience that generally, by going through a very clear clinical evaluation, adolescents understand why they need to take this medication. They then have no difficulty understanding the need for medical management and, in fact, are excited to accept it. It is important that adolescents feel they have a choice and that they are choosing to take medication by understanding why, when, and how they need to use it. When there are extenuating issues, it becomes important to identify all of the underlying emotional issues contributing to their actions and reactions. It is not enough to just diagnose ADD. Especially in adolescence, we must consider all the factors that may be operating to produce the behavior and academic problems that occur.

It is so critical to identify exactly what happened in an individual's development to provide adolescents with the rational side, the reason for their emotions. Only then can they take control of their lives.

11.4.4 Enhance Self-Esteem

It is highly important to enhance the self-esteem of adolescents during this particularly vulnerable time in their lives. The stakes are high and it is difficult to keep up with their peer group. The idea is to find those areas of competency and for the adolescent to pursue them, whether in sports or a particular area of learning. This is also the time to give them responsibility and jobs that are within their range so that they feel competent, important, and as if they have accomplished something. Finally, it is very critical to teach the adolescent about failure. They need to know they can make mistakes and still keep working toward their goals. Too often, adolescents tend to give up too easily.

The overfocused subtype of individuals tend to easily give up due to their fear of failure. Sometimes, they are so afraid of failing that they don't even begin the task. Unfortunately, this results in not being able to experience new things in their environment due to the fear of failure and criticism if mistakes are made. It becomes so important to know that one can learn from one's mistakes, that failure simply makes us smarter and we learn every time we fail. Instead, ADD individuals, especially the overfocused group, tend to regret failure and condemn themselves for failure, and thus create such a negative situation that they never allow themselves the opportunity to learn that they can fail and recover from failure. It is impossible to know everything to avoid failure. We have to be able to fail to learn and to experience new things in life.

11.4.5 We Need to be Empathetic

It is easy to become frustrated with the ADD adolescent, who, by this time, has tried our patience to the max. We are tired of picking up the pieces. However, the point at which we are most exhausted is the exact time that children may need the most empathy and understanding. Because they are so vulnerable at this age, if we blow up about what they have or have not done, it contributes to the increasing feelings of hopelessness and helplessness about the ability to control their futures. This is a time of life when adolescents are questioning their ability to make a future and withstand adult pressures and, thus, they are too vulnerable for us to become upset with them and to question their abilities. It is important that we are not deceived by the outer hard-shell appearance, which the adolescent adapts to make us think they can handle anything — the truth is very different. They are actually quite afraid and fragile. They are far too vulnerable to handle the criticism that their cool exterior makes us believe they can handle.

11.4.6   Need for Control

Being an adolescent feels much like being on a runaway horse. Everything feels out of control; emotions, thoughts, body, eating, and sleeping are all confused. There is a need for control over something, anything. ADD adolescents feel even more out of control as they feel they do not have adequate abilities to accomplish the task. There is a great tendency toward low self-esteem and general inadequacy. They have entered into adolescence already feeling out of control only find that feeling exacerbated. To foster self-esteem, we need to point out the areas where adolescents are in control and can impact their destiny and what happens to them. Identifying and maximizing their areas of strength is absolutely critical. It will help them to move through this particularly difficult time with some hope and not fall victim to the feelings of total hopelessness and despair that so characterize this population. Providing structure and a method for them to accomplish their goals can be extremely helpful.

Everyone needs outside help sometimes to get from point A to point B. But, despite good intentions, not everyone can always follow through on the necessary steps to achieve their goals. Adolescents are no different. Thus, outside help is important to provide the environment, structure, or training necessary to attain their goals. An example would be to help adolescents increase their academic skills by placing them in a situation of structured study time, library time, tutoring, computer time, and so on. The idea is to arrange a course of action that adolescents can begin without placing them in the position of having to set up a situation that they are not sure they can complete.

11.4.7   Think Win-Win: Provide Opportunities for Success

Working with the adolescent ADD population, the goal is to develop the areas in which they are good and to transfer those feelings of self-esteem to areas that are more difficult. Due to the avoidance, procrastination, and tendency to give up, a belief in self must be fostered, as well as the idea that one needs to keep working at something until it works — they can always develop competence but they need to make mistakes to learn and grow. Teaching adolescents opportunities to find success, take responsibility, make something happen, or help someone else will foster confidence in their abilities to make decisions and choices, to fail yet learn, and to generally feel more powerful. It is well known that if people truly feel internally powerful they will take action, seize the moment, and use it. Adolescents tend to approach life with a puffed-up chest, trying to make everyone think that they can do something about which they have doubt. The idea is to help them build a sense of self — who they are, what they can do, and what they can't do — and to help them feel proud of the whole package, not just the success and the assets.

This is a time of establishing an identity with the goal of acceptance of the self, who and what they actually are, accompanied by the choice to make the changes to be who they want to become. Resolution of adolescence is the emergence of an identity wherein the individual can say, without the judgment of being good or bad, this is who I am and these are my strengths and weaknesses. When these issues remain unresolved, adolescents may emerge from this time period feeling they are good enough, there is identity diffusion, they exist as others or situations define them, and they are only as good as their most recent deeds.

11.4.8 Driving

It is difficult to surrender the wheel to an individual who can be impulsive, out of control emotionally, and who may very well have a spatial problem. Spatial problems create the inability to perceive the whole, and thus, to predict and anticipate accidents happening. ADD persons tend to put the brakes on too quickly because all of a sudden they realize that the car has stopped in front of them. Spatial problems create parking difficulties and the tendency to have difficulty getting out of semi-enclosed spaces without hitting or scraping something. Sometimes, providing double driver training, so the adolescents take training classes twice to make sure they have all of the concepts down pat, can be a useful device. Another idea is to spend at least 1 year with a learner's permit and to teach adolescents about all types of driving situations before they drive the car by themselves.

12

The Impact of Attention Disorders Within the Family System

12.1 Introduction

Often, the ADHD family is divided: family members band together and exclude the ADHD member who, by the very nature of the disorder, tend not to collaborate and refuses to honor borders and boundaries. The ADD child tends to also be excluded from the family structure. This type of child becomes lost, cannot keep up with other members, and, as a result, is left behind. Both types of individuals operate outside of the family structure, however, one is due to behavioral opposition (ADHD) and the other is due to being unaware (ADD).

The household can easily revolve around the ADHD child, who demands attention and is continually causing a problem in the home, school, and community. There is unpredictability in living with ADHD individuals — no one knows at what moment they may decide to do something or act a certain way, and there is no viable rhyme or reason for their behavior. Isolation can occur, with extended family members, grandparents, aunts and uncles refusing to accept the family because of the child's behavior. Parents who spend much of their day disciplining children have little energy left for intimacy and fun. Parents continually inform us that they have little private couple time since no one else is available to help care for their children. Marital time, extended family experiences, and vacations become a distant memory.

12.2 So What Do We Do?

The family must work together to cope with the disorder, whether it be ADD or ADHD and to view it as a characteristic of the family, not the specific member. (Families as a whole should attend support meetings to learn about the disorder.)

12.3 Suggestions for Coping

Family meetings tend to be the most important tool used to foster collaborative problem solving and specifically target cohesiveness of the family. This is where members get to air their feelings without worrying about someone becoming hurt or angry, or a consequence occurring because they speak up about what they do not like. Sometimes families will sit down and take 15 minutes or so to write down their thoughts and what bothers them. They then read them to the group. Another method is for children to write down their feelings and give them to their parents so their parents will be aware of what is happening in the relationships among their children.

12.4 Specific Suggestions for Family Meetings

1. It is suggested that family meetings be held at the same time each week to provide consistency. Too often, individual family members are very busy and it is difficult to get them to agree to a time to be together. Thus, require that the group meetings be conducted on a regular basis to lend an importance to the meeting. Attendance is mandatory and, if for some reason one member cannot meet, then the meeting is rescheduled. Two positive outcomes occur from agreeing to meet regularly.

   a. Members do not feel pushed to meet as a family since the meeting has been established as a tradition and integrated into the weekly schedule. In general, anything that is established as a routine simply becomes part of our lives and therefore part of our expectation for that particular day. We cease to have feelings about the meeting, given that it is now simply part of the day. If feelings do emerge, at that point it is a positive experience as family members look forward to addressing certain issues and are therefore very happy that a meeting is going to occur that day, the next day, or that week.

   b. Members will continue to be present on a regular basis as they have agreed to attend. If family meetings are held on a crisis basis only, then all that occurs is crisis management. It is like just continually trying to stop a flood from occurring. It becomes easy to move from one crisis to another as things are never truly fixed, just managed or temporarily corrected. This does not help to achieve a long-standing tradition of working together and operating as a cohesive group or learning from each other as part of the process. Finally, if there is a meeting each week and a problem cannot be handled or resolved in a meeting then it can be scheduled again for the next week, at which time everyone might see things a little more clearly or have new ideas for solutions.

2. It is important for all members of the group to feel some sort of equal status, regardless of age. This allows and promotes freedom of speech without fear of repercussion. One way of ensuring that everyone feels equal is to allow each of the family members to take a turn in running the meeting and taking notes of meeting results. Whether for young or old, such positioning promotes self-esteem and a sense of power and uniqueness.

3. Everyone should be taken seriously and allowed their time to speak. Borders and boundaries need to be honored. Members should not interrupt nor should they react with emotional outbursts. When working with the attention-disordered it is important to maintain a sense of structure and rule regulation. Those taking medication should make sure that they have taken their dosage prior to the start of the meeting to ensure full participation in the discussion. Meetings should be free from distractions. (Conducting a family meeting in front of the TV set pretty well ensures that members will not participate.) A sense of ceremony and ritual underlines the meeting's importance to family members.

4. Seek unanimous agreement on solutions. There are times when this simply will not occur and the matter should be tabled for later discussion. Further, it does not hurt for members, especially adolescents, to exhibit appropriate arguing skills as long as both parties listen to one another's viewpoints in a calm, nonreactive manner to eventually arrive at a decision. A principle to remember is that usually when someone is adamant about a topic it is due to some unseen value or emotional experience tied to the issue in question. In other words, something else, rather than the obvious, is happening to produce the reaction they are presenting to the group. Determining why the person is so adamant is an effective means of breaking a stalemate. Good family therapists are worth their weight in gold as they help the family to accomplish this task. The empathetic response of the parent and good problem-solving skills can do much to alter attitudes and build or increase self-esteem. It is crucial to the healthy development of the child.

EXAMPLE

One of my major goals as a family therapist is to "get fired," states Dr. Beckley. Part of my first interview with every family is to determine what either they need to do or I need to do, so that they will "fire" me. I tell them that I don't want to get fired too early or too late, but I do want to get fired. They can rehire me at any time. One of my goals is to teach or to model a family meeting. If your family meeting is not going the way you want it to go, treat yourself to a few trips to the local family therapist. He or she can help to put your meeting back on track.

The common misconception about therapy is that you must be sick or at least unable to run your family or your emotional life and you must return once a week for years. The truth is that most family therapy cases consists of six or fewer interviews spread over a period of months.

5. Finally, establish housekeeping at the beginning of family meetings; describe the rules of not interrupting, not correcting, not lecturing, and agreeing to disagree. Set a time limit of less than 1 hour and a general format to follow (such as opening the meeting, listing the concerns, who needs time, setting priorities). Simple, direct, straightforward information exchange aimed at behavioral change and household management is needed. Personal calendars must be present as well as the family calendar.

6. Changing someone's behavior is a very doable but short-lived deed. We can train someone to do something (such as straighten the mess in their rooms) but too often what we miss with behavior-management programs is that the attitude does not change and, consequently, the behavior will reappear in another form or when the behavior is no longer monitored.

Family meetings provide the opportunity to instill true attitude changes and connection with the parent. As a group, the attention-disordered tend to lack internal motivation and rule regulation and thus require external motivation. Connectiveness allows parents to become external motivators and to teach a value system. Children will respond if connected with parents.

12.4.1   Agendas

- Agendas can be developed throughout the week and displayed on a bulletin board placed in a common area. A white board on the refrigerator will work well. Sundays tend to be a great time to meet.
- Planners are in hand as all family members assemble.
- A household "administrator" collects the existing agenda and presents it to the person who is running the meeting.

- After a moment of absolute silence (don't press your luck by asking for more than a moment) to calm the group, the chairperson opens with, "Are there any additions to the agenda?" If so, they are then stated and added to the bottom of the list and will be addressed should time permit.
- Once the agenda is accepted, discuss each topic and focus on the solutions. Stick to the agenda. Do not vary. Do not sermonize, moralize, blame, lecture or criticize. Do not fall into the trap of telling children how it was when you were a kid. Nobody cares.

12.4.2   Rules of the Meeting

- No personal-attack statements.
- Everyone has the right to pass and say nothing.
- Speak only from the "I" position.
- Follow a win-win philosophy. For this to be successful you have to win and so do I.

12.5   External Organization Aids to Cope with Life in the ADD Household

1. External organizational aids allow the ADD individual to remain focused and record things in one place. Many types of planning systems employ the notion of continual goal setting (completing tasks the next day that one could not do the day prior). Thus, it keeps ADD individuals on track and focused on completion, from which they tend to wander (whether it be due to an out-of-control problem for the ADHD individual or the confusion of the ADD without hyperactivity).

2. Blended families tend to be very sensitive to familial issues. Scheduling between their work hours, appointments, and their former spouses' households keeps them on their toes. Add in sports, especially traveling teams, and the schedule can become very overwhelming in a hurry. All things need to be detailed visibly on both family calendars, e.g.,

   - Work schedules.
   - Family meeting times.
   - Kids' lessons.
   - Little League sports programs and sports in general.

A 2-month calendar works well with everyone having a different color for their activities. The rule is, if it is not on the board, it does not exist.

3. It is a part of life that we must repeat our directions and wishes to our children. An ADD household is especially susceptible to the frustration and rage that comes with constant repetition of requests and before long the anger becomes as natural as brushing one's teeth. Following parental wishes and directions can be discussed and processed at the family meetings as part of a conversation. It is not barked or ordered but part of an understanding that is struck between parent and child.

4. Colored sticky notes as a visual aid are wonderful backup systems to the auditory modality. We often advise the attention-disordered family to communicate in a multimodal fashion, verbally communicating, nonverbally communicating (with eye contact), and following communication with visual reminders. In translation, after giving a direction also write it on a sticky note. Upon completion, the child returns the sticky note.

5. Beepers (inexpensive pagers) provide for children a means of always being able to reach family members.

12.6 Suggestions for General Maintenance

1. Daily life can be very strained in an ADD household. It is helpful to plan frequent and regular family outings or short trips out of town to provide relaxation and escape from daily routines. This may also allow family members to reconnect with each other. These trips need not cost a lot, only the expense of time to reconnect, given the everyday frustrations of living in a normal household, much less an ADD one.

2. A major liability in the ADD household is communication or, rather, miscommunication. Members miscue, fail to understand each other, or make incorrect assumptions. The result is often chaos. Missed meetings, forgotten pickup times, and even the simplest exchange of words necessary to run a smooth household can become confused and misunderstood. Establish eye contact prior to communication, follow verbal messages with written messages, and use feedback to prevent these constant errors.

A recent Gallup poll reports that 35% of American families with children under 12 participate together in the evening meal. What it doesn't stress is that 65% of us do not even have dinner together.

We are doing other things. We eat in the car, or standing up, or on the way out the door, or in front of the TV set. Family meetings focus on the family as a group or unit that might not occur otherwise in our busy hectic lives. The goal of the family meeting is to emotionally and cognitively connect with each other. It is designed to ensure what many child experts have determined as necessary for positive development of self-esteem.

- The idea of being connected to something
- The idea of being unique and special
- The idea of having some degree of power to voice one's opinion
- The idea of having a positive parent after whom to model oneself

3. Self-esteem is basically a concept suggesting that one feels good about oneself, that one can internally reward oneself (e.g., thinking, "I feel good about the job I have just done or the paper I just completed or the problem I managed to solve, and I am proud of myself") without needing the constant reward from the external environment (without needing the teacher to say, "good job," the parent to say, "well done," the spouse to okay things). While we need the feedback, it is important not to rely solely on that feedback to feel proud about ourselves or powerful as individuals. If that occurs, we are only as good as our last deed, we will continually need our ticket punched by someone or something and there will come a point where nothing is good enough and we are never okay enough.

ADD individuals are at great risk for developing a distorted and negative view or sense of themselves. Biochemically, they are more vulnerable to coexisting disorders such as depression, anxiety, bipolar, and addictive disorders. Kids without a clear sense of connectiveness, specialness and uniqueness (whether as a member of the Cub Scouts, Mrs. Cooks' third-grade class, the Falcons, etc.) are more prone to join gangs, cults, and other groups that collect and feed on people who don't feel connected or who have been discarded from those groups that appear more accepted by society as a whole.

Let's not generalize by saying that without a family dinner your child will join the Devil's Disciples. What is clear though, is that the person without a sense of connection are much more susceptible to later development of a whole host of depressive or personality disorders, and a skewed sense of social participation. In general, family meetings, family outings, and family time are viable tools that you can use to take responsibility for the direction of your children's lives. They will make a difference in their choices over their life spans. Sometimes, taking a day off and playing hooky with your child can establish a connection that lasts much longer than just the 6 or 8 hours that you might spend. Recent research points to the idea that while we cannot change the genetics of this disorder (nature) we can have a more positive outcome by working with the problems (nurture) and change things from this respect.

Children who had parents with a strong sense of direction and discipline and isolation of right vs. wrong, and who delivered this information to their children with warmth and connection, had far more positive results in the way their children developed, as opposed to the more-critical and negative parent who continually communicated to their child that *they were more trouble than they were worth*. Sometimes what happens with ADD kids is that parents can become focused on the children's schoolwork, completion of their chores, and responsibility as individuals that they forget to just spend time with their children.

13

Living With the ADD Adult: How Does ADD Affect A Marriage?

13.1 Living with an ADD Partner

Living with an ADD spouse can be a very difficult and trying experience and can leave people easily embittered and eventually wanting to leave the marriage. Partners of ADD spouses tend to be co-dependent individuals and they specialize in picking up the pieces of their ADD partner. As a result, the ADD people tend not to address issues and cope with the consequences of the disorder themselves, and their partner aids in this process. They begin their marriage as equals but become locked in a situation where one person is more powerful than the other. As non-ADD spouses care for ADD people and assume more of their responsibilities and duties, the ones who are needed become more powerful, which unfortunately is what co-dependent individuals are truly looking for (which is why they would foster such a situation in the first place). The non-ADD spouses are needed and critically important to their mates, which alleviates any fear they may have of being abandoned. It is a boost to their self-esteem (aren't they wonderful) and all goes well for a while.

Eventually the non-ADD spouses may become tired, overwhelmed, and no longer able to pick up all the pieces. If they have a job and/or children they find it increasingly difficult to take care of everything and if they don't take care of it themselves no one else will. Children add to the burden of non-ADD spouses and as the needs of the children increase, these spouses have less time to devote to caring for their ADD partners. The ADD partners, who were used to being taken care of, have come to view such caretaking as a sign of love and caring. When the caretaking is diminished and pulled back, ADD spouses feel abandoned, no longer important, and discarded. Sometimes there is jealousy of the children, who still receive the attention and nurturing ADD spouses so desire.

Distance is established in the relationship and everyone becomes lonely. A depression ensues, followed by anger and bitterness on both sides. Finally, to correct the situation, non-ADD spouses may say to ADD people "Okay, I want you to do more." The ADD individuals are ill prepared for this endeavor because the co-dependent spouses have covered for them for so long. They have learned *not* to take care of themselves. The old system is falling apart, the old roles are changing, and no one knows what to do.

When couples can't recover it is because the non-ADD spouse has allowed problems to continue for too long. They have become too angry at that point or too fearful of slipping back into old patterns of doing tasks themselves just to get things completed. What also may happen is that the ADD individuals cannot shift, they feel too abandoned and too wounded by this sudden (it appears sudden to them) swing or shift in behavior and thought pattern of their spouses and thus they cannot make the necessary adjustments. Either the couple works together to develop a whole new relationship as equal partners, helping one another, or the relationship ends.

EXAMPLE

One sad example of this is a man, diagnosed as ADD, who started a landscaping business. He was very good at landscaping and did excellent work. When he was a child, his father had a landscaping business and it meant a great deal to him to follow in his footsteps. So he started this business and did quite well at first because he was a hard worker. The business grew as customers liked him and referred him to other people, but as the business grew, he found that he could not handle all of paperwork. Details that were part of owning a larger business became increasingly overwhelming for him. So as he tried to grow and expand the business to become more successful, he became increasingly entangled in one mess after another due to his own inability for task completion and follow-through. Eventually, he was unable to handle the several crews he had, missed appointments with customers and took 2 to 3 months to complete a job that should have been done in 2 weeks. He began to lose customers as a result. At that point, his non-ADD wife stepped in because the finances had turned into a disaster area. She was very organized, did quite well at task completion and knew accounting. She seemed like the perfect choice. However, her stepping in and taking control made the man feel very stupid and useless. He lost confidence and feared that he would lose her and his new family (they had begun to have children) due to his incompetence. She began to say "no" to decisions he knew he should make, such as hiring people, or buying certain equipment he needed. Before long, she was running the business, making decisions about an area about which she had known nothing. Meanwhile, he became more depressed, anxious and confused. He withdrew because he was afraid of making more mistakes. As a result of this pattern and his continued withdrawal, the business began to slide (even with her help) and remains problematic to this date.

This is a sad example of one partner taking over and ultimately losing respect for the person rescued. The one rescued (in this case, the adult ADD) can become more dependent, less efficient, and less capable as self-esteem wanes and eventually becomes virtually nonexistent.

13.2 Traits of ADD and Results Within the Marriage

13.2.1 Information Processing Problems

The loss of information and the miscommunication that results is probably the most problematic aspect of ADD. In general, marital disputes are often caused by communication problems. With ADD, the communication problems are exacerbated. Communication problems are consistently related to an issue of missing pieces of information; the non-ADD spouse does not feel heard and takes the response of the ADD spouse personally. Finally, non-ADD spouses decide that the ADD spouses don't listen because they are no longer in love with them.

What becomes so frustrating in the marriage is the confusion that occurs because of the missed information. The adult ADD will constantly state that they "never said that," "were never told the time or date," were never talked to about that issue." They look at their spouses with the blank stare of "unknow-ingness" and then proceed to blame them for their lack of communication.

EXAMPLE

A woman who was involved with an adult ADD individual had a wonderful relationship until they got married. Things went from bad to worse as her husband failed to follow through on business dealings, which led them into financial problems. He then attempted to blame her. As her husband continued to experience failures while she became more successful, he continued to blame her, and further, began to be angry at her. She started to avoid him and spend less time with him. He became more angry and frustrated and further targeted her. When she would broach this issue with him he would deny it and state that she was the one causing the problem between the two of them and asked when was she going to "change." Arguments grew more heated and, for the first time, divorce became an option. This occurred in a relationship that was supposedly the "love of the century." Between these arguments and periods of isolation and avoidance, they would have a fantastic weekend or trip that helped the relationship continue for a longer period of time. Eventually, the woman was in such a state of depression that she could no longer remain in the situation. Her self-esteem had deteriorated and her health was becoming a problem as well. Anxiety and panic attacks increased and finally it looked like the relationship would have to end. While the relationship was being renewed by the out-of-town trips the couple continued to take, they would just return to the negative homelife they had created. He was caught in the tangled web of ADD symptoms. She was addicted to him, loved him, and was therefore caught in the symptoms as well. She couldn't live with him and did not want to live without him. The story does have a happy ending. Fortunately, the couple began to work together to change the system in which they had both participated. They sought help in the form of a family therapist, established family meetings and began to take nightly walks to talk about the issues that bothered them before things grew out of proportion and anger set in. They began to manage their household and to share in the duties. Life became less negative and less chaotic. Their love and commitment for one another was sufficient to persevere through the problems. Miscommunication always occurs when people feel bad (anything that has truth to it feels okay whereas if something causes pain it may actually be an untruth or illusion).

Information gets so messed up (due to the information-processing issue) and to such a degree that it continually amazes us. Often in completing ADD evaluations we will explain something to the ADD person who will then call 1 day, 1 week, or 2 months later to ask me what I had said. For this reason, several years ago we began to tape our sessions and at the end, we would hand the tape to the ADD person who was just evaluated to make sure he or she wouldn't call later all confused. Things still become mixed up and in the followup interview it is not uncommon for the ADD person to say something like, "I don't remember you telling me that," only now they may say "I don't remember you telling me that but I am sure that you did."

We can laugh about this but in real life this loss of information and/or confusion can be excruciatingly frustrating when someone is prepared to go somewhere or do something and adult ADD individuals look at their spouses with that blank stare and ask they are doing or talking about." Because of the information processing problem the information is actually being lost and a complete lack of knowledge exists. If there was a true memory problem, there would be partial recall with a vagueness attached to it, such as, "Well, I think you may have said that but I am not sure," because in all likelihood they received part of the information. With a memory problem you will not find a clear denial of knowledge of dates, times, events, and things discussed with regard to the family and children.

13.2.2   Private Conversations or Self Talk

ADD individuals, especially those without hyperactivity, tend to have more conversations with themselves than with anyone else. They don't have to wonder and figure out what anyone said and nobody talks back. The racing thoughts result in continual conversations in their heads, making it too hard to talk with others. It is easier to withdraw and talk to themselves. The more traumatized the person is, such as with PTSD, the more this will occur due to the additional issue of trauma (and the tendency to duck inside for safety, protection, and comfort).

Overall, finally, ADD adults are generally unaware of their feelings. The brain is sleeping, they are too busy just trying to function and so do not have the time for feelings. ADD adults dislike parties (too much chaos and commotion) or they don't have the time to schedule social activities. There appears to be too much work involved in trying to hold meaningful conversations. Thoughts come and go so fast they can't catch them, much less explain them to someone else. Thus, adult ADDs tend to have lots of private conversations. Their social life can become diminished as a result.

13.2.3   Distractibility

Adult ADD persons do not maintain eye contact for very long if they are vulnerable to being distracted. What happens is that the visual stimuli of the face are so distracting to them that they cannot, *absolutely cannot*, look at someone and think at the same time. Everyone has been in the situation in which they look away for a second or two to think a thought and return to the conversation. It is as if they needed to stare into space to collect their thoughts and formulate them enough to share them with someone else. But adult ADD individuals can't look at the person at all. They continually stare away and totally avoid eye contact. It is painfully obvious to anyone observing and often very embarrassing to the spouse. One doesn't need to explain why it becomes difficult trying to carry on an animated conversation with someone while they are looking at the back of someone else's head or studying their shoes. Some ADD persons who are in sales and are trained to maintain eye contact will establish a fixation point, either at the person's forehead or something behind them to appear to be actually maintaining eye contact.

EXAMPLE
Recently, Dr. Fisher had an ADD evaluation with a young man who continued to look down at the floor while she explained the test findings. She found herself becoming somewhat disturbed, questioning whether the young man was actually getting the information and understanding what she was trying to say to him. She took the opportunity to explain to him and his wife why it was difficult for him to look at her. While talking about distractibility she was aware that his scoring reflected an enormous amount of distractibility and that he was, in fact, highly vulnerable to being distracted. His newlywed wife was relieved to understand that this thing that she had been battling — not being able to get him to look at her and establish eye contact — didn't have anything to do with her.

13.2.4   Moving from One Unfinished Task to Another

Adult ADD persons tend to move from one unfinished task to another and rarely complete things. This can happen for a number of different reasons.

- There might be a capacity problem, a true sustained attention disorder, and they can only focus for so long on one task.

- They may have wandering distractibility where they are working on something while thinking about something else. They then leave that task to do what they were thinking about.
- The distractibility may be that fast-moving, fast-paced shifting from one thing to another, almost like a firefly in motion.
- They may not want to finish the task and may leave one small thing undone, for fear that it is not perfect and they would rather have it unfinished than less than perfect.

For whatever reason, the result is unfinished projects.

Basements that were started as a refinishing project are left midway, rooms are half painted and never completed. The minute a problem erupts, it becomes difficult to finish the job because the ADD symptoms get in the way. They go to buy the tool they need and find it is not in stock. The clerk tells them it will be there in two days, but they forget to go back. The job does not go as planned and negativity sets in it. The thought is that this is never going to work. Everything becomes overwhelming. The ADD person takes a break and never returns.

When household tasks, projects, and so on, do not get completed, the non-ADD spouse becomes frustrated and feels powerless, especially if there is not enough money to hire the job out. ADD adults feel more worthless and become more negative and turn inward and away from their loved ones. The idea of going back and completing the project becomes more scary and disturbing with each passing day. So these people are left in a no-win predicament. They feel guilty about not completing what they started and yet they can't bring themselves to do it. Eventually they display avoidance, procrastination, guilt, and anger (getting mad at — guess who? — the long-suffering spouse). The spouse appears more competent and the power struggle begins. The non-ADD spouse, on the other hand, remains frustrated, unable to even bring up the project lest the ADD spouse become more upset. The project, consequently remains unfinished. The non-ADD spouse is also in a no-win situation, unable to take care of the problem, unable to talk about it, and having to continue to see one more unfinished thing as an example of the inadequacy and incompetency of the person he or she married.

EXAMPLE

After seeing one couple for quite a lengthy period of time it became increasingly obvious that the husband had an ADD disorder. So we evaluated him and sure enough he did. It existed primarily in the area of distractibility. At the time, he was a manager with a fairly large corporation and had approximately 20 people report to him who he was expected to evaluate for work performance. Each day he went to work prepared to work on these evaluations but became distracted by the business at hand and each night he returned home with the evaluations still hanging over his head. So he purchased a computer program designed to complete evaluations in the hope that he could accomplish this task. Unfortunately, he continued to remain distracted and couldn't focus long enough on the program to complete the evaluations. This resulted in a great amount of frustration, low self-esteem and anger, which he initially directed at himself but eventually turned on his wife who, in fact, was able to finish what she started. There is a postscript. One of the reasons, besides distractibility, that he allowed his ADD symptoms to interfere with the completion of the evaluations was an emotional issue — he was fearful of someone becoming angry and if he was to be honest and fair, some people would not like what he had to say. An emotional issue can result in the ADD symptoms becoming worse, increased or exacerbated if it touches a hot spot for the person.

So is it an ADD symptom or the emotional reaction? Both. If you ask any ADD people, they will tell you that any form of task completion is gratifying, particularly for those who do not complete much. Emotional symptoms in the form of avoidance and procrastination are often seen with ADD, usually that of ADD without hyperactivity. Often, the reason behind their avoidance is the fear of failure, which develops in ADD people because they grow up experiencing failure after failure. They attempt to do something only to find that they can't for some unknown reason. They look at their classmates and things always seem easier for them, they don't have to study and get good grades. They become determined to succeed where they feel they can suceed. They want to be perfect at the things they feel they can do and to ultimately avoid the things they don't think they can do. A pattern develops, they leave at the first sign of trouble: the going gets tough and they're gone. It becomes an issue of perfection vs. noninvolvement. Life becomes quite limited. Failure is absolutely not tolerated. Low frustration tolerance develops. Life continues to be restricted and they cannot learn from their mistakes. It has to go right the first time or forget it. They really hope things will go well because there is no second chance. Everyone is on pins and needles hoping things work out, knowing that if not, ADD people will give up.

13.2.5 Slow Cognitive and Speed-Slow Performance in General

Slow thinking speed can easily translate into slow speed, period. As a result, the ADD without hyperactivity person tends to take a longer time at most tasks. If the person is bright and attempting to compensate for symptoms of the disorder, thus developing the need for perfectionism, tasks will take even longer to complete. Slow speed in combination with perfectionism will result in few tasks being completed because they take far too long. Eventually adult ADD people become so tired that they just give up. There can also be a capacity problem and they lose their focus after a period of time.

Unless one has a lot of time, conversation with ADD individuals can be very trying as you wait for their response and then wait again and again. Often people find it much easier to just answer their own questions, make their own decisions and not have this whole detailed discussion. It is quite difficult to have a short and efficient conversation with adult ADD persons who have slow thinking speed, for a variety of reasons.

13.2.6   No Regard for Consequences

The tendency to not care about the consequences of their behavior is more common for ADHD adults. Since the frontal processes are down, there is no brain mechanism to consider consequences and utilize feedback from their behavior. ADHD individuals make the same mistakes over and over. They have no error utilization. In other words, they are unable to use information to learn from their mistakes.

ADD without hyperactivity individuals may also seem as if they have no regard for consequences, but their seeming indifference is different from ADHD people, who truly do not care. ADD people do care. They appear to not care outwardly because they are spacey, out to lunch, and unaware of their behavior. It is their total lack of awareness that makes them seem to have no regard for the consequences of their behavior. They miss the big picture. They do not see the ramifications of how their behavior will look down the road. The frequently heard "Oh!" of surprise means *I did not know that this would happen or that would occur.* And they really didn't.

Disregard (or the appearance of) for the consequences of one's behavior is problematic in marriages, as ADD individuals cannot foresee or meet the needs or feelings of their spouses. Like Mr. Magoo, they go about their business unaware of the impact of their behavior upon those left behind, namely the marital partner. Think of the famous Mr. Magoo cartoon where the whole building caves in behind him as he walks out the door, blissfully unaware of what is occurring. This not only frustrates the spouse but it is easy to assume that one is not thought of, not loved, and not appreciated. Sentences automatically run through one's mind: if they loved me they would think of me and not do that or if I was important they would not be doing that. The marriage does not feel like a partnership, instead it feels like a rather one-sided arrangement run by the actions, reactions, and belief system of the ADD spouse.

Finally, when dealing with someone who has no regard for consequences, it is difficult to guilt them, implore them to do things differently in the future or successfully use any technique to get them to see someone's else's point of view. They just can't see that their behavior is eventually going to lead to unhappy consequences. So in the marriage, spouses may threaten their ADD partners that if they continue with their behavior, it will be the end of things. ADD people really do not believe them, because they cannot see it or identify with what their spouses are talking about. They continue their behavior just as before and are astounded when their spouses finally end the marriage. However, it's sometimes not too late. ADD individuals, if they finally realize the full implications of the situation and are now ready to make changes, can still turn the situation around.

EXAMPLE
We spent 3 years working with a couple where the wife kept saying, "Okay, this has got to change," over and over. Over and over her ADD spouse said "Okay, I can make those changes" and over and over, he didn't. Finally, we struck a 30-day agreement where he would make those changes. We devised a plan that he could easily comply with and accomplish. If he didn't, then it would be time to call it a day. Unfortunately, it became time to call it a day and he still couldn't understand what he had done to cause the divorce.

More often than not with ADHD, the brain's inability to consider the consequences leads to spending money these individuals cannot afford to spend, or loss of a job. They spend the money and think somehow it will all work out or they don't care if it doesn't. It becomes difficult for ADHD individuals to hold down a job because they have to yield to the decisions of others. They have to be followers at times and not always leaders. Many are self-employed for this reason, being unable to work for anyone else. If fired, they think they can find another job. They get fired because they do not perform the job as required, do not place all of their energy into the job, do not produce positive results or alienate or fight with their superiors. Again, the lack of regard for the consequences allows them to take that extra step into the danger zone and to exhibit unwarranted behavior or speak that inappropriate statement. Either they think they are too important to be fired or they don't worry about losing their jobs. They are not concerned that they can't be counted on to contribute to the family income.

13.2.7   Poor Planning and Poor Sense of Time: Late Appointments

ADD individuals are often late for business meetings, appointments, school events, to pick up the kids, for dinner, for the airplane, or for dates with their mates.

EXAMPLE
One mother was always late picking up her kid. She was always apologetic and always late again due to the inability to plan her time effectively. She would be walking out of the house, become distracted and attempt to do just one more thing: e.g., make one more phone call or tidy up one more time. Then she was always late to where she was going. As a result, her children could not count on her to be there for them. Her husband felt totally neglected and mistook her lateness for lack of caring about him. Her poor time management meant less time for him (and quality partner time is crucial). Her spouse began to feel less than okay and very taken for granted within the marriage. It seemed there was no place for him. Because she was always late for something else, she rarely spent time with him. When she finally was with him, her mind was elsewhere (another ADD symptom — distractibility).

ADD individuals have difficulty planning their days, their goals, their lives. ADHD individuals have no sense of time and frequently over- or underestimate how long something will take them to complete. In both ADHD or ADD without hyperactivity there is distractibility that makes people late. If distracted they get lost in the task, move off to another task, or become preoccupied with one aspect of the task and just get lost in general. Distractibility results in a lack of focus because they always find just one more thing that has to be done before that meeting or this appointment. Something *always* comes up. Something will always come up because their minds are always in a million different places. Or they become so over-focused on one aspect that they miss the big picture. Or there is a spatial problem and they can't see or visualize the whole picture of things. They can't see how long it will take to get from point A to point B and often underestimate their time. Spatial issues are more characteristic of ADD without hyperactivity.

So what is it like living with this? Well, if one takes their behavior personally, non-ADD spouses could be hurt much of the time when their ADD spouses are late for appointments. They will see that as an insult to them rather than the result of ADD symptoms.

13.2.8   Disorganization — The Continual Piles

Everyone jokes about the ADD piles. And there are piles and piles of them everywhere.

EXAMPLE
One woman told her husband that the piles were not moving with them when they relocated to a new home. They could not eat at the table because there were so many piles on it during income tax time. One woman described to me how she could barely crawl into bed at night because there were so many piles in her bedroom. It took this man's whole family to come and clean up the piles all around his apartment before he could move.

Whenever ADD people go through their piles they are amazed to find all of this stuff they had no idea they had. They find all sorts of missing items they had been looking for at one time or another.

13.2.9   Restlessness

ADD persons are restless individuals. Whether they are restless due to the ADHD constant need for movement or the pervasive anxiety of ADD without hyperactivity, it is still restlessness.

Anxiety is often misdiagnosed as ADHD due to its symptoms of restlessness. ADD without hyperactivity individuals participate in a lot of outdoor activities such as biking, running, swimming, and skiing, as they offer a sense of vista, land that stretches out before them providing arenas to alleviate anxiety. These ADD individuals find it difficult to relax and sit still. They can't do just one thing at a time. When talking on the phone they are flipping through the newspaper, washing dishes or reading a magazine. They eat standing up or walking around the table. It is hard for them to have a conversation without moving. The only time they tend to sit still is while watching TV, which can become incredibly addicting as it is one of the few things these highly anxious people can do while sitting. But they don't just watch one program. They channel surf, which can be awfully annoying if people with them are trying to watch a program or spot something they would like to watch further. However, it just flashed on and off the screen before they could open their mouths to say stop. ADD persons will sit for hours staring at this screen, sometimes a couple of screens, clicking the remote over and over until it drives their spouse crazy. In fact, this is a major complaint from non-ADD spouses.

13.2.10   Boredom

Spouses of ADD adults have to constantly keep up, keep going, keep moving so the ADD people do not become bored. With ADHD everything is boring because of the lack of internal stimulation. The satiation center of the brain is down so they never get their fill of anything. Frontal processes that regulate motivation and internal stimulation are absent, which forces these individuals to rely on external stimulation. ADHD adults continually crave external stimulation and feed off the excitement happening around them. It is this constant quest for more and more excitement that leads them to some of the gutsy, scary, inappropriate and, at times, illegal activities in which they become involved. This, in part, is why ADHD adults tend to fill our prisons and jails. Another factor of the high incidence of imprisoned ADHD people is their inability to weigh consequences. They think that they won't get caught or they don't care if they do.

However, ADD without hyperactivity individuals compose more of the delinquent and prison population than we think. Working with the court system for a period of time, as Dr. Fisher did during the early years of her career, she realized that those in jail are not very good at being criminals. They were in the wrong place at the wrong time. They could not anticipate the consequences of their behavior, they had nothing to do at the time and it seemed like a good idea. The group wanted to do it and they just went along. Criminals who are crafty and hardened (like that true oppositional defiant personality disorder) rarely get caught. It is the ADD persons who didn't anticipate the cops arriving.

With ADD without hyperactivity, things usually become boring if the person has trouble doing them. Think about the times that you find yourself bored with something. This does not always mean that you are truly bored, it may be because it is something at which you are not competent. It's easier and safer to say that you're bored than to face the fact that you don't think that you are up to the task. These individuals will do this in work settings, at parties, games, or sports — they will say they're bored and leave rather than show their inadequacy.

Spouses of ADD persons frequently complain that their mates will not go to parties or stay at parties for any lengthy period of time. This leads to couples participating in fewer social activities and isolates them from friends and acquaintances. *Fear* is perhaps the most problematic issue affecting the ADD population and is perhaps the reason behind the lack of follow through. They do not follow through, they quit or give up because they feel they just can't do it. Thus, they do not attain their goals. Sometimes I wonder which is worse — the symptoms of ADD or the emotional consequences that result.

Many adults I've evaluated, when they are clearly not achieving at their potential, say they are "bored" and quit. They may be afraid of failure or they may not know how to do something but the answer they always give is "boredom."

13.2.11   Hot Temper, Outbursts of Anger, and Moodiness

13.2.11.1   Moodiness

ADD persons are moody individuals, perhaps because they are frustrated and feeling bad about themselves. Maybe they are moody because there is an assignment hanging over their heads that they are avoiding. Maybe they are moody because they are worrying about money. Maybe they are moody because they have a meeting with the boss and they are unprepared. When they are moody, and because they won't talk about their feelings, they can get even moodier.

There is depression associated with ADD (generally ADD without hyperactivity — ADHD are upset *only* if they can't get what they want) due to the grief and loss over what could have been. This is seen quite often in the adult ADD without hyperactivity population. The depression creates more negativity, low self-esteem, as well as a loss of energy which, again, results in moodiness.

13.2.11.1   Hot Temper

Temper outbursts and anger occur with ADD without hyperactivity when they are feeling particularly incompetent and useless. It is easier to blame someone else and blow up and become angry when feeling bad. Anger, by definition, is sadness turned outward. The grief and loss over symptoms of ADD can lead the adult to be continually sad and thus, angry. When angry toward themselves, they become angry toward others. They expect you to be upset so they get angry before you do. The temper provides a means of protection against the critical onslaught of those around them. They anticipate rejection and criticism and are sensitive to this. They have the reaction toward another that they perceive would be directed toward them.

A hot temper is significant of individuals who react and do not think. They live more in the "right brain" and react out of emotions rather than logic. This would make the person very difficult to live with. Often it is ADHD people with hot tempers who begin the abuse cycle. Whether physically or emotionally, they abuse anyone around them, usually their spouses. They may abuse the spouse and not the kids, or the kids and not the spouse or they'll abuse both. The household goes through periods of tension building, eruptions, abuse, and guilt afterward that leads to the "making-up" period. Often, there is a family history of abuse that has already sanctioned this behavior.

13.2.11.3 Outbursts of Anger

Outbursts of anger usually occur in the marital system when things do not go as planned. Outbursts of anger occur when the ADD person feels overwhelmed. This is the person we see who blows up at the airport for no apparent reason. However, what we don't realize is that the chaos is overwhelming to them. ADD people are inundated by stimuli — noises, smells, people moving frantically — they cannot think, much less get to the correct gate in the chaotic surrounding of the airport facility.

Outbursts of anger may also be blamed on a total lack of tolerance and the inability to control reactions when things do not go their way. Especially with ADHD adults, who want what they want when they want it. They will be quick to anger and erupt in a rage, if they don't (or think that they will not) get what they want immediately.

13.2.12 Low Frustration Tolerance: When the Going Gets Tough, They Get Going

Low frustration tolerances are predominant in the ADD population. When the going gets tough, they all disappear. ADHD adults exhibit a low frustration tolerance because of their inability to gate the brain mechanism responsible for inhibiting instantaneous reactions. ADHD adults tolerate little. They do not put up with noise, chaos, problems, and the learning curve. They don't stay in any situation long enough to learn toleration. For example, every new job means a period of learning — the learning curve — when new hires do not know what to do and are inadequate at the task until training takes effect and they master the job. ADHD people cannot withstand the learning curve. They leave or quit when things become difficult because they are unable to tolerate a period of time of not knowing. They give up before learning the task.

Thus, ADHD people quit jobs, or lose jobs on frequent basis. Imagine how disturbing this is for a marriage as it threatens the financial stability and security of the home. And once they do quit, they are done and there is no hook to get them back. There is no way to guilt them because frontal processes are down. Once they have decided to give up and leave, that's it.

ADD without hyperactivity individuals may also show signs of low frustration tolerance. Theirs, however, is vastly different from ADHD. ADD persons will hang on and pursue something until they do finally learn or acquire something. Sometimes they hang on for too long and become obsessed. When frustration tolerance decreases in this group it is the consequence of too many painful failures. It's not until they've tried hard and long and failed again, that they finally give up. You can see this pattern through these people's lives. You can see how, over a period of time, they had so many failures and made so many mistakes that now, like a wounded and frightened animal, they curl up in a corner and just give up.

13.2.13 Procrastination and Avoidance

ADD persons are more the procrastinators and avoiders. ADD without hyperactivity individuals are so fearful of failure that they avoid the situation or put it off as long as they can until it evolves into a crisis. Crisis works better for them because once something has reached this critical point, they are forced to swing into action without the time to ruminate, obsess, or worry about the results. Crisis supersedes fear and also allows for the external stimulation that will bypass the symptoms of ADD. Not only do the ADD people work better under pressure but they impress others with their seeming ability to work miracles.

While this is all well and good for ADD people, their spouses, on the other hand, develop panic attacks, heart attacks, and stress-related disorders from constantly living on edge waiting to see whether their ADD spouses will pull things off at the eleventh hour. The stress becomes unnerving. Are the bills going to be paid or will the electricity be shut off? Is the house going to be put up for sale in time or are we going to have two mortgages? Is the job going to get done for the boss? Is the lack of follow-through going to preclude the promotion?

Then there are the minor issues that become increasingly annoying until finally it feels as if these people no longer care about their spouses or families. If a job is started, it becomes doubtful if it will ever be completed. Sometimes, the final touches are left undone — this in case the job is not perfect. If criticized, ADD people can say that it is not completed. Spouses find themselves asking the same types of questions over and over. Are the drawers ever going to be cleaned out? Is the mess in the closet going to be addressed? When can we ever find anything in this house? What is going to be done about those piles in the corner? Are those newspapers from a year ago being kept for a special purpose? Is the kitchen project ever going to be completed? When are the finishing touches on the deck going to be done so that it can be used? And so on and so on.

You really do not see this pattern with the ADHD person, they simply tell you that they are *not* going to do something, and that is that.

13.2.14 Perfection as a Method of Coping with ADD Symptoms: Cover the Inadequacies

So what do ADD people do when they hope that they can do the job but really are not too sure? They know they are smart but oftentimes they appear stupid and at the worst possible moment. Then they begin to wonder if they really are smart. Or did they somehow lose their intelligence as they got older? Things seemed easier when they were younger. Life did not seem this difficult. Mistakes are very embarrassing. People expect so much more. How do you continue to feel worthwhile when everything you do turns into such a disaster?

Their answer is often to do *only* what they think they can do well and then do it perfectly. They learn to cover up inadequacies by completing the tasks they choose in the most perfect manner possible. The more they care and the brighter they are, and the more severe the ADD symptoms, the harder they fall. The greater the discrepancy between their actual functioning ability and their intellect or possible potential the more they need to appear okay. The best way for them to do this is to do things perfectly when they can. In this way, they can continue to be viewed as competent and adequate. This way, they think, no one knows how bad it is, how serious things are, or how incompetent they really are. Perfectionism becomes more and more a part of the ADD person's life.

It would seem as if perfectionism provides the answer to maintaining self-esteem and continuing to operate at higher levels of functioning. There is a problem, however. It is inherently difficult to always complete a task perfectly. For someone to manage to come close to completing a task perfectly will take a long period of time. Task performance becomes almost impossible to complete. Things must be done so perfectly that they often cannot get done at all.

Spouses wait forever for the additions on the house to be finished or other home projects to end. Things take so long that by the time they finally do get completed it is anticlimactic, no one cares, including the ADD people's spouses. So here are the ADD individuals happy as a clam, waiting to be properly commended, applauded for finally finishing the task, while their spouses are so angry that it took so long, they can hardly muster up a thank you. As a result, ADD people feel unappreciated, their self-esteem lowers, and they get angry. They are caught in a double bind. If they empathize with the feelings of their spouses, they too feel bad that it took so long and more negativity ensues. If they feel their spouses are wrong, they feel angry and abused. Either way, it is a mess.

EXAMPLE

One woman diagnosed with ADD without hyperactivity talked about how she sought to surround herself only with "needy" people, who would need her and provide her with a sense of importance. It is not acceptable for her to need anything: she has to appear perfect at all times. It helps her image to have others "need" her. Often ADD people will fulfill this desire to have others rely on them by embracing people outside of the family. They'll spend more time helping others than being with their families or spouses. It becomes so necessary to feel important that the marriage is sacrificed.

You will not tend to see this pattern with ADHD. They feel they are already perfect and if they aren't, who cares? Their opinion is more important anyway.

13.2.15   Responsibility

ADD adults have a difficult time taking responsibility for their behavior. ADD without hyperactivity people have such a fear of failure that they avoid taking responsibility at all costs.

EXAMPLE

One woman summed it up quite well in her response to instructions on how she could institute a behavioral program with her children, some of whom were diagnosed with ADD. "My instant internal reaction was to run far, far away from this responsibility. I felt afraid to talk, to think, or even to respond. My whole body stiffened. Cramps hit my legs, back, neck, and arms in waves. All of that stuff about setting up your house and life in certain ways being so important for the welfare of the ADD child rose up like a threatening giant. I couldn't handle it. I wanted someone else to do it. I knew I didn't have my own act together enough to set it up for anyone else."

She looked to her spouse to handle the situation, which he did but she remained feeling inadequate. This happened to be an extremely competent woman who does not believe herself capable of handling such situations. She is unable to acknowledge her assets and is focused on her liabilities. She talks of feeling stupid, inadequate, incapable, and immature. She constantly feels at war within herself, fighting back so many tears and hurt feelings that it is wearing her out mentally and physically.

Generally, when ADD people do not take responsibility it is not through laziness and not caring, which is what others assume. It is due to a fear of failure. It is better not to try at all.

The case with ADHD is different. They will take responsibility for something if they feel like it. If they don't want to do something they won't, whether they are requested, asked to take responsibility for it or not. There is neither sufficient loyalty nor binding ties present in ADHD relationships to promote the taking of responsibility.

13.2.16   Blame

Both ADHD and ADD without hyperactivity blame those closest to them for their problems. It is easier. They don't have to face their own feelings. They don't have to take responsibility for their behavior. They don't have to change their behavior, since you can't change what you don't acknowledge. They don't have to feel bad and their ego can remain intact.

Someone else is always to blame for the difficult lives of ADD adults. Usually, it is the spouse. When ADD couples fight the argument ends with it always being the fault of the non-ADD person. Later, when the ADD members try to resolve the situation, they approach their spouses and say "I'm willing to accept your apology now." The spouses respond, "*My* apology! What about yours? What have *I* done?," and so goes the cycle.

This is one of the most frustrating issues for non-ADD spouses, who eventually start to doubt their own integrity. They begin to believe ADD individuals and question their own value systems, their beliefs, their "okayness," and their abilities. Depression hits and self-esteem plummets. This may be the point at which they leave their marriages. If they stay, they risk deeper depression and falling into a state of nothingness — much like an abused spouse.

When the blame becomes extreme and when it is combined with name calling, it falls into an abusive situation. Finding fault in others tends to become a trigger for physical abuse in an abusive household. Physical abuse is seen more with ADHD than with ADD without hyperactivity. There is often a typical family history related to alcoholism and abuse.

13.2.17   Impulsivity

ADHD adults suffer from true impulsivity — they think of something and then just do it. They don't think of the consequences. When an idea comes into their minds and the "stop sign" of the frontal processes is not functional, they just do it. Generally, we all think of doing absurd things but we realize this or that might happen and cause trouble and so we don't do it. ADHD people do not go through this process, they don't have the brain function. So, as a result, they just act impulsively. Impulsively, they tell off the boss and get fired. Impulsively, they quit their jobs. Impulsively, they disappear for several hours and forget their responsibilities at home. Impulsively, they break the law.

ADD without hyperactivity adults may appear impulsive but it is not that true impulsivity seen with ADHD. They will commit an impulsive act only after repeated trials and failures, extreme anxiety or some other extenuating circumstance that drives them to lose restraint. If the person is attempting perfectionism on a continual basis this can become a very negative and upsetting experience. They try so hard, yet experience failure time and time again.

They climb almost to the top of the mountain only to miss a step and slide to the bottom, then have to start again. The frustration, the helplessness, and the sense of depression and unworthiness create the impulsivity. The "I don't care anymore" attitude leads to "let's just do it." In a similar manner, the ruminating will create impulsive reactions to shut down the brain and stop over-thinking things.

13.2.18   Total Sense of Underachievement and Chronic Dissatisfaction with Their Lives

Dr. Fisher recently met with a couple. She had diagnosed the man several months earlier with ADD without hyperactivity. What he talked about was his sense of loss and total dissatisfaction with his life, as he'd never attained the goals he had set when he was younger. At the age of 40 he felt life had passed him by. It was too late. His father was right when he said he would amount to nothing. Everything seemed impossible. We talked at length about his need to pursue his goals. He expressed the extreme feelings of inadequacy regarding his present employment as a janitor. Yet he was grateful for the steady income it provided, having been laid off so often in the past. This man truly felt beaten. His wife attempted to be supportive and encouraging, but she too was tired. She was tired of the outbursts of anger and rage displayed by her husband. But more than anything, she was sad from watching the effects of his total dissatisfaction with his life because of his own underachievement and failure to make use of the high level of intellect he knew he had.

It is important to understand the frustration of having the ability and yet not being able to put it into practice. ADD people can have the best of intentions but somehow their plans never materialize. This is probably the most frustrating of experiences: to want to do well and not to be able to. To continually have things not happen as you desire and to deal with that disappointment time after time. I tend to liken ADD symptoms to going to bat: sometimes these people hit a long home run and other times the best they can do is swing hard and pray they connect with the ball. ADD individuals never know when their brain will work and when it won't.

13.3 The ADD Spouse

Despite their difficulties, ADD people can be full of life, funny, witty, and exciting. They can make the party, make the trip happen, and make everybody feel alive. They can be highly addictive due to some of their extreme traits (when it is good, it's real good and when it's bad, it's awful). When they are in their element, feeling good and "on," it is like a little piece of heaven for those around them. This is what keeps their spouses hanging in there. It is hard to stay, but harder to leave. Everyone is caught in the tangled web of ADD.

14

ADD in the Workplace

14.1 Introduction

We have found that ADD individuals truly have difficulty sustaining and maintaining a job that is the least bit demanding of them. ADHD people have little or no frustration tolerance and if things do not go their way, they leave. Thus, ADHD individuals perform better in self-employed positions or, if employed by a company, in a position where they can operate primarily by themselves.

ADD without hyperactivity individuals tend to procrastinate and avoid any situation in which they fear they may fail and thus often do not complete tasks and projects. They tend to develop low self-esteem, which compounds their already precarious position either with customers or within their company. This is due to their failure with follow-through and accomplishment of set goals. They make promises they can't or don't keep and eventually people tire of this (and of them).

Thus, ADD individuals saturate the legal profession (they run their own show and the secretarial staff takes care of the details), become business owners (others take care of the details, paperwork, and follow-through) or go into teaching (lots of structure to their day).

There is a lot of emotional reactivity in ADD persons as a whole. However, they lack the ability to follow it with action. All talk and no action. For example, they will complain about a job situation forever yet not do anything about it. One of the reasons ADD individuals lose their jobs is that they become upset about things in the workplace, complain, and yet do nothing. As a result, their feelings fester and pretty soon their performance drops as they stop putting as much energy into the job as they once did. It is only a short trip from there to being fired.

ADHD people cannot follow a sequence of events to reach a goal and therefore constantly tend to be moving and out of balance with their own productivity. They look busy, but don't get much done. They may also go off on an idea without the proper groundwork to make it happen. ADHD persons come up with great and exciting ideas but they are only ideas. They have no notion (due to frontal processes being down) of how to make these ideas reality or how to make them happen. They remain, however, the movers and shakers. Their exuberance for an idea compels others to join in the venture, which is a critical component to success. It is the "joinees" who must do the work because, more often than not, the ADHD person does not produce. ADHD persons tend to forge a system of caretakers who balance them and provide the necessary follow-through.

The ADD adult population as a whole can become bored easily and require constant change and stimulation to remain interested in what they are doing, no matter how well they do it. Although they need routines, routine behavior can become very boring. ADD individuals dislike close supervision. It induces anger in the ADHD person and fear in the ADD person (ADD without hyperactivity). ADHD persons tend to explode while ADD people keep everything inside and become more anxious. Both will erupt in time. Both groups are in need of freedom of choice. ADD persons easily become distracted in a crowded office or workplace, which can provoke intense irritability and frustration. They must, therefore, be forced to create a setting that works for them. Both groups simply cannot complete their paperwork. This can lead to noncompliance and problems. Careless errors are made through lack of attention to detail. ADD people cannot do simultaneous tasking and tend to become easily overwhelmed when things involve multiple factors.

Finally, both ADD without hyperactivity and ADHD have poor organizational skills for various reasons. For example, ADD without hyperactivity would have planning and organization problems due to distractibility — it may take too long and cause overall confusion — while ADHD cannot plan and organize at all due to the shut-down of the frontal processes. There is a slow learning curve for ADD people due to the lack of a time frame and slow thinking speed. With ADHD people, there are true learning disabilities and problem-solving issues; thus, they have trouble learning the simplest lessons from their environment and will require more repetitions.

Therefore, it is the task of ADD individuals to find the job or career that will best benefit them, given their specific symptoms of ADD. By highlighting their strengths and not focusing on their weak areas, they can be successful. It is important to weigh employment opportunities to ensure selecting the one that will best provide success. It is imperative to choose a line of work that will be interesting for the individual.

14.2 How to Find the Job or Career that Most Suits the ADD Person

The most organized means of finding a suitable job for the ADD person includes the following steps.

1. Undergo a complete clinical evaluation detailing all ADD symptoms to determine what is most problematic or severe. Determining the level of severity of distractibility, information processing, confusion, slow thinking speed, planning and organization, impaired or immature social skills, cognitive flexibility, problem-solving skills, and other learning problems, as well as a low frustration tolerance, helps to highlight strengths and weaknesses. Decisions can then be made based on how the adult specifically functions and the greater or lesser degree of impact of the symptoms of the attentional disorder. The degree of the following symptoms is then used to determine the type of job position that would best fit the individual.

   - *A severe information-processing problem* would impact the person's ability in a job situation that demands numerous meetings and considerable interaction with staff, ongoing communication, and absorption of information. Management positions would not be suited for this person, particularly middle-management positions.

   - *Severe confusion* will cause more difficulty with heightened pace and multiple tasks. Positions in large companies running at a fast pace, a number of things happening at once, and lots of moving parts for which the person would be responsible would not be suitable. These individuals will perform better with more structure, less stress, a slower pace, and fewer operating variables.

   - *Severe distractibility* means that positions in large-company settings would not be suitable. A setting that contains a large amount of external stimuli, many responsibilities, and a number of job duties would prove to be highly upsetting. Settings like a bull pen with several modular spaces would be very disturbing due to constant stimulation and noise factors. Unless ADD adults were highly interested in the external setting (thus bypassing the disorder), they would have a particularly frustrating time in a place such as the stockmarket floor. These individuals would function better in an atmosphere that has a great amount of external structure and is somewhat, but not completely, quiet (total quiet is upsetting as well because they can become distracted by their own thoughts or hear small sounds others would never notice — like ants on the ceiling).

   - *If thinking speed is very slow,* a job that requires them to produce things on a short turn-around would create a great amount of pressure for ADD individuals. Short time frames and deadlines create a great deal of anxiety and thus subsequent avoidance and procrastination for ADD people. So any sort of job position that requires continual deadlines would be too traumatic for them. They would fare better in settings that require quality, not quantity.

- *If the planning and organization problem is severe,* ADD people would have a problem in a job situation where they must rely on themselves for their own structure, such as self-employment or sales. They would perform better in settings where there is extensive external structure built into the job situation, such as teaching.

- *If social skills are severely underdeveloped or inappropriate,* ADD people would experience problems in positions that are managerial, sales oriented, or have a high degree of interaction with others. They would fare better in settings that are more insulated, so they can work by themselves and are not dependent on other people to perform their jobs, such as in a scientific laboratory setting.

- *If the problem-solving issue is severe* and individuals cannot think on their feet, they would do better in a more structured setting where there are few surprises and greater predictability. Also, other positions requiring more problem-solving skills such as self-employment or managerial positions would be problematic for this same reason.

- *If there are other learning problems, such as reading, writing, or spelling,* job situations that require high usage of language skills should be avoided.

- *Low frustration tolerance* would mean that positions such as self-employment or sales in which individuals make their own schedule and fill their day with difficult activities would be the most fulfilling. These individuals would not perform well in a setting that is monotonous, structured, or repetitious.

2. Relate ADD symptoms to the individuals' intellectual potential and rank their strengths and weaknesses. *The more intelligent the people the greater their ability to compensate.* There are issues of frustration intolerance based in their lack of performance compared with their known potential. What they achieve is not commensurate with their abilities. Individuals who are very bright and have an extreme ADD experience more emotional problems than their more average intellectual counterparts because of the impact of the disorder on their functioning and their realization of the impact. Emotional symptoms tend to result when there is a greater discrepancy between the intellectual ability and the severity of the ADD symptoms. Mostly, the discrepancies serve to exacerbate the ADD symptoms.

3. Evaluate to find the individuals' interest areas: what do they like to do, where do they see themselves, what holds value to them, what can they be proud of in terms of a career choice?

4. Relate personality traits to the job situation: *More outgoing, gregarious individuals will do better at sales* than clerical positions especially if they are anxious or restless. This type of position will prevent boredom and allow the movement they need. Furthermore, these individuals will perform better around people with whom they can utilize their social assets.

Shy, fragile people will work better tucked into a job that they can do pretty much by themselves while still being part of a large company. Being part of a large company provides stability, as they feel taken care of and provided for. These individuals would have difficulty in positions such as self-employment or sales where they must rely on themselves to produce income and stability.

Fearful, anxious people tend to avoid and procrastinate and will *experience difficulty in a job setting with a boss who closely watches them* or whose demands are extensive. They will function better in a setting that continually puts them at ease, still sets limits and deadlines and yet allows for some latitude.

Perfectionistic individuals have more impatience with themselves (as well as with others) and *do not tend to work well in team-oriented situations* nor are they supportive in managerial or supervisory positions. They do better in positions of self-employment or something similar as their high expectations drive them to overachieve. Often the result can be that they will not be able to complete the amount of work required for the job. If they do complete all of the work, they can become burned out quickly as a result of over-working to accomplish the work while still maintaining their high standards. These positions require both quality and quantity work. And the perfectionists who will work and work until the job is done just right will do great on quality but quantity will suffer. If they try to accomplish both quality and quantity they will not last long in a position that does not necessarily reward quality. The consequence of overworking, trying to do the perfect job, will result in the need for positive reinforcement and feedback that will not be forthcoming because quality is not valued to the degree of quantity. The person eventually quits, feeling spent, having given too much with too little in return. However, the system never asked for the quality they demanded of themselves.

People who are negative and self-defeating obviously will not perform well in self-employed or sales-type ("self-starter") *positions.* As they will continually be exercising a negative self-fulfilling prophesy, they won't be able to muster up the necessary self-esteem and belief in-the-self system to make it when things get tough. Once things don't work (which is often in these types of positions) instead of continuing to try they will give up. These individuals would do better in a setting that is structured and job duties are clearly laid out for them. They may experience problems in settings that require a great amount of social interaction.

Passive, dependent individuals are the best people to have on a team and do extremely well in large companies, where they can operate as team players. These individuals go along and do not buck the system and therefore are wonderful assets on a team or in a middle-management position. On the other hand, they do not do well in settings that demand that they think for themselves and make decisions, such as sales or executive positions. These individuals will not be able to rise to the occasion and make decisions for fear of upsetting someone by making a decision that someone might not like.

Aggressive individuals, on the other hand, *do rise to the top of large companies* as they are not afraid to make someone angry by their decisions. They will take the bull by the horns and make changes when needed and thus can operate well in management positions or in self-employed situations because they will persevere until things work. They are not afraid and they don't give up. Their aggressiveness can cause them to ignore the advice and suggestions of others, therefore they do not make good team players or middle managers. They do better in the role of leadership.

14.3   Strategies for the Workplace

14.3.1   General Rules of Thumb

- Break tasks into smaller more manageable parts.
- Take breaks at one- to two-hour intervals to refresh yourself.
- Use exercise as a form of relaxation. Exercise either in the morning before going to work or at lunch time. This allows for relief of tension and some meditative time to plan the rest of the day.
- Write everything down, leave nothing to chance — Back up all decisions on paper and with memos, noting reasons behind the decision.
- Your planner is your best friend — it goes everywhere, to the bathroom, next to the bed, to the office, and home again. Or use other items like the small hand-held computers that can accommodate dates, times, phone numbers, notes to remember, and just about everything you would want or need.
- If allowed, tape recorders provide a great means of obtaining or "getting" all of the information so you can participate in the discussion fully and without worry. This is a very big issue because ADD adults as a whole are unable to fully participate in business meetings, much less interact and think creatively because they are so preoccupied with the idea of missing information.

- Don't cramp yourself for time — Leave extra time to allow yourself to arrive calm, mentally refreshed, and ready to participate in meetings or appointments. Being late places you in a "one-down" position and does not allow you to fully participate as you're so busy concentrating on the fact that you arrived late.

- Use medication at strategic times and plan ahead. If a meeting is going to take four hours and there may only be a few breaks, find out the breaks in advance or calculate as much as possible to allow yourself to remain medicated without dropping during the meeting. Feeling yourself slide downhill can be particularly upsetting during a business meeting.

- Remember that your body is subject to such things as low-blood-sugar reactions — Hypoglycemia, or low blood sugar, increases with stress. Do not allow yourself to become hungry during the business meeting or you may suffer a reaction, resulting in total confusion. Have little snacks available for yourself in the drawer of your desk.

- Request feedback from your peers and immediate supervisor to continually monitor your performance. One of the downfalls of being ADD is not always knowing and being able to assess how you are doing and how others see you.

- Make sure you have your instructions and directions down pat. It is easy to misconstrue or make mistakes about what you are being asked to do.

- Find a setting that is not distracting or use "white noise" to block out common distractions so you are able to complete paperwork. Be prepared to use your portable CD player, offering instrumental music for increased concentration.

- Do not take phone calls while in the middle of something that demands your total train of thought, focus, and concentration; this can be seriously disrupted. Provide some means via a secretary or business partner to hold all calls or interruptions to complete the types of work that require total undivided attention and sustained concentration. When attempting to complete these types of tasks, interruptions become highly frustrating and can lead to either non-completion of the task and/or irritability and anger with whoever has dared to interrupt you.

- When work requires enormous amounts of attention and concentration, arrive at work early or stay late to complete those tasks that you know need amounts of undivided attention not subject to interruptions. You need not worry about interruptions or having the time to contemplate and can consider issues in depth without the fear of losing your train of thought.

14.3.2   Use Positive Traits to Maximize Performance and Enhance Your Career

- ADD persons who use their assets and strengths in their job protect themselves by being very good at what they do, so that when the little things occur, like the paperwork not being completed properly or promptly, it is overlooked.

You will hear supervisors overlook some of these issues, or complete the paperwork for individuals who are so skilled at what they do that they benefit the organization far more than any losses due to task noncompletion.

Sales supervisors will cover for salespeople who are so good that they rack up volumes of sales, by often completing their paperwork for them, so that they will get paid for their efforts. Salespeople who do not turn in their volumes, do not turn in their expense reports, go months with high amounts on their credit cards, are disorganized in their paperwork, are intent on the volume of sales, often forgo the paperwork that is necessary to turn their hard work into financial gain.

14.3.3   Assert Legal Rights If Things Get Out of Control and There Is the Probability of Demotion or Job Loss

The right to be free from discrimination in the workplace is provided under two critical federal laws.

14.3.3.1   *The Americans with Disabilities Act (ADA)*

The ADA applies basically to businesses employing more than 15 full-time employees. The ADA act of 1990 protects those individuals with physical or mental impairments that result in a substantial limitation of one or more of their major life activities. The Equal Employment Opportunity Commission (EEOC) defines mental impairment to include mental or psychological disorders that would substantially limit someone's functioning. However, the disability cannot limit their functioning substantially enough to prevent their meeting the job requirements.

Disorders such as depression, anxiety, PTSD, and schizophrenia as well as learning disabilities, attentional disorders, and neurological disorders are included in this impaired category. Major life activities are defined as the ability of the individual to interact with others, concentrate and sustain attention, care for oneself with regard to physical hygiene and basic everyday activities, and the ability to maintain and sustain employment. Recognized professionals must provide proof that individuals are able to do their job, as well as document the impact of their specific impairment on that job.

Reasonable accommodations can be made on a case-by-case basis to account for the disability that these individuals have proven exists and which, when implemented, will substantially improve their ability to perform their jobs.

Some of the following accommodations are specific interventions that can be easily and readily employed to address substantiated disabilities as suggested by the EEOC.

- Unpaid leave or accrued paid leave can be used for necessary time off to provide treatment in an inpatient or outpatient setting.
- Work schedules can be modified to meet the individual's needs.
- Accommodations can be made to the workplace or in the equipment provided to enhance the individual's ability to perform (soundproofing, visual barriers, use of CD players, advanced computer equipment and other technological aids).
- Workplace policies can be modified to allow the use of tape recorders or detailed notetaking during business meetings.
- Supervisory methods should be provided that best fit individuals to communicate in writing, verbally or by electronic mail what they need to know to do their job.
- Increased feedback or structure of task performance or chunking of major projects into smaller jobs can be made available.
- Job coaches can be employed to temporarily assist the individual in getting back on track in terms of job performance.

14.3.3.2 Rehabilitation Act of 1973 (RA)

The RA follows federal money and applies to federal government, federal government contractors, and federal grant recipients. These statutes provide protection for those disabled individuals who are discriminated against in job promotions, benefits, or privileges based on the symptoms of their disorder if they are otherwise qualified with or without reasonable accommodations for the job in question.

Otherwise qualified means that the person can perform the essential functions of the job with or without the reasonable accommodations. A *reasonable accommodation* is an accommodation that does not create undue hardship for the employer and yet alters the nature of the job to allow maximum performance. *Undue hardship*, however, would imply an accommodation that would result in an essential change in the nature of the job or job setting at considerable difficulty or expense for the employer.

ADD falls under the heading of a disability. The learning and thinking problems associated have been clearly documented and are legally recognized as a disorder that impairs one's ability. The hitch is how much and to what degree a person must be impaired in order to qualify. Also, it must be clearly proven that the disability of ADD was the reason for the employer's discriminatory action.

This is difficult to prove as the employer will work around the ADD symptoms to find other reasons for the action. The best that ADD people can probably do is ask for special accommodations but, by so doing, they must expose themselves. Therefore, the general rule is to wait until all other avenues have been exhausted before doing this.

14.4   For What Accommodation Can the ADD Adult Ask?

- Reduced distractibility in the work setting — Perhaps ask to move your space or rearrange divider and cubicles to do paperwork. Or request to work out of your home.
- Request oral and written instructions — Explain that you work best when written instructions follow oral instructions.
- Ask that tasks be assigned in small chunks with clear and reasonable timelines.
- Request constant provision of feedback and warning if performance becomes problematic.
- Request special training in useful aids such as the computer to help you in job performance — Ask for additional data on the job requirements to help you maximize your job performance.
- Ask for job restructuring or job re-assignment if a particular position does not prove conducive to your talents and is compromising your productivity due to the negative interaction with symptoms of the ADD disorder.

The idea is to try to work out whatever is possible to provide the best career choice for you without compromising your potential or ability while, at the same time, limiting the negative effects of the symptoms of ADD.

15

Legal Information: IDEA, Section 504, and ADA

15.1 Information

Three federal laws currently exist for the benefit and protection of ADD students and family. They are briefly discussed in the following sections. These statutes and their corresponding application seem to go on for pages and fill volumes. We have attempted to provide the reader with at least enough information to handle most cases regarding ADD schoolchildren. Many parents may skip this section because it often does not have a "here and now" consequence. However, when the school district is aware that parents know the basics of these three laws, parents will be amazed at how cooperative the school can become in a relatively short period of time.

15.2 Individuals with Disabilities Education Act–Part B

IDEA was formally known as 94-142. When children are tested and placed into categories of disabilities with names like "Specific Learning Disabilities," "Emotionally Impaired," "Speech and Language Impaired," "Mentally Impaired," or "Physically and Otherwise Health Impaired," school districts receive federal funds. To qualify for those federal funds under IDEA, the school district must comply with certain rules. The other laws that will be discussed later in this chapter are not as stringent or specific. Under IDEA, the federal government says to the school districts that if the government is going to shell out money for kids with disabilities, they want the schools to follow stringent guidelines. There are good reasons for this for all involved.

15.3 Basic Concepts Under IDEA

1. Services are designed for those with handicapping conditions who "have a physical or mental impairment that substantially limits one or more major life activities such as caring for oneself, performing manual tasks, walking, seeing, hearing, speaking, breathing or learning."

2. Children must be between the ages of 3 through 21 years and have not yet graduated from high school.

3. The child must be evaluated by a multidisciplinary evaluation team (i.e., a school psychologist, a teacher, a social worker, and a person to do the academic evaluation).

4. If the necessary criteria are met and the child qualifies for special education services based on specific standards, the student receives supportive education services in a free, appropriate public-education atmosphere (FAPE) in the least restrictive environment.

5. An Individual Educational Planning (IEP) committee is established to decide whether a handicapping condition exists, what to do next, and to set achievable goals. The committee consists of a school psychologist, school administrator, a teacher, any professional having pertinent test results, parents, and the student, when appropriate.

6. The IDEA was re-authorized on June 4, 1997. The law now includes several changes. Generally they are as follows: School districts are no longer required to perform the standard 3-year reevaluation of a child with disabilities. Students who violate the law under weapons, drugs, or rape charges can be expelled without benefit of an IEP but can be placed in an "interim alternative education setting" for up to 45 days.

15.4 Basic Concepts Under Section 504 of the Rehabilitation Act of 1973

1. The general aim of the Section 504 rule is to provide "regular or special education and related aids and services necessary to meet

    the individual educational needs of handicapped students as adequately as the needs of non-handicapped students are met."

2. Procedural safeguards mimic IDEA's safeguards: the right to attend all decision-making conferences, to examine records and protocol, to dialogue/disagree, to an impartial hearing, and to appeal.

3. Traditionally, Section 504 involves cases of ADD, ADHD, AIDS, asthma, a broken leg, alcohol and chemical dependency, allergies, diabetes, epilepsy, and heart problems, among a long list of other maladies.

4. FYI: Think of "handicapping" the way golfers handicap. Strokes are awarded so that, when implemented, all players will have an equal chance of being "on par"— or what a "normal" golfer *should* score when the game is played as it is designed. Theoretically, everyone should have an equal chance at shooting par.

Section 504 tends not to involve new services and operates as an amendment of the disability that is already defined, recognized, and established. It is not special education, it does not have an IEP. It is part of the Rehabilitation Act, that is, a federal statute that states one cannot discriminate against someone because of an impairment or handicap. Section 504 operates more as an adaptability and an accommodation under general education services.

15.5 What about Gifted Children with ADD?

Gifted children with ADD have had difficulty receiving services within the school system. They do not qualify with learning disabilities due to their scoring on the intellectual and achievement testing. Typically, these children have a number of discrepant scores due to their tendency to build their strengths while neglecting their weaknesses. Even though their scores fall under impaired status when compared with their potential, they still remain in the average range and would not qualify for special education services. These children have the ability to progress through school and achieve. Their intellectual assessment does not reflect their true abilities and the result is that they often appear average and learning at the rate of average, thus not qualifying under IDEA.

    They can, however, request special accommodations related to the attentional disorder under Section 504. There is a section under IDEA for which the gifted could receive services. The category, Physically or Otherwise Health Impaired (POHI), would require documentation from the medical field. Under this category, the ADD would be determined a physical disorder and qualify the child for services.

15.6   College Students Can Receive Services that Make all the Difference

The legal rights of college students fall under two federal statutes, the Rehabilitation Act of 1973 (RA) and the Americans with Disabilities Act (ADA). These statutes provide that students with disabilities must be free from discrimination in college, which includes courses they are required to take and testing and activities in general. The ADA act can be utilized provided the student meets the requirements of having a disability. They must be qualified to participate in college studies with or without reasonable accommodation and if there is no other valid reason for denying admission or continuation of admission. There is an issue that the ADA must apply to that particular institution. ADA applies to all Title I colleges (public) and Title II (private) colleges and universities, as well as other places of extended education such as bar-review courses and licensing courses. The two basic mandates of a general prohibition against discrimination and specific requirements for the provision of auxiliary aids and services allows ADD individuals to be tested under special conditions and utilize aids such as tape recorders or a notetaker in class.

Legally, examination must be structured to accurately reflect students' learning or achievement level and may not reflect their disability or impairment unless the purpose of the examination is to measure those factors. Students who have a language disability that might interfere with written examination are entitled to oral evaluation unless the specific course of study is designed to teach writing skills. The issue of testing accommodations has resulted in court cases where universities have argued that students needed to complete the examination like everyone else as a measure of their ability to complete the total course program. A legal precedent that occurred in 1994 granted students to be directly involved in the right decisions concerning which methods are educationally effective. Required reasonable accommodations include taped examinations, large-print examinations, large-print answer sheets, qualified readers, transcribers, interpreters, taped texts, and so on. Alternative arrangements that can be utilized include videotaped lecture cassettes and prepared notes. Accommodations that are not required are services that focus on increasing the skill level of the student in the area of the disability such as developmental reading courses or remedial tutoring. Colleges and universities may not charge supplemental fees for services required by law to be provided to students with disabilities. They may charge for services beyond what the law requires.

Colleges and universities are making every attempt to provide services for the ADD population. They offer

1. Support staff and services of professionals who are aware of ADD and are available to help students.
2. Substitutions for required courses available for ADD students who have a problem in a particular area due to symptoms of the disorder.
3. Examinations that can be given orally, in a separate testing environment without distractibility, and without the pressure of time. Students can also request the opportunity to seek clarification of an exam question in addition to extra time, a quiet room, and possibly an alternative format if needed.
4. Services that provide either a note taker or use of a tape recorder in class. When there are services of a note taker provided, students may be requested to sign an agreement that they will appear at all of their classes with full participation to continue to receive services of the note taker.
5. Sometimes there is the availability of recorded materials, possibly lectures that have been recorded or books on tape.
6. A number of technological tools are provided to aid the student, such as use of computer-designed training programs to increase word-attack skills, reading skills and so on.
7. Tutorial and assistance programs are available when a class proves particularly difficult for the student.
8. The availability of reduced course load and strategic scheduling and planning of classes to facilitate study time. Students may be allowed access to registration prior to the normal time period to allow them to plan their courses and ensure that they will receive what they need.
9. Individual counseling, support groups, and assistance with educational and vocational decisions are provided to allow the student a smooth transition from high school to college and from college to the working world.
10. Students can request that instructions be repeated both orally and in writing as well as frequent and specific feedback from their professors and instructors.
11. Students may request other in-class accommodations such as priority seating.

To receive services students will need to produce documentation of the presence of ADD and to show that its presence and symptoms are impacting their ability to learn to the level of their potential. Further, students will need to document that they can participate in a college program with reasonable accommodations that can be instituted without undue cost to the institution. Finally, if given the requested accommodations, this will result in their being able to function to the level of their potential and will make a difference in their ability to learn and participate in the college program of study.

Issues that have not been addressed specifically are the degree of required detail documentation and the issue of confidentiality. Documentation is labeled "reasonable" and would probably depend on specific requirements of the college or university, but should be enough to establish the presence of a disability. The issue of confidentiality is more complex. Some students have reported that documentation of special services for testing of the college entrance exams is noted and others have indicated that the testing service had no notation that the examination was taken under special conditions. This is a concern of practically all of the ADD student population. Many applying to very specific programs are afraid of being "blacklisted" if they note that they have a disability and require specialized testing services. At this point, we do not know of a way to resolve this issue due to the lack of uniformity among the different programs and the differing responses received via the students. Some students report receiving excellent care, support, and consideration while others are made to feel as if they should not apply to the program at all, much less utilize any sort of specialized testing procedures for their entrance exam.

16

How to Work with the Schools to Get What You Need

We look for so much from the school system, don't we? As parents, we demand that the local school honor, protect, defend, and educate our children. We expect them to play a host of roles — police officer, psychologist, diagnostician, coach, nurse, on-site parent, and, oh yes, teacher. However, as long as we observe, rather than participate, we will always remain on the outside. Parents have been assigned the primary responsibility of providing an education to their children. All too often, parents charge into school with righteous indignation, fueled by fear or their own unresolved issues around personal school experiences, only to meet with the same kind or degree of resistance that they faced may years prior. As consultants to school districts for many years, we found it terribly disheartening to watch a completely outflanked parent attempt to simply be part of the school team, having no idea how to go about it and walking away from the school meeting feeling angry and frustrated because they did not understand why their few simple requests met with so little success. When approaching your local school district regarding planning and/or placement of an ADD youngster, follow these tips.

1. Be an expert on ADD — Read recent articles and publications on the subject. Bookstores and local universities are excellent places to start to educate yourself on the topic. Local support groups, C.H.A.D.D. or professionals speaking on ADD can also enhance learning. Be sure to contact state or county intermediate school district personnel and ask for guidance. An expert on ADD is employed on their staff. Your job is to find them and pick their brains.

2. Don't ACT like an expert — You probably know the irritation of someone entering your place of business and telling you how to

do your job. Whether they are right or wrong, no one appreciates such intrusion. As parents, we do the same thing to the school teacher on a regular basis. Knowing that we are former teachers and consultant, many people request that our services be even more intrusive and combative than they perceive themselves. Much to their disappointment, they are directed to the latest research and the next Dale Carnegie meeting for a few tips on making friends and influencing people.

3. Request a meeting to talk about the present situation.

   • *Hint #1*: Early morning meetings, before school, work much better than those scheduled during or after school hours.

   • *Hint #2*: After requesting a meeting and securing a time, date, and location, follow it up with a typed (if possible) letter confirming your conversation. In the letter, briefly reiterate the telephone conversation and include the necessary personnel (the principal is an absolute must) and the agenda you wish to discuss.

   • *Hint # 3*: Keep your agenda extremely focused and brief. After "meet, greet, and seat" get down to business. If you've done your homework up to this point, school personnel will be feeling a bit defensive and (often) wondering where you are coming from. Do not make small talk. Be direct and honest.

   • *Hint # 4*: Do not under any circumstances:
     • Whine
     • Moan
     • Bitch
     • Complain
     • Fault find
     • Condemn
     • Play victim

   Should school personnel begin to engage in any of the above behaviors, politely and firmly interrupt them (before they build up a lot of steam) and refocus the meeting to its original objective: "What is needed for school success for this child?"

4. Make your agenda as simple and clear as possible — An example of an agenda item would be: Student doesn't begin tasks in a timely fashion or does not complete tasks in a timely manner. Student lacks necessary organizational skills. Agenda items must be both countable and observable. The idea is to shape behavior, not attitude or emotion. "I'd like my child to feel more like a part of the group" may be a sentiment that can't be disputed, but has little value as a behavioral objective. Also, how will you know when this objective has been successfully met? However, "My child will

participate in group activities three or more times per week without fighting," can achieve a similar objective, has success criteria built in, and is stated in one sentence. *Rule of Thumb*: If you can't speak your message in less than two (yes, two) sentences, you are not yet ready to meet with school personnel.

Always bear in mind how you would like your meeting to end, that is, what results will demonstrate you are successful? Is it a certain grade in the class? An increase in the number of completed tasks in a day/week/month? A certain achievement level in a certain subject? (e.g., Bob will be reading at his grade level by February with a 90% mastery level.) Remember, the key here is focus and brevity.

Another extremely important issue or question to be discussed before leaving the meeting is what the teacher's role is in your child's behavioral change. Also, what is your child's role and what is your role as parent in the proposed change? Further, how will success criteria be measured (remember to include numbers in your success criteria). Use words like "specifically" and "exactly."

After the task has been formulated, roles have been specifically and clearly assigned and success criteria spelled out to the letter, your task is almost complete. You must specify the follow-up date and a Plan B, or Screw Up Plan (in case our well-laid plans go awry).

- The follow-up date keeps everyone honest and on task. It allows school personnel to know that you value your child's education highly and that you are absolutely determined to be successful. No one will come to a follow-up meeting unprepared or not having completed the tasks that were previously agreed to at the meeting. Keep in mind that with the principal in the picture (you know the teacher's boss, right? the one who fills out the teacher's evaluation), the job is more likely to be successful. A follow-up date ensures that follow-through will occur and a change will be made.

- *The Screw-up Plan.* What if for some reason the well-intended, well-laid plan that this committee has set forth falls apart? An ace in the hole can be The Screw-up Plan. Here's how it works: After all is said and done and after the next meeting has been set, you simply wonder out loud, "Hey, what happens next if this well-laid plan goes down the tubes and does not work? Then what?" The secret is that the answer to this question is not nearly as important as asking it. Asking "Then what?" puts the school district on notice that failure will not be acceptable as a response. It also implies that you are not going to go away and that you have the necessary perseverance to accomplish the task.

At the follow-up meeting (no longer than three to four weeks from the initial meeting) return to your original brief and focused question and its accompanying success criteria. If necessary, repeat the process. At this juncture, send the principal a letter of thanks and recognition regarding the teacher and ask that the letter find its way to his or her personnel file with a copy to the teacher. Let's face it, none of us get enough positive strokes, least of all public ones.

Bear in mind most school problems come in pairs — behavioral and academic. As you formulate your child's school issues, separate one type from the other. Further, what appears in your household comes under the heading of emotional. It is where your child knows that the behavior or academic fallout can safely be felt and emotionally discharged. For the ADD child, feelings are terribly unpredictable, do not make sense, and are potentially dangerous to one's self-esteem, self-worth and self-image.

16.2 Examining if the School is Right for Your Child

It is helpful to go to the school you are considering and speak with the principal and other school personnel. Attempt to determine from this interview if there is an awareness of ADD in the school, if there are a number of children receiving medication, or there are in-services regarding this disorder. It is also helpful to determine if there are individuals interested in understanding exactly what it means to be ADD and what these children need.

Look at the sizes of the classes and whether teachers are being overwhelmed by students, which may make them unavailable to the special needs of your child. Check to see if the school is prepared, funding-wise, to offer special services, such as a resource room, or if it is limited in the extras it can provide to your child.

Finally, are teachers accustomed to working with the parents with such things as daily assignment books and to developing a continual communication regarding your child? Is this a priority and do they have the capacity and time to maintain this type of communication on a regular basis? The above are mandated by law. However, the reality of school reminds me that it is silly to reinvent the wheel. That is, don't look for education skirmishes if other options already exist.

16.3 Parents of a Child Who Has Been Identified as ADD and Recognized by the School as ADD

If the child is identified as ADD, refer to any "parent–kid" model. School (and many institutions) seem to work best under a guise of informality.

Often, at this stage, the opportunity to succeed is still very evident and failure is distant. School authorities are also motivated at this point. They know that, should failure occur, the formal process of Section 504 or IDEA looms in the not-too-distant future. One of the major difficulties in getting school systems to test and diagnose children as ADD is that once a school district has pronounced a label of ADD it becomes responsible for treating it. A school district should not order that your child needs individual or family therapy for much the same reason — it becomes either liable or eligible for the cost of the treatment. Conversely, a school district will diagnose a learning disability because it knows how to treat a specific learning disability and can absorb the cost for treatment. However, in most cases, the school district becomes responsible for anything that it diagnoses. A very familiar retort to parents of potential, yet undiagnosed, ADD children, is that ADD is a neurobiological and/or medical disorder and that it certainly isn't in the area of school. The authorities then recommend that the parent deal with the problem privately. Those concepts are common and have been carefully chosen. The school district is not saying that the child is or is not ADD nor is it taking any responsibility for diagnosis and treatment. It is washing its hands of the entire question.

One must better understand the school disrict's position. Loosely translated, Section 504 and IDEA both state in grand and glorious terms that anyone with a "handicap" should receive assistance to help them become a more productive citizen and to achieve their potential. The Education For All Handicapped Children Act was passed in Congress in 1975. After 15 years and much debate the updated version of this statute became IDEA. In Michigan, original sponsors of the state's bill first proposed that "handicappers" should receive attention from age 0 through age 26 or on graduation. Knowing that a compromise would occur in the 26-year span, many expected the current 10-year age span (6 to 16 years compulsory) to also apply to special education. Surprisingly the 26-year age span passed with little debate and was signed into law. However, the lawmakers forgot to sign into law by whom and how this educational mandate would be financed. This oversight has caused serious confusion and fear between the well-intended, good Samaritan, pretty-nice-guy-lawmakers and the local school-district administrators, who are now in a position of implementing a grandiose plan and looking like the bad guys.

When looking at the application of Section 504 or IDEA, almost any person can/may qualify for assistance: from glasses that are too thick to diabetes to not necessarily having a handicap but merely being suspected of having one. This translates to a person who has been evaluated or tested in the past, regardless of the reason or outcome, is or can be, considered handicapped and eligible for *services*. To your school district, *services* equals money spent. The school officials certainly want control over who spends it. As private practitioner psychologists, our clinic provides a test battery that is clear and concise. What we advocate is the idea of cooperation with the school for children and adolescents but not at the expense of either the local school district or the student. The "us" vs. "them" dichotomy is not helpful, but is counter-productive to all involved.

Many parents have a needlessly bad attitude regarding a Section 504 plan. The process can often lead to the labeling of a child, as does the special-education labeling of "learning disabled" or "emotionally impaired" students. My experience reminds me that teachers have little or no opinion regarding labels and that children all label each other anyway. Ask your child who is the smartest, dumbest, fastest, slowest, roundest, tallest, brightest kid in the class and most will agree on the designated student. The truth in labeling kids in this process is a funding label. That is, with a funding label, one student might receive funding that another might not receive. Our goal is to shift the reader's perspective and perception of the word "label." After high-school graduation, this often negatively viewed label translates into a form of financial assistance with post secondary education or training. What was a *label* in high school can mean *financial help* in college.

EXAMPLE

In high school, Dr. Beckley had a diabetic condition. In the pre-Section 504 days, little was done to accommodate special-needs students. He was extremely private about his health (unlike today) and deciding that he didn't want the added attention, chose to struggle with school. A unique and very caring teacher/coach gently steered him to a state agency of Vocational Rehabilitation where he got the good news–bad news. As a diabetic, he was handicapped and the state agency paid for half of college tuition and books. Feeling as if he had won the lottery, the term "handicapped," for some reason, seemed incidental.

One last point, teachers and school personnel are no more (and no less) equipped to deal with the subject of ADD than anyone else. They do have motivation to learn about it and know it better than the average person if for no other reason than that they are in the business of teaching. In our 20-plus years of experience working with the schools, kids, and teachers, we have found that the overwhelming majority of teachers are still very interested in doing a good job with their students. Also, no formal training for ADD has come to my attention in our last four graduate degrees. That is, we expect teachers to be the reigning experts on ADD and to have serious training and education on the subject but none exists at the university level. Current training methods are available via teacher in-service lectures and/or commercially produced workshops, most of which are available to the public.

17

Medications

17.1 From a Clinical Perspective, Why Take Medication at All?

17.1.1 We Need Medications as a Fine Tuner to Allow the Coping Mechanisms to Work

When one understands that ADD is a biochemical disorder you believe in the need to correct it chemically. Stimulant medication does not treat the ADD symptoms, it allows the individual to have the necessary awareness to use the coping mechanisms to address the symptoms. Stimulant medication cannot be relied on to complete the job, it merely allows the person to get from point A to point B. The stimulant medications tend to be the best course of action for treating ADD primarily because they can be used as a fine tuner, especially at those times when it is necessary to address ADD symptoms. That may be three to four times per day or only once a week.

The job of Ritalin as a stimulant medication directly increases the availability of dopamine and norepinephrine at the receptor sites where the neurons talk to one another. Ritalin will decrease symptoms of distractibility, improve the speed of one's performance, and improve the ability to process information. It will not impact spatial deficits because this is not due to ADD, but is due to the lack of use, and requires re-training instead.

Ritalin is the most widely used and widely researched medication for ADD. It has been shown to have the fewest side effects, to work the best, and to be the easiest to use. Long-term studies of more than 30 years have substantiated that there are no long-term height, weight, and overall growth side effects as a result of the use of Ritalin for that period of time. Thus, this is always where we suggest that both the ADD child and adult begin. If Ritalin does not work after a decent trial, there are alternatives. However, before discontinuing Ritalin, in our opinion, one should try all possible options to remain on this medication.

Individuals can vary the dose of the medication. Some small children commonly take 5 mg per dose while, although we do not suggest this, others can tolerate as high as 20 mg. Incorporating nutritional supplements may make it possible to prescribe a lower dosage of Ritalin to produce the needed changes in thinking abilities, and to improve the ability to tolerate the medication. ADD people must assert their options. It requires a great amount of creativity, perseverance, and general knowledge about medications to adequately treat this disorder.

17.1.2   So Why Does Ritalin Work?

Ritalin is a stimulant and as such it excites the production of both dopamine and norepinephrine. There are two types of Ritalin, short-acting and a longer-acting, sustained-release version. Generally, even though everyone is different, the short-acting takes 20 minutes to kick in and lasts for hours. The longer-acting takes anywhere from 45 to 90 minutes for effect and lasts for 6 to 8 hours. We find that the longer-acting lasts about 6 hours and takes about 1 hour to gain effect. The short-acting types comes in a dosage range of 5, 10, and 20 mg and the tablets are scored to be cut in half. Sustained-release type comes in two dosage ranges, 20 and 40 mg. The 20 mg tends to act as 10 in the system and the 40 mg as 20 within the system. We suggest that there is a cap at 20 mg per dose of the short-acting Ritalin and 40 mg per dose of the longer-acting Ritalin. This is because, at higher levels of Ritalin, people tend to develop nosebleeds, headaches, and sleep disturbances.

The brain is aroused with the stimulant medication and then it does its job. There are other types of stimulant medications besides Ritalin, such as Adderall, Dexedrine, and Cylert. Other medications impact the neurotransmitter system of dopamine and norepinephrine, but not as well, nor in the direct manner that the stimulants do. Other medications, such as antidepressants, allow for more of the neurotransmitter substance to be available. They do this by taking *less* dopamine and norepinephrine into the system. In other words, the antidepressant operates by leaving more of the neurotransmitter behind, while the stimulants actually excite or stimulate the production of these neurotransmitters. So which is the more powerful of the two types of medications? The stimulants, of course. The antidepressants, however, *do* impact the symptom of distractibility and provide increased control over one's vulnerability to being distracted by both internal and external stimuli. The antidepressants do *not* impact the issues of slow thinking speed or information-processing deficits. Only the stimulant class of medications can address all three of these issues.

Of all the stimulants, Ritalin is suggested as the first line of defense, because it is short acting and can be taken with greater monitoring ability. This means that the medication can be taken and results can be seen within 20 minutes. There is no need to take this medication on a continual basis for it to build up within the system. You can hold off taking the medication for a month and then take it and again see results within 20 minutes. Due to its short-acting qualities, studies generally report no long-term side effects.

Original Ritalin is what we suggest. This means that you have to have the letters D.A.W. (dispense as written) on the prescription otherwise you will receive the generic version. You will know you have generic if it has an MD engraved on the pill and you have the brand name if it has CIBA engraved on the pill. It is our belief that the generic does not work as well and, in fact, can create tremendous problems. There are several reasons for this. First, the generic is cut with different chemicals and therefore works differently in the system. There are two types of generic forms of methylphenidate, which results in the dosage on the pill not always being the dose that you actually get nor what is metabolized in the system. Obviously, this can quickly lead to rebound problems (the medication stops working with a thump), inadequate dosing, and over- or underdosing. You may think you are getting 10 mg and you are actually getting anywhere from 6 to 12 mg. This makes it very difficult to titrate (increase) doses or figure out what the best dose is because, unbeknownst to you, the actual dosage keeps changing. So you may think that 10 mg works, but you actually had 12 mg that day, or now the 10 mg no longer works because you actually had 6 mg, but you think it is due to something else.

The ADD person keeps playing around with the dosage, never being able to actually regulate it because every dose may be different. We see ADD persons become more irritable and cranky, and have lower blood sugar. Overall, the generic just does not work as well. So the child or adult takes more only to begin to overdose themselves in an effort to make something work, that simply will not work. Ritalin will take approximately 20 minutes to have an effect and lasts for only about 4 hours. Everyone is different. For some it may take 10 minutes to kick in and last for 3 hours or less. These people are the quick metabolizers who may do well with the combination of sustained (longer-acting) Ritalin and the short-acting Ritalin. Ritalin works very well for 60% to 90% of the population, in general. As a short-acting medication it can be closely regulated and tailored to one's day. People see the best results with this medication if they are creative and willing to tailor the dosage to their exact level of sensitivity and timing of the day's activities.

As stated before, Ritalin does not need to be subjected to a rigid schedule of 3 times per day and the dosage *can* be changed. Ritalin need not be maintained in the bloodstream to be effective. It can be taken when needed. Ritalin is a "thinking" pill not a "happy" pill or a "behavior" pill, and should be used whenever anyone needs to think: sports, studying, homework, and generally anywhere or anytime someone needs to focus, attend, use sustained attention or not have the interference of slow thinking speed, information-processing deficits or distractibility.

When an individual believes that Ritalin does not work, we suggest that other interfering variables that may be conflicting with the medication be ruled out prior to changing to another stimulant medication.

17.1.2.1 Variables We Have Seen That Can Interfere with the Use of Ritalin

- The person is not taking enough of the medication — If someone is not taking enough medication then there will not be a change in thinking speed, information-processing deficits, or distractibility.

- The person is not eating and hypoglycemia or low blood sugar creates symptoms that confuse the reaction of Ritalin — Adolescents complain that Ritalin makes them tired. It is difficult to imagine how a stimulant medication can make someone tired, however, if taken without food, low blood sugar sets in and can make them feel tired. Therefore, we always suggest that the stimulant medication be taken with food either before or after the dose. If the blood sugar drops, confusion can occur, vision can become blurry, thinking can be difficult, and tasks can take longer. They begin to think that Ritalin is not working. Hypoglycemia causes the person to feel shaky and anxious due to a drop in blood-sugar levels.

- There is a suppression of appetite — The child, adolescent, or adult is always advised to take the medication with food as previously noted. When someone does not feel like eating, we ask them to eat anyway. We ask them to snack and nibble all day long on whatever they like as long as it is healthy and has only a minimal amount of sugar. If they refuse to eat, they cannot take this medication.

- The person is anxious and Ritalin makes them more anxious — This is a stimulant medication and ADD persons are a very anxious group. It is not surprising that many of the ADD population would become increasingly anxious with heart palpitations, anxiety and panic attack symptoms becoming apparent. Generally, if this is going to occur, it happens with the adolescent or adult population and rarely with the child population. Taking the medication with 250 mg of calcium (nutritional supplement) will tend to relieve the anxiety. The calcium is either taken at the time of taking the medication or in suggested dosages at bedtime. Nutritionists usually recommend 800 mg/day for children, 1000 mg/day for adolescents and males and 1500 mg/day for females.

  When anxious people take Ritalin they become even more anxious. As a result, they say they can't tolerate the medication and stop taking it. Or they can't tolerate a high enough dose to make a difference in the ADD symptoms and decide it really is not working. With these individuals we found that taking calcium with Ritalin can help them tolerate a higher dose and use the medication properly. Sometimes it helps to start at a low dose and work up to a higher dose in small increments. This is also true for individuals who are sensitive to medication. One can shift upwards at a level of 2.5 mg, having started at 5 mg, a very low dose. Adults start at a low dose and gradually increase it over a period of days or weeks. With children, lower doses are used at younger ages and increased as the child matures. These pills can also be divided in half and thirds.

- There is a disruption of sleep patterns — We suggest that stimulant medication not be taken past 6:00 pm or a minimum of 4 to 5 hours before bedtime. If disruption of sleep continues, the person may be taking too much stimulant medication.

- There may be stomachaches or headaches that do not stop with continued usage — If this continues then the person needs to switch to another stimulant medication or may not be able to take stimulant medications at all.

- The person is taking generic Ritalin — They can't get their dosage regulated. They are irritable and cranky. They need to get brand-name Ritalin. However, in making the change, they may need to take less Ritalin initially until they are used to the real thing.

- The person is taking the sustained-release version of Ritalin — We have found that taking sustained-release alone has not produced the necessary thinking changes the person is looking to have with the medication. Due to the overall mild impact on symptoms and general loss of effects, this type of medication tends to be overdosed. Increased doses are prescribed in an attempt to evidence some type of improvement in thinking ability or decrease of ADD symptoms. This is how a child becomes quickly overdosed and tired in school as a result. Sustained-release does not appear to make as much of a difference in symptoms nor work as well due to its long-acting, milder properties.

- Ritalin can accelerate the heart rate but not enough to promote long term cardiovascular effects — The use of stimulant medication can eventually result in a decrease in the amount of blood pressure medication needed in those diagnosed with hypertension or high blood pressure.

- Ritalin, belonging to the class of stimulant medications, stimulates all underlying disorders — Ritalin, as a stimulant, will excite or exaggerate anything that lies below the surface, whether it be hypoglycemia, hypertension, seizure disorder, schizophrenia, tics, Tourette's Syndrome, and so on. Should these disorders occur on the introduction of Ritalin one should consider the notion that the medication does not cause the symptoms but rather acts as a catalyst for them to surface from their dormant state. However, typically when other symptoms surface, our first reaction is to take a person off the medication, and treat the newly emerged disorder, then we never go back to the use of Ritalin. A better idea is to diagnose the secondary problem, control it with another medication, or some other means, and re-institute the stimulant medication. Creative approaches can be used to combine the stimulant medication with other medications and even vitamins.

The concerning side effect is tics. Transient tics will diminish with a lower dosage of the stimulant medication. If they persist, further investigation into the possibility of a seizure disorder or seizure-like activation is warranted. Even a mild or latent seizure disorder can be triggered by stimulant medication, and cause untold effects. However, as problematic as the impact of seizure can be, it can be addressed with antiseizure medications (alone or in combination) and can be administered with relatively few side effects, working well with the stimulant medication.

It is common for tics or symptoms of Tourette's Syndrome to emerge while on stimulant medication. The person is often pulled off the stimulant medication and treated with antiseizure medication for the Tourette's. Then, unfortunately, the ADD goes untreated.

EXAMPLE
Dr. Fisher spoke at a Tourette's Society meeting and found this to be the case over and over with individuals. Members at this meeting were all taking medication for the Tourette's but the ADD symptoms whose previous treatments with stimulant medication helped discover the Tourette's, was no longer being treated. Therefore, they continued to have trouble with work and school functioning due to a lack of sustained, focused attention.

Medication can enhance the emotions of the ADD individual and bring increased depression and anxiety to the surface. If grieving for the loss that occurs after being diagnosed with an attentional disorder and its impact on their lives, ADD people may find this grief sharpened by stimulant medication. The ADD individual and family members need to be aware of and prepared for the seemingly sudden onslaught of emotions that accompanies diagnosis and medicinal treatment.

17.2 When to Use Stimulant Medications

The general concept is to use stimulant medication when you need to focus, maintain sustained attention to task, and control symptoms of distractibility, information-processing deficits, and slow thinking speed.

EXAMPLE
During the summer, sometimes our son will take Ritalin and sometimes he won't. It depends on what he is doing. If there is a family activity, he may take Ritalin just to allow him to participate more fully. We have found it helpful to have him take Ritalin

during sports activities. We went to see him play basketball and during a game noticed that he was at one end of the court while everybody else was at the other. So he took his Ritalin and, although not a star basketball player (hockey, golf, and skiing turned out to be his sports), at least he was with the other kids and not where he shouldn't be. These are the issues that lead to the shame, embarrassment, and feelings of failure. Now, when in school and doing homework he always takes Ritalin.

Many individuals are frightened that they will lose their creativity or their personality will be affected with the use of Ritalin. This rarely occurs because they can regulate the dose to certain settings. Thus, they would take Ritalin only in settings in which their creativity would not be compromised.

We also find that *people don't know how to use Ritalin* correctly. They discontinue it when they are having problems, side effects and so on without examining reasons for the side effects, addressing those problems, and then returning to the Ritalin. We have seen terrible consequences when children are pulled off Ritalin and not put back on the medication. They then suffer as adults.

It is important to observe specific problems with stimulant medication and then attempt to fix them. If there are tics, examine the idea of a seizure disorder, whether due to head injury or mild seizure-like activation, which tends to be associated with the severe ADD without hyperactivity, overfocused subtype population. An EEG is one possibility, however, this only has a 15% detection rate. Even the video EEGs and 24-hour-monitor EEGs cannot show evidence of seizure when in fact the person is actually experiencing seizure activity. One should not assume that because some event does not show on a measure such as the EEG that it does *not* exist.

Neuropsychological evaluation tends to reveal evidence of seizure and other types of disorders long before they are severe enough to be measured by a neurological evaluation with the EEG or MRI. The SPECT scan or brain mapping, while not particularly successful in diagnosing ADD (due to the problem of differentiating the two subtypes and not being able to specifically define symptoms) has been very successful in identifying seizure activation and brain problems. Another measure we have found helpful is the QEEG (computerized EEG) that has been around for some time, offering a much finer approach and tending to isolate abnormal responses that characterize a seizure-like activation that would result in tics after stimulant medication has been used for some time.

The individual can be trialed on an antiseizure medication (many of them have surprisingly few side effects) and then put back on Ritalin while continuing to take the antiseizure drug. This is true with any other disorder, schizophrenia, bipolar, etc. that may erupt. Again, the idea is to take individuals off the stimulant medication, medicate the underlying problem, and put them back on the stimulant once the underlying problem is under control.

Ritalin is used as a fine-tuner, not a panacea. It is not typically seen as a pleasure drug, but we have heard of at least one teen who was selling it and another man who kept trying to take Ritalin to produce a high. Generally, though, addicts and individuals as a whole don't overuse or overdose on Ritalin because the use of the medication solves the problem and thus reduces the predisposition toward that kind of behavior. Despite worries and a lot of controversy, Ritalin has been found by both physicians and psychiatrists to be an excellent medication and very safe to use without fear of toxicity.

17.3 Tips on How to Maximize Use of Ritalin or Correct Problems

When using short-acting medication, individuals may find that when the medication wears off (after 2 to 4 hours) they have a severe rebound effect. They may become very irritable, depressed, and angry. In that case, the combination of sustained-release and regular Ritalin tends to be very effective. Just as the regular Ritalin is leaving the system, the sustained kicks in, and just as the sustained is leaving, another regular is taken to maintain the balance. A regular and sustained are taken together at the beginning of the day, and, later in the afternoon, a regular is taken by itself. Sometimes when an individual is taking high doses of Ritalin (over 30 mg per dose) and still does not see an effect, using sustained Ritalin as a backup to provide a low, continual stream works quite well. Thus, these people would take their normal dose of Ritalin three or four times per day, and then, one to two times per day, take a sustained-release. This can provide not only continual coverage but also result in the person seeing an effect without continuing to increase the dosage of short-acting Ritalin. The following is an example of how this would look in a given day:

Pairing the sustained release and the short-acting Ritalin

8 a.m. Ritalin short-acting and sustained-release

noon Ritalin short-acting

2 p.m. Sustained-release

4 p.m. Short-acting

Total coverage from 8:00 to 8:00, no rebound — a gentle way to increase or augment the level of Ritalin beyond 20 mg.

17.4 Stimulant Medication Does Not Increase Alcoholism or Substance Abuse

The use of stimulant medication will tend to help the person increase their self-esteem and, if possible, prevent the negative and hopeless feelings that lead to the need to escape into abuse of alcohol or drugs. In the case of ADHD individuals, this is a more-complex issue as their brains may be more hard-wired toward the development of some sort of addiction (alcoholism, gambling, drugs, workholism, and so on). What we are learning is that the brain of the ADHD individual is different. Because brain processes are operating differently due to genetic reasons, they are more susceptible to the kind of behaviors that would result in alcoholism.

17.5 Other Stimulant Medications

17.5.1 Adderall

If Ritalin does not work, for whatever reason, another stimulant is Adderall, with which some people have been quite pleased. The company that produces the drug, Richwood Pharmaceuticals, claims that the medication lasts approximately 8 hours. We find that it actually lasts some 4 to 6 hours. This medication proves a comparable alternative when Ritalin has been unsuccessful.

Problems may occur if someone has a poor appetite. This is a new medication on the market but is actually the revival of an old medication that used to be called Obetrol®, which was utilized as a diet drug. Adderall contains a form of amphetamine (similar to Ritalin) and dextroamphetamine (similar to dexedrine). The compounds of the mixture apparently dissolve at different rates, giving Adderall a timed-release quality with a therapeutic effect that people describe as smoother than Ritalin. Adderall tends to have a longer, slower rise without the jolt of Ritalin. Some individuals report that Adderall is more effective than Ritalin for reducing distractibility and impulsivity. Some have combined the use of both stimulant medications in varying dosages throughout the day.

17.5.2 Dexedrine and Cylert

Other choices are Dexedrine® and Cylert®. These last two medications do have side effects and a greater impact than Ritalin. Dexedrine can work quite well for both young children and adults. There is a standard form that lasts for about 4 hours and a sustained form that lasts 6 to 8 hours. Dextrostat is an updated version of Dexedrine that has a greater capacity for flexibility in dosing. For some individuals, it is too strong and can result in the release of uncontrollable emotions; it also could be abused for weight loss.

Cylert has not been shown to work very effectively and can cause damage to the liver. Cylert is given once per day and remains effective for approximately 8 to 9 hours.

17.5.3   Dopamine Agonists

There are other forms of stimulants called dopamine agonists that trigger the release of dopamine. We expect to hear more about these in the future. One of these, Amantadine®, has been found to benefit cognitive function and reduce agitation. Another is Fenfluramine (Pondimin) which has been shown to produce good results among the mentally retarded and head-injury populations. Side effects include drowsiness, body odor, halitosis, and significant reductions in heart rate, blood pressure, and body weight. Finally, s-adenosyl l-methionine (SAM) used in adults with ADHD, revealed *some* evidence of improvement but there is very little data at this time regarding this medication. A recent type of agonist used for weight loss, Redux®, has been pulled off the market because of side effects.

17.5.4   Modafinil

This is a recently released medication being targeted to treat narcolepsy and may in the future be used to address ADD. This medication might accomplish the same task as the stimulants by using another neurotransmitter system.

17.5.5   The Antidepressants

Antidepressants can be used to treat attention disorders in addition to bed-wetting, migraine headaches, eating disorders, and obsessive-compulsive disorders. Antidepressants work to block the re-uptake of neurotransmitters and increase their concentration, enabling more-efficient brain transmission. In terms of helping the ADD symptoms, the area affected most is distractibility — both the vulnerability to being distracted by the environment and the tendency to operate in a behaviorally distractible manner.

17.5.5.1   Tricyclics

Imipramine (Tofranil®) has had a beneficial effect on bedwetting, anger, and aggression. There are a number of side effects and overdose can be toxic for the individual. Most common side effects in children are nervousness, sleep disturbance, fatigue, weight gain in later years, dry mouth, and overall fatigue. The risks associated with the above-named medications are greater than stimulants.

Desipramine (Norapramin®) is similar to Tofranil but with fewer side effects. It blocks the reuptake of norepinephrine and can be subject to overdose. Currently, in psychiatric circles, use of this medication is being discontinued due to concerns of toxicity to the brain and negative effects on the central nervous system. At one time, this medication was commonly used to treat adult ADD.

17.5.5.2 Atypical Antidepressants

Bupropion is unique in that its primary action is to interfere with the uptake of dopamine. It stimulates the central nervous system and is four times as likely to produce seizures than the tricyclics. Due to the stimulative properties of this medication, Wellbutrin®, it has been suggested for ADD. However, there is not a great amount of research to support its impact.

Remeron® is a relatively new medication that is having excellent results and operating similarly to the monoamine-oxidase inhibitors. This medication has been clinically useful for addressing overwhelming anxiety.

17.5.5.3 SSRIs

The SSRIs are third-generation antidepressants, which include Prozac®, Zoloft®, Paxil®, and Luvox®. They work by selective inhibition of serotonin uptake rather than through the norepinephrine system. These medications target depression first and then can have an impact on anxiety. They do make a difference with ADD symptoms, however, only in the area of distractibility.

Zoloft has been found to be a very effective medication for all populations — children, adolescents, adults, and the elderly — for relief of symptoms of both depression and anxiety. It helps to relieve the constant feeling of sadness, worthlessness, and fear and allows ADD people to feel like connecting to those around them. This results in their becoming more social and more willing to participate in activities. Some side effects may appear with the use of decongestants and antihistamines, the most common being dry mouth, increased sweating, dizziness, sexual dysfunction (males more than females) and restlessness. Zoloft usually does not cause an increase in anxiety, nervousness, or agitation.

Paxil is another antidepressant that has been used successfully with the elderly as well as children, adolescents, and adults. The aged population should always begin at a decreased level (10 mg) per day with a maximum dose of 40 mg per day recommended. Medication is usually taken in the morning so as not to interfere with sleeping. Some problems may occur when taking other medications such as Coumadin®, Tagamet®, or Lanoxin® as well as the possibility of some interaction with Imitrex®. Some side effects may appear with the use of decongestants and antihistamines. The more common side effects are a generalized feeling of weakness, sweating, nausea, dry mouth, constipation or diarrhea, decrease in appetite, drowsiness, insomnia, shakiness, nervousness, anxiety, and sexual disturbance (males more than females).

Luvox has been excellent in addressing symptoms of obsessive-compulsive disorder, and even symptoms of obsessive-compulsive personality as well as panic attacks and anxiety. It works quite well with the stimulant medications.

17.5.6   Anti-Anxiety or Anxiolytics

Buspirone (BuSpar®) can be used to augment the action of the SSRIs as it occupies the presynaptic serotonin receptors, reducing the release of serotonin into the synapse while at the same time competing with serotonin for postsynaptic receptors, thus reducing anxiety and enhancing the antidepressant action of the SSRI drugs. BuSpar is a mild antianxiety medication that helps to calm and relieve the constant feelings of edginess, tension, and fear. Sometimes, if this is given in the early stages of anxiety when symptoms are first noticed, the person can be calmed down enough to prevent the development of panic attacks, which are very frightening. (With a panic attack, people feel as if they cannot breathe, as if they are having a heart attack.) BuSpar can be slow acting and may take more than a week to become effective. This medication can be helpful in treating agitated behavior. Common side effects are dizziness, drowsiness, restlessness, headaches, tremors, insomnia, and nausea.

Ativan® is another medication used for all groups — elderly, children, adolescents, and adults — for relief of symptoms of anxiety. However, his medication can cause agitation in the elderly. Drowsiness, lethargy, and fainting can be other side effects. This medication can interact with smoking and needs to be closely monitored if used with Digoxin®. Dosage should not exceed 2 mg in the elderly.

Xanax® is a similar medication often given for quick relief of anxiety. It is often taken during the day in small doses to quickly relieve symptoms of anxiety. It has rather immediate effects. It may cause drowsiness, lightheadedness, headache, confusion, hostility, dry mouth, nausea, vomiting, and constipation. There needs to be close monitoring if used with Digoxin.

17.5.7   Lithium Salts

Lithium is the treatment of choice for Bipolar I Disorders and is helpful for some forms of recurring unipolar depression. It may also intensify the action of tricyclic antidepressants and MAO Inhibitors. Lithium can be a very difficult medication to take due to its severe side effects.

17.5.8   MAO Inhibitors

MAO inhibitors show much promise for very impulsive ADHD children and adolescents. It prevents the enzyme MAO from breaking down the neurotransmitter norepinephrine. They must be taken very carefully because they can be fatal if mixed with particular foods. This could become quite problematic given the difficulties of food maintenance with children and adolescents.

17.5.9   Serotonergic Interventions

One medication that seems to enhance Ritalin effects is a novel antidepressant, Effexor®, used with children, adolescents, and adults at this time. Effexor tends to target the serotonin as well as the norepinephrine system.

This provides backup to Ritalin resulting in even more of an impact of the medication to help the ADD. As well, it produces good effects on symptoms of both anxiety and depression through its impact on serotonin. When used with adolescents, this medication could work quite well, but the enhanced actions of the drug (in combination with the normal high anxieties of adolescence) might be too much. When this medication does work, it is very effective and really seems to help the dramatic, overfocused subtype of ADD without hyperactivity. Serzone® emerged subsequent to Effexor to address the problems of impotence in males, and, although occurring less often, the problem remains in existence. Serzone works extremely well at lower levels of dosage to address symptoms of ruminating that plague the overfocused subtype — when used with Ritalin dosage needs to remain between approximately 50 to 150 mg to avoid the serotinergic effect.

We heard from one man who stated that this medication not only helped his Ritalin to work better, but he felt more focused, more aware and more in control of his emotions than ever before.

17.5.10   Antihypertensives

Clonidine (Catapress®) has been used often with the ADD population to help highly aroused, overactive children who responded poorly to Ritalin or Dexedrine or have persistent side effects from these medications. This medication has also been found to be beneficial for children who exhibit signs of conduct disorder, oppositional behavior, aggression, and explosiveness. It can be used alone or in combination with stimulant medication.

Clonidine treatment has resulted in improvement in both ADHD alone and ADHD with tic symptoms. Those with ADHD with comorbid tic disorders enjoy a more frequent positive behavioral response to Clonidine. Clonidine has been quite helpful in reducing symptoms of aggression, overactivity, and impulsivity, especially in those individuals who have other disorders such as Tourette's. It is beneficial for overfocused sleep-deprived children. When given a few hours before bedtime, Clonidine allows them to sleep more soundly, and wake up in the morning with less irritability. Overfocused children and adolescents who experience an adverse effect with stimulants benefit as well from this medication. Clonidine used alone, however, has not been shown to alleviate the symptoms of ADD. Side effects tend to be fatigue, headaches, dizziness, stomachaches, and nausea. Blood pressure should be monitored for rebound hypertension if the medication is suddenly withdrawn. Otherwise, this medication tends to be tolerated quite well. With the recent advent of all of the new medications, the antihypertensives are being used less often.

17.5.11   Antipsychotics

Risperdal® is a medication that can be used for psychotic symptoms in the child and all the way up to the elderly population. It can be used when individuals become very paranoid or suspicious of everyone. They may be hearing voices or seeing things that are not there. This can be very frightening for these individuals. The recommended initial dose for the elderly is 0.25 to 0.50 mg daily and not greater than 2 mg per day. Risperdal tends to operate as a milder form of medication and is, therefore, suggested for use with the elderly rather than the traditional antipsychotics. It eventually can provide an effective treatment and maintenance program. Risperdal treats the outward symptoms or positive symptoms of schizophrenia, such as delusional thinking, hostility, hallucinations, feelings of persecution, disorganized thinking, incoherence, or excitement. It also treats the negative and more hidden symptoms of emotional withdrawal or isolation, apathy, social withdrawal, lack of emotion or display of inappropriate emotion, as well as an inability to follow the flow of conversation. Treatment is based on the lowest and most effective dose for that individual. Certain antihistamines may have an additive effect on the severity of some of the side effects. When used with medications such as Sinemet®, Levadopa®, and Tegretol, this medication may become less effective. Predominant side effects are dizziness, agitation, anxiety, sleep disorders, weight gain, headache, constipation, nausea, drowsiness, tiredness, sun-sensitivity, and sexual dysfunction. There is now an oral form of this medication, Oral Solution Risperdal.

Zyxepra® is a recent antipsychotic medication that is being found clinically useful for the anxious type of individual who suffers from a loss of reality.

17.5.12   Antiseizure

Tegretol-XR® is a newly released sustained version of the antiseizure medication Tegretol and may be more suitable for the elderly, although no systematic studies have been completed. Seizure activity, which is quite common in the elderly, will occur at various stages of the aging process, even early stages depending on the degree of damage to the brain and progression of the disease. Side effects are aplastic anemia, *agranulocytosis, thrombocytopenia,* dizziness, vertigo, drowsiness, fatigue, ataxia, and a general worsening of other symptoms, as well as the aggravation of coronary artery disease.

Neurontin® is a relatively new antiseizure medication, originally introduced to augment the major antiseizure medications available, however, recent studies are showing that it can be used by itself. There are fewer side effects than with the older antiseizure medications. Side effects are dizziness, *ataxia,* fatigue, *nystagmus,* and somnolence. It is, however, usually well tolerated.

Lamictal® is a rather new medication. Originally it targeted the adult population; however, recent studies are showing use for children and the elderly. Its potential for use with the elderly is in a chewable tablet form. Side effects are rash, headache, nervousness, *asthenia,* ataxia, *diplopia,* nausea, blurred vision, dizziness, vomiting, and somnolence.

Still used are the old standbys for treatment of seizure activation, Dilantin®, Tegretol®, and Depakote®. Depakote has been showing great results to treat the out-of-control conduct-disordered behavior seen in children, as well as explosive personality disorder and mania. However, liver function and general health need to be well maintained with the usage of Depakote.

Newer antiseizure medications now being used with children are Gabitril® and the recently released medication Topirimate®. Generally the newer medications have fewer side effects, but a note of caution is in order, as often they have side effects that we do not know about until used with a large number of people over a long period of time.

17.5.13   Sleeping Medications

Ambien® allows people to fall asleep fast and to get a full night's sleep. It has a rapid onset of action (within 30 minutes) and does not cause sedation the next day. Ambien works quite well as a mild sleeping medication. However, it is intended to be used for only short periods of time. In the elderly, dosage is reduced to 5 mg immediately before bedtime. Side effects are daytime drowsiness, lightheadedness, abnormal dreams, amnesia, dizziness, headache, hangover effect and sleep disorder, nausea, vomiting, diarrhea and dry mouth.

18

Treatment Does Not Mean Just Medication

18.1 Determining the Needs of Our Children

Determining the needs of our children is based on the knowledge of what their particular age in their developmental cycle means for them. To begin, we need to understand the needs of our children: what the issues for their age are and what the expectations of normal development are. What do the experts say to expect in terms of thinking development, emotional development, and social development? The following represent some general developmental themes.

Ages 3 to 5 years

- Thinking abilities take a big jump at this age.
- Ability to be verbal increases as they emerge from the toddler stage.
- There is the belief in magical thinking and magical powers greater than themselves.
- They are likely to blame themselves if something traumatic occurs in the family, such as divorce.
- Egocentric; self-consumed; see self as center of the universe; exaggerated belief in their own power.
- The development of their inner or internal sense of security comes from the stability of their environment (the more stable the environment, the greater their internal sense of security).

Ages 5 to 10 years

- There is the need for family and to belong to some type of group that provides definition as an individual as well as a sense of being connected to something.
- This is a time of learning to socialize, the art of being social, and the building of social skills.

- This is also a time of academic abilities and a focus on learning. These very important years of academic learning are called the building-block years because what is learned each day in grades 1, 2, and 3 (and even beginning in kindergarten) becomes the foundation for all future learning. Difficulties during this time period make it particularly hard for ADD children to catch up to their peers.
- There are fears of abandonment, being left and the child needs to have an intact bond with both or at least one parent.
- Children this age remain egocentric in their thought processes and thus will still tend to feel responsible for divorce.

Throughout childhood

- Parents need to accept and encourage their feelings.
- Time needs to be allowed to express and address their feelings with some type of solution (the solution may be simply to hear their feelings).
- Assist child to express anger appropriately so they do not need to feel guilty later.
- It is important to avoid power struggles with the child during this age. They are attempting to flex their muscles and cannot back down without a loss of self-esteem, thus they need to win to develop a sense of competency in themselves.
- Set structure and routine for children at this age to provide security and stability.
- If there is a divorce, the child needs the parent to support the child's relationship with the other parent to avoid becoming polarized and aligned with one parent against the other.
- The parent needs to be available to talk about what is occurring with their children in their daily lives.

By knowing the needs of the child at each developmental age, the parent can address those needs and provide a good base for the child to then cope with the symptoms of ADD, which become less overwhelming when the child is not addressing other family or individual issues at the same time. By having a supportive family atmosphere and parents who understand their needs children can handle more adversity and difficulties in their lives than they would be able to do otherwise.

18.1.1 Recognizing the Symptoms of Depression for Early Treatment

There is a depression that naturally occurs when someone attempts to do something only to find themselves not up to the task. The result is failure.

There are certain universals in life, meaning these are things we can predict will occur given a certain sequence of events and this would be the reaction to expect from most people. Universal principles, however, will not remain true for special populations such as autism, schizophrenia, bipolar, and obsessive-compulsive disorders, as well as, genetic, biochemical disorders.

Universal principles will tend to apply to the population at large. For example, it is a universal principle that people want to be told they have done something well. It is universal that people want to be touched and hugged and made to feel special. Given the presence of ADD symptoms and the impact that such symptoms can have on one's ability to function academically, as well as socially, it is not surprising that a great amount of depression would be seen in the ADD population. In fact, anxiety and depression are probably the two most common disorders seen in the ADD population, whether we are talking about children, adolescents, or adults. Consequently, in terms of treatment, it becomes important to know what depression will look like at the different ages of the individual so we will be able to spot its existence. Depression can then be treated chemically with medical management (depending on the severity), nutritional supplements, and either individual, joint, or family therapy.

Infants and Toddlers will show depression with the following signs

- Decreased motor activity — they move less, more stationary
- Withdrawal from friends and family — not wanting to be close to anyone
- Too little or too much crying
- Excessive whining — upset all of the time
- Failure to grow and thrive in life — not participating in the world around them
- Lack of social interest in things in general
- Sad or bland — deadpan facial expression, no emotion shown on their faces

Preschoolers will show depression with the following signs

- Frequent stomachaches and headaches
- Fatigue, tiredness
- Overactivity, excessive restlessness — anxiety increases with depression and leads to increased activity
- Sadness
- Low tolerance for frustration — when they cannot do a task in the manner they expect they become agitated and want to quit
- Irritability, general agitation
- Loss of interest and joy in the activities that they used to enjoy

School-age children will show depression with the following signs

- Frequent physical complaints, stomachaches, headaches etc.
- Refusal to go to school or avoidance of school
- Weight loss or gain — depending on their tendency to gain or lose weight
- Hostility or aggression — the child is more angry, more snappy and irritable
- Grades drop from where they were — the child studies less and appears to not care as much about academic studies
- Hopelessness — tearful much of the time

Adolescents will show depression with the following signs

- Grades drop, poor conduct, more argumentative, more out-of-control behavior
- Fatigue — they often spend a lot of time sleeping
- Low self-esteem — the idea that nothing they do is right
- Sleep and eating patterns change depending on the tendency to lose or gain weight
- Self-destructive behavior — actions that have very negative consequences
- Careless about their physical appearance; different from a prior concern and obvious caring about how they dressed and looked

Adults will show depression with the following signs

- Listlessness, overall fatigue, malaise
- Loss of interest in activities that used to be fun and bring pleasure
- Sleeping and eating problems — cannot control and regulate food or sleep
- Tend to be a victim of the disorder
- True depressive — always predicts the worst, highly negative
- Limited by fear of failure and lots of avoidance
- No interest in anything, loss of hope for the future
- Others find themselves tired when with them
- They tend to predict disaster striking; they see only the worst
- They don't hear anyone else and listen only to their own often crooked thinking
- When they have an idea about something, they become stuck in it

- They isolate and insulate, they don't allow any new ideas, information or events to happen in their lives that might be more positive or rewarding

Knowing the signs of depression will *allow parents or spouses to take some type of preventive action* before things become too problematic and disaster strikes. Besides medication and nutrition, treatment can involve some type of activity, even if these individuals resist and complain. These people should be pushed toward doing something, preferably some type of activity with people, even if it is only for an hour. Going to the movies provides an escape from depressing thoughts (maybe not *Titanic*) and often can change the person's outlook on things, at least temporarily. Sometimes just to laugh at something, find anything funny provides a relief. Exercise on a regular basis helps to release tension. It is difficult to be anxious or depressed and still exercise. Therefore, although these individuals may balk at going, and initially things are difficult for them (depression really depletes your energy) by the end of the workout, they feel good.

The idea is to *change the point of reference*. When the person is tired, at the end of their day, things look pretty black and bleak. However, a workout, on a sunny morning, listening to lively music, things may look a little more promising. What this does, however, is provide only a temporary relief, not a cure. The possibility exists though, that during this time of temporary relief, people may then take the risk they have been avoiding, do something different to change their lives and this will eventually treat the depression.

18.2 "I Just Forgot"

One of the more frustrating things that occurs in the ADD household is that it is quite common for the ADD child, adolescent, or adult to forget something important. When they forget something that the parent wants them to do it impacts the parent's life. When they forget to do something that their spouses want, the spouses' lives are affected. It does not always impact someone else, sometimes it impacts only the ADD person. However, then their life becomes more chaotic and confused, without resolution.

The more important the task the ADD person forgets to do, *the more frustrated you will feel* and the more guilty they will be as a result. Try to prevent this from even occurring as all it does is lead to anger, frustration, and upset with the ADD person. You will find yourself liking them even less. (You always love them, but often you don't like them.)

If you have something that is very important to you to have done, set it up for the ADD person to be geared toward success. Plan it so failure will be virtually impossible. This may mean writing sticky notes. This may mean reminding them of what you need in the morning and then again just minutes before you need them to actually accomplish the task. If you want your spouse or child to be available for a social event, write it on the calendar, remind them the night before, and remind them the morning of the event. Set up all kinds of stop-gap measures, such as telling them they need to be there 1 hour before they actually need to be there. The idea is to make things so foolproof that failure is not a possibility.

18.3 Learning is "Boring"

The more exciting things are, the more ADD children or adults are *likely to learn, retain,* and *be able to recall* what they have learned. The less exciting, the more material is subject to interference from other, more interesting information. The brain tends to zero in on the information that most important. Due to under-arousal, the ADD brain will tend to choose what is exciting because that is naturally arousing. In fact, if something is externally exciting, it seems to bypass the ADD symptoms and you will not tend to see ADD. As stated before, ADD symptoms appear when things are boring, so the idea is to work at making the mundane exciting.

This is where the multimodal process is helpful. Using different modalities, such as touch, sight, sound, and taste, can render the material or stimuli salient or important, despite being intrinsically boring. This is what occurs when a movie is made about a war that, if read about in a history book, would put us to sleep. Suddenly the war comes to life, the historical material that we have read becomes something with which to identify, because it's been given a story line with lots of sound effects and colorful costumes. Many people had heard of the *Titanic* and what happened, yet knew relatively few details about this major event. Now, thanks to a movie of epic proportions, the *Titanic* tragedy has become real for us.

It is not exciting for children to sit in a classroom all day long and listen to someone talk, especially when verbal language is the most difficult type of information for them to process. It is particularly difficult for ADD children due to spatial issues and the inability to visualize spoken words, which is what most people tend to do naturally. Due to the difficulty of assimilation, verbal information is highly susceptible to information-processing deficits and the loss of details. The answer is to augment verbal learning with some other type of modality that makes the material stimulating.

Another problem can occur with new learning. An outer structure needs to be developed that will allow new information to be accommodated and assimilated. Due to the spatial problem, the development of an outer structure with which to relate new information to old is not always present internally. It, therefore, needs to be applied concretely and specifically. Generally, the structure is automatically implemented with the provision of new information. With ADD people, this is not always the case and if they do not specifically create a structure, they have no way to process the information and make sense of it.

The computer uses multimodal approaches, using several systems, visual and aural, to increase the odds of the user getting the information via input and then processing that information. In this day of high technology, the Internet has provided a critical link for ADD people. It is an excellent information resource that can aid in the enhancment of self-esteem and pride in their accomplishments.

18.4 Fostering Self-Esteem

Obsessive-compulsive behavior, or perfectionism in the ADD person, is their attempt to do something well and gain some sense of self-esteem to make up for how terrible they tend to feel about themselves. Thus, the brighter they are, and the more serious the ADD, the more upset they become when they can't do things as they expect, and the more they need to do something, *anything*, perfectly. Hence, perfectionism becomes a necessary part of their life. By fostering increased self-esteem people can come to accept the symptoms of the ADD disorder and understand that it is a part of life, like wearing glasses. It is when they don't accept the ADD, determine that it is bad or terrible, and become somehow *not* okay, that the need to be perfect in a few specific areas occurs and people can get out of balance. Rather than attempting to be perfect in a few areas, they should concentrate on building weaker areas. In this manner, they can become more balanced as opposed to the tendency to do a few things extremely well, which often limits the risk-taking that new learning would require.

As children build their strengths and neglects their weaknesses, they can develop such large gaps in their learning and abilities that they appear to have been involved in a head injury or have brain damage, as opposed to the ADD. The gaps that are created as a result of a lack of learning can have a tremendous impact on an individual's life. Reading is an example of this. When reading becomes difficult, it is easy to abandon. Often ADD person will inform you that *reading is boring* and that is the reason they do not read.

The impact on the self-esteem as a result of the ADD often tells a very sad tale. The brilliant person who never went to college. The person who stays in the same job, hating it, yet fearful of making the necessary changes to move to a different type of work. The low self-esteem results in tremendous losses, experiences that were never encountered, tasks that were never completed, and lives that were not quite lived. ADD persons remain frustrated with themselves and their own lack of accomplishments. They bemoan what could have been and ultimately feel frustrated and angry at those around them.

EXAMPLE
We recently evaluated a 45-year-old full-time nurse and mother of two children. We were going through the results and the woman began to respond with rather derogatory statements about her performance that we were just beginning to go over. She made statements such as, "Oh, I didn't think I did badly on that, did I do bad on that?" "Oh this is terrible, well I had a headache that day." Finally, we asked her if she was going to continue to beat herself up and defend her performance throughout the whole evaluation. She indicated that she was not aware she was doing this and yes, she was a perfectionist and wanted everything to be correct.

18.5 Use of the Computer

We cannot say enough about the use of that interactive, CD ROM computer and the difference it has made in our household. Our son feels so different about himself. He has learned countless new factoids. He uses the word processor and can finally read what he has to say. For the first time in 7 years, this year there was no summer school yet he actually learned more.

Truly, this appears to be a major helpmate for the ADD individual. Computer programs are stimulating and, therefore, bypass the ADD symptoms. Computers use several modalities at one time, making the material both interesting and easier to comprehend. By using several modalities such as sound and visual, the ADD person is able to take in the information and make use of it. Computer programs can be individually tailored to meet people's needs and provide instantaneous monitoring. Users can go at their own pace. The computer holds their interest and allows them to learn in a setting that meets their specific needs.

Retraining the brain and enhancing the spatial areas can occur through the use of the computer. There are many programs employing the parts-to-the-whole concept, which automatically forces the person to train that often unused area. The key is to identify those programs that the individual finds difficult. Generally the more difficult the task is for the individual the higher the probability that there are spatial factors involved. We tell children they are going on a weight-training program for their brain using the computer.

Programs are available to target weak academic areas. There are programs to learn a language, improve math skills, and explain math concepts. Reading benefits tremendously from use of the computer. There are programs where a word slides across the screen, the computer says the word, defines it, and spells it. Using different modalities, the computer is able to make the information interesting enough for learning to occur. Saying the word allows people to memorize their words through a sight vocabulary that is necessary for reading due to the problem with phonetics. Research is confirming that people can learn to read and improve their knowledge by memorizing words. The better that they are at memorizing words, the better the reading skills, the less likelihood that they will misread the word. The computer becomes a teacher. And it does all of this in a fun way.

Learning is made fun through the encyclopedia program offered on the computer that allows people to learn and enjoy themselves. What a wonderful way to learn something — dancing figures on the screen accompanied by words, music, and action.

The newest thing is voice-activated computers that are going to become more common in the very near future. What this means is that you can talk into the computer and it will type the words for you. No more spelling errors. No more typos and phrasing that does not make sense. These computers are already in use by the learning-disabled population and are soon to be available to the general public.

18.6 Building Social Skills: What is Appropriate and What is Not?

It is important to provide social knowledge or information directly to your child. ADD children generally do not pick up all of the social nuances in their world and often miscue situations due to this lack of knowledge. When you are out with your child and see someone doing something inappropriate, discreetly point this out to your child. Talk over the situation in depth, who did what, when, and where. Talk about the why of things. Help the child to understand what the problem was or is and how it could have been handled in a more effective manner. Thus, as a parent, you begin to provide the type of information the child may not see and to teach that child in a very concrete and specific manner how to relate well to others socially.

Groups can be a very effective means of teaching social skills and allowing ADD children and adolescents, and even adults, to interact with each other in a positive manner. In these groups, examples are provided of behavior that will become problematic and behavior that is a more positive approach to a given social situation. Modeling provides a concrete example for the people to commit to memory and add to their repertoire of social responses.

Identifying exactly what is problematic socially for the individual provides the direction for treatment. Working with the child, adolescent, or adult on rearranging what is appropriate, what will fit and what will not, provides them access to increased information on how to approach or address social interactions. By teaching a number of procedures, solutions, and approaches in a concrete manner, individuals are provided with a number of social interventions that they can apply to any given situation.

18.7 Nonverbal Interactions and Tone

ADD persons are unaware of their voice and tone becoming louder than the norm or not in keeping with a situation. Their voices may accidentally rise with their excitement. Sometimes that voice modulation may become difficult as a result of spatial issues. They may miss the whole picture of the social situation, or the whole of the conversation, or the whole of their own conversation and, thus, voice modulation. Their voices may trail off as they become lost in another thought while still completing the thought they were presenting at that point in time.

Sometimes just talking and working things through with these individuals helps them to figure out what happened in a social situation that resulted in their being rejected or ignored. Showing them how they may be presenting themselves negatively with nonverbal behaviors by modeling the tone of their voices, facial expression, and body posture (leaning forward or backward means different things) provides a concrete understanding of a very painful experience. We cannot fix what we don't know or understand.

ADD persons need to understand that they cannot take all comments literally. Explain that sometimes one thing can be meant when it is said, but the tone of voice can make those words sound quite different, often not what was intended. A simple tone of voice can upset someone in a hurry. Leaning forward can show that you are interested, although sometimes it can be threatening. Leaning backward or folding one's arms tends to communicate disinterest or intimidation. Softening one's voice can communicate empathy and compassion. However, making one's voice too soft may communicate fear or vulnerability. Speaking in a strong and definitive voice filled with commanding authority may make people feel as if they are being parented, so they become resentful over being told what to do. Once again, the key is balance and the understanding that social relationships can be highly impacted by tone of voice and body language.

18.8 Empathy Skills

How can we teach empathy skills? Sometimes ADD persons, unintentionally, are not particularly empathetic. They don't realize how the little things create warm feelings that pass from one individual to another. Social nuances can be specifically taught. It is those little things that make such a difference in relationships. Describing things like how a pause of silence between someone finishing a sentence and another person speaking indicates a more thoughtful response can be very helpful.

When someone says something like "Boy I am having a hard day," and the person immediately responds, "So am I," the first person does not feel as if they have been heard. Everyone likes to be heard and pausing is a great social tool that can be used to foster good communication. Repeating back part or all of the sentence also communicates to others that they have been heard.

Little things contribute so much to a personal relationship. The development of social skills that ADD people do not necessarily pick up in their world and that we can teach and give to them directly helps them communicate more clearly.

18.9 Awareness of Personal Space

People have spaces that should not be invaded unless one is invited to do so; learning to gauge the boundaries of a person's space is very important. Similarly, one type of touch may be appropriate and another may not. The intensity of the contact or touching the wrong spot can make people uncomfortable. Touching someone in a way or place they do not like can set off a reaction that is not expected and create a rather traumatizing social situation for the ADD child, adolescent, or adult. Knowing the difference between a positive (light and soft) and negative (harsh, poking) touch and what it will communicate to others is critical for anyone in a social situation. These are things that we can teach directly to ADD children. They may not have learned these things, which can contribute to their being socially outcast or neglected by their classmates.

18.10 Dressing for Acceptance

It may sound snobbish, but there is something to be said about the way one dresses. Style of dress can communicate moods, such as dressing for the evening when going somewhere during the day, or clothing that is overly tight or loose. Children, and especially adolescents, can easily be labeled a if their style of dress is unlike their peers.

When ADD children are among their classmates, their tendency is not to compare themselves, to check out everyone else to see what they are wearing and to want to be in tune with them. This is probably more true of boys than girls, but girls often lack awareness as well. Things begin to change in pre-adolescence and adolescence. There is almost a type of awakening that occurs for ADD children who, several years behind their peers, all of a sudden wake up and become aware of themselves in comparison with their peers. This early lack of awareness may be due to either spatial deficits, information-processing deficits, or both.

18.11 Hygiene

Taking care of one's hygiene becomes increasingly critical as the child gets older. Often ADD children are unaware of why they need to bathe more often, when it is time to begin using deodorant, and how this may be a factor in ostracizing them from their friends. This is not true of all ADD children. Sometimes this issue is not related to ADD at all, but rather is a cultural value. Many parents, depending on where they were raised and how, do not believe in bathing on a daily basis. The care of teeth and the number of visits to the physician fall under the same category. Children believe and follow what is taught in the home, having no idea that things are supposed to be any different, until encountering someone outside the family system who either teases them, makes fun of them, or, in a professional position, communicates a need to change those habits.

18.12 Parental Anger and the Need for Anger-Management Training

There is a cyclical pattern involving the anger of the parents of ADD children. The children misbehave and the parents feel helpless and inadequate. The parents, who may be ADD as well, inconsistently set limits, overindulge, and then overreact when the children misbehave again. The parents feel increased failure and frustration and ultimately anger. They express that anger and then feel guilty for doing so. This sets off the cycle and things proceed all over again.

Overall, parents tend to misinterpret their children's misbehavior as a sign of their own inadequacy as parents. They become angry with themselves, angry with the children and their guilt grows. To alleviate their guilt, they overindulge the children. This inconsistent behavior is confusing to the children, who may misbehave again to see what will happen. At times, the feelings of frustration parents experience lead to depression and even less structure and limit-setting in the home. This promotes more problem behavior on the part of the children and the cycle is repeated. All of this is to say that parents need to remain consistent and firm. However, many parents of ADD children are ADD themselves and consistency is, therefore, difficult for them.

Sometimes parents see the child's behavior as aimed at them. The child is perceived as deliberately trying to upset them, to make them feel bad, to embarrass them. They see the child's behavior as the way the child gets back at them for imposing some previous disciplinary action. These parents may not be connected with their children. They may see their children as a job or duty for whom they are responsible. Those parents want their children to behave all of the time. They tend to want their children to be like wooden soldiers — seen and not heard. These parents may be addicted, participating in the addictions of alcohol, food, drugs, work, or shopping and the child impedes what they want to do.

One of the hardest things to do is to remain consistent as a parent, whether you are ADD or not. As life becomes more busy, more hectic, more demanding, it becomes more difficult to impose the punishment that you have told the child that you would do. Sometimes you are too tired to impose the punishment or too tired to put up with the child being upset and whining at you. So you let it go, thinking that tomorrow will be different — only it isn't.

Behavior-management programs will become successful by defining the types of punishments that the parent can consistently impose and implement. This cuts down on the anger in the household. If the parent is not angry about having to impose the discipline they feel pressured to do and don't want to do, they do not foster anger in the household.

The best time for parents to discipline children is when they are not angry. Parents are instituting something that is going make the children uncomfortable, not them. Therefore, the ideal situation is when parents can tell children they are sorry that this has to happen, and mean it. They communicate empathy to the children, while the children have to experience the consequences of their behavior, which, hopefully, will decrease the likelihood of the behavior recurring. Teaching parents how to impose sanctions that will have more of an impact on children than on themselves is the utmost in behavior management and discipline. Children learn right from wrong, and there are consequences to their behavior, without the whole process having to be so negative and filled with anger. Teaching behavior-management programs that work without a great amount of effort on the part of the parent can be fun for both parent and child and can ease the tensions in the household. Using a "goodie" menu (see Figure 18.1), rewarding for good behavior, allows parents to shape and mold the behavior they desire from their child without anyone having to be upset or angry. Giving the child a job to do around the household promotes self esteem. Later, the parent can be proud of what the child has accomplished, while still imposing the discipline. The idea is to not be angry while disciplining and that will accomplish the goal of shaping the child's behavior more effectively.

Parents must give an ADD child more attention and give it so that the child will attend to the parent. With ADD, the child makes the parent attend to them. Parents of ADD children need to be managers, implementing a higher degree of attention and management than parents of children who do not have ADD. ADD children respond better when they are attended to in the way that they need. The problem is resources: there is not enough of the parent to go around, especially when there is more than one child in the family. This problem becomes more intense with several ADD children in one family or some other type of disorder demanding equal amounts of parental attention.

18.12.1   Anger Management for Both Parents and Children

Anger-management training is designed to create problem-solving skills and to improve information processing. Its goal is to modulate the reactions of anger, improve our thought (cognitive) processes, and lessen the effect of physical symptoms (physiological) symptoms. Methodology is to train the person to recognize when they are angry, interpret the situation correctly, and cope with both their own anger and of the anger of others.

1. First recognize your own anger and know that when people get angry they move into a "right brain lock." This means that anger is such an all-encompassing emotional reaction that we immediately move into the emotional area of the right brain and then get stuck there (the left brain is our thinking, or rational area). We cannot be emotional and rational at the same time. That is why it is impossible to talk to people when they are crying or screaming. They are so stuck in their emotions they can't think, let alone relate to you. So recognize that either your own anger or someone else's anger will produce that right brain lock.

   To get out of that lock it is necessary first to be aware of it. The symptoms include a tingling sensation, the heart starts to thump, the face feels warm, tone of voice is raised, sweating increases, and breathing quickens.

2. Using a method of relaxation to move out of the anger is important. Count, breathe in and out deeply, or imagine a beautiful scene, any of these will work.

3. Review the situation objectively. Look at the whole picture to understand what is happening. Maybe someone has jumped to a

conclusion without evidence. Look at what someone has said or done from a different perspective, rather than seeing them as someone who wanted to hurt you or be unkind to you. Also, realize that it is easy to misinterpret what someone has said.

4. Use "cool-down" statements, repeating things that allow you to work the situation out

- you can handle this
- it will be okay
- the anger does not scare me
- I can make it
- I am in control
- I can do it

Cool-down statements allow us to remain logical and to handle the situation without getting into that right brain lock.

Remember that we can get angry and control it. Others can get angry and we can handle it. Anger management is especially critical in adolescence. Adolescents need assistance in recognizing their angry feelings, and in understanding what events or things will trigger anger in their lives. Point out and warn against the strong tendency to misattribute (misinterpret the anger) and help them develop their coping skills to deal with anger.

18.13 Stress Management

Staying in control means managing stress. This does not mean allowing things to build inside until they burst forth like a volcano. When one feels out of control and totally overwhelmed, stress increases and becomes a problem. Plan effectively, know the limitations of both yourself and of time. Set goals that can be met and know when to stop and relax. We have sayings such as "stop and smell the roses." But who has time?

One of the things that we unfortunately learn as we get older is that being superwoman or superman becomes increasingly harder to do. We think that we can burn the candle at both ends, stay up all night and function effectively the next day, and we can't. We think that we can accomplish all of the tasks that we set, no matter how large or how small and sometimes we can and sometimes we can't. The idea is to look at things, size up the time factor, see what can be delegated and what can't. Take a few minutes to assess the situation before plunging in with both feet and going under. And last but not least, do take the time to smell those roses, and to do just nothing.

18.14   The Structured School or Boarding School

Private schools with smaller numbers in their classrooms may be beneficial to ADD children by offering increased monitoring and one-on-one attention. Sometimes we provide our children with so many choices that they are overwhelmed and cannot make a decision. Generally speaking, these schools offer fewer choices: finishing your homework is not a choice, it is expected. There surely are stories to the contrary but the 50s taught us that children can have choices without being militaristic. Many of the private structured schools, if for no other reason than to stay in business, will make accommodations for the ADD student.

Some private schools remain dated; they are unaware of the new research on ADD and still see it as a childhood disorder. They may make accommodations by allowing the child to do less work, which only teaches the child to get along with less. Thus, they may make accommodations to appease the parent without understanding what is truly needed to accommodate the ADD child. The public schools have spent thousands of dollars learning about this disorder, sponsoring conferences for their teachers to attend and learn what the ADD child truly needs.

The boarding school focuses the child's attention on academics; there are fewer external distractions present in this type of educational environment. There is no one right answer. Sometimes a new setting and the opportunity to start over allows the child the freedom to be a different kid, and a different student. This can become positive in that they are able to make the changes they always wanted to make without encountering the negative feedback or anticipations others may have of them, based on their past behavior. They have a blank slate to be whatever they always wanted to be. They can "turn over a new leaf."

18.15   Finding the College that Fits Your Child

Colleges now offer ADD students untimed evaluations, individual testing rooms, and permission to use tape recorders or note takers. It is very exciting to see the accommodations that are being made for the ADD student. Prospective college students must assess strengths and weaknesses, then determine which college can most meet their needs. Visiting the college, meeting some of the faculty, and interviewing with the dean can help in making the correct decision. There may be a range of support services offered, such as degree-requirement substitutions, alternative examination, note-taking services, recorded reading materials, technological tools and auxiliary aids, tutorial and learning assistance, support groups, self-management instruction, individual therapy, strategic schedule planning, reduced course load, mentorship and assistance with vocational choices.

18.16 The Specific Coping Mechanisms

Specific coping mechanisms (see Chapter 9) provide relief for individual symptoms of ADD and help ADD people to effectively manage symptoms and their lives.

18.17 Behavior Management Training Programs for Parent and Child: The Position of the Parent in Today's Culture

The current youth culture is so drastically different from any other culture in our history that the parent of the ADD child is in a position that has never been seen before. This is one of the first times in history where our culture means more to our children than their parents and their family do. Adolescence is now fraught with diametrically opposed value systems between their parents and their peer groups. We have never seen this phenomenon, we have no parenting models to provide expertise on how to cope with today's youth. Our parents never had to contend with the loss of more and more control over their children as do today's parents. It is no longer a surprising and startling fact when a teenager runs away from home. In the past this would have been a major deal for both parents and the community.

Therefore, it takes special parents to raise an ADD child. They may need to try parent-training methods and a few sessions with a family therapist. This does not mean that they are poor parents, only that they require a variety of methods to attempt to cope with today's requirements. What we have found is that ADD children benefit from a multiple approach, designed to facilitate a higher degree of success. Those families who work with one or more educational strategies and alternatives aimed at approaching many of the different ways that a child can learn attain greater success. Parents need to be up to date on medication and aware of the ever-changing need for medication shifting that occurs as the child grows. Today's parents are forced to cope with the trials of managed care and to demand medication that is not generic, and to prove the need for more-extensive evaluation than their health insurance plan routinely has to offer. Parents need more help from the psychiatric and psychological community during a time when managed care is designed to cut costs by offering only short-term crisis treatment, thus making it more difficult for families to obtain services for longer treatment. Parents become caught in the battle between their insurance agency and their doctors. The primary-care physician from their managed-care plan, who apparently is instructed to approve only absolutely necessary procedures, will tend to discourage any alternative treatment approaches parents would like to try for their children.

Parents are faced with situations for which they have no parenting models because their parents were never placed in such situations. Further, most families now need two incomes to support their household given the increased cost of living. Therefore, where previously one parent was in the home to make phone calls, doctor appointments, and keep the house intact, now no one is there to do this full-time job. It has to be split between two full-time working parents. Children, unable to obtain the time they require from these busy, harassed parents, turn to their peer group for comfort and the cycle continues downward. Parents realize the need to attend to ADD children and see the positive results but feel caught between the needs of the other children in the home. Siblings become understandably jealous that their ADD brother or sister receives attention for noncompliant behavior, i.e., the kid who does not follow the rules gets more attention. Parenting becomes a balancing act between the needs of the ADD child and the needs of the other children in the household. This whole problem is increased if there is another ADD child or some other type of disorder present. Thus, parents are facing the toughest issues of all time without models or experience or education in how to work their way through this often overwhelming, rather hopeless, maze.

18.18 Parent-Training Programs

Parent-training programs provide education for the parent by suggesting various behavior-management programs for the child, presenting new information on medical management, revealing extensive information regarding ADD and other issues that may impact their children. All help to enrich parents' knowledge and supplement their coping skills. To provide clear diagnostic information about the child, a very specific diagnosis of the attentional disorder and a psychological evaluation is performed. This allows parents to have some degree of predictability regarding their child: by knowing the child better, so they are better able to predict his or her behavior.

We have developed a very effective parent-training program that provides pertinent information to its graduates. Long after the program is over, they still utilize the information to cope with the demands of their ADD child, adolescent or young adult. The program, which consists of six sessions, addresses the following areas and provides the latest research findings.

- The first session outlines the differences between the two subtypes of ADD without hyperactivity and ADHD. We talk in depth about symptoms that may be similar between these two disorders, but for very different reasons.

- The second session spends time discussing and providing a clear understanding of some of the correlated disorders that go along with ADD without hyperactivity and ADHD. Examples are presented of how the presence of these related disorders can impact the ADD symptoms in a cyclical spiral, at times making ADD symptoms worse.

- The third session deals with behavior-management strategies and the evaluation process. It deals with how to employ coping mechanisms based on the findings of the evaluation and the delineation of the child's strengths and weaknesses.

- The fourth session provides information on medical management. The different types of medications available to treat ADD symptoms are presented as well as symptoms related to other related disorders. This includes information on nutritional supplements.

- The fifth session addresses family treatment suggestions: how to conduct family meetings and settle conflicts that occur within the family. This session also discusses how to address the school system and your child if certain accommodations become necessary. This includes a discussion of Section 504 and various other mandated federal policies.

- The sixth session makes time for parents to provide specific examples of problematic situations or behaviors that occur within the home. Suggestions are provided as to what can be done to cope with these issues.

Shaping the Behavior of the Child

The following is a behavioral program utilized in a rather successful manner by Dr. Beckley over the years to address problems in the school setting and with the child at home. The idea of this program which utilizes a "goodie" menu and a contract, is to teach the child how to behave, not to punish or reward behavior. This allows the parent to be in the position of *teaching* rather than *controlling* child behavior.

Certain General Issues are Critical to the Success of This Program

1. It is important to reward "good" behavior as soon as possible. Otherwise, you will have lost the connection between the behavior and the positive consequence of that behavior.

2. During a vacation, most contracts or programs are suspended unless you want to take the program with you.

3. Be prepared to put the contract or grid in a place where the child does not have access if you believe that the child will want to rip up the program or tear up the contract.

4. If you are not concerned with any aggressive act on the part of your child, place the grid or contract on the refrigerator or where it is most likely to be seen by family members.

5. Be careful to not have a punishment turn out to be a reward, e.g., having the child clean the kitchen when you are there, which provides time with the parent rather than a punishment.

6. Pick punishments that will fulfill some type of task or job that needs to be done around the home so the child can then be proud and the family members can give the child credit for task completion. The length of time a task takes is dependent on the age of the child. There should be an increase of 2 minutes for each year of life. So a child of 5 years can do a 10-minute task. A child of 6 years can do a 12-minute task and so on.

7. Pick rewards that are actually what you already provide for the child and that are easy for you to give. Rewards must be things that you can provide immediately and that do not cost a lot of money or time on the part of the parent. Thus, the reward is something that the parent is willing to give and that is easy for them to give.

8. If attempting to use any of these programs in the classroom, always pick the best, most complacent child who you know will be successful at a given task. This child's response can be presented as a positive reinforcer so other children will want to participate.

Step One

Develop a good, clear-operating, written goal of what you want to change or have the child do differently. Goals need to be specific in terms of days, time, task, and criteria for completion. Criteria for completion are set by the parent *not* the child. Remember that parents and children are not equal.

Step Two

Develop a goodie reward menu. You should choose a reward that the child will work for and that the parent can comfortably provide. Consider what you already give away as a reward for good behavior. Ask children for their input and discuss the kinds of things they would want. Rewards should be tangible, approachable, and easily implemented. Low-cost items, with a minimum of three items and maximum of six items. Examples are uninterrupted time with the parent, choosing the evening meal, extension of bed time, watching their favorite TV show that night, or special privileges. The reward has to be instant, something such as going to a movie is expensive and not easily implemented right away. The delivery system has to be easy on the parent and needs to occur shortly after the completed task behavior.

Step Three

Develop the punishment menu. Think of all the things that you want to have done in the home, any job that the family needs to have done, from which the family will benefit, and of which the child can be proud. Examples are cleaning a common area, mopping the floor, cleaning the kitchen, weeding the garden, and so on. Again, be careful the task does not become rewarding in some manner other than pride of accomplishment.

▨ Goodie Menu
(What are you giving away?)
1. Free time minutes
2. Gum/Candy
3. Choosing activities
4. Stuff...

▨ Punishment Menu
(What do you need completed?) *2 min per year of life*
1. Clean
2. Polish
3. Sweep
4. Physical task

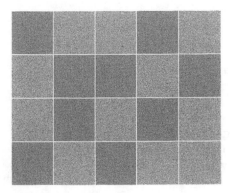

1st = 50% +1
2nd = 25% + 1
3rd = 10% +1

Goal:
Who
Does what
How well

FIGURE 18.1
An example of the grid that a parent can create to employ the behavior-management program.

Step Four

In this step the grid is made for either 20 or 30 days. There are 20 or 30 squares. Half of the squares plus one extra are colored in at random. Remember this is a recording device, not a calendar.

Step Five

Day One

After clearly setting the goal, parents determine that the child has successfully completed the predetermined criteria.

- parents put their initials in the box for day one. The child moves to the next square.

Parents determine that the child has **not** successfully completed the predetermined criteria.

- parents do **not** put their initial in the box for day one. The child remains in the same box in the grid, frozen on the game board until successful at task completion. The child chooses a punisher from the punishment list for that day.

The child is successful with task completion and for **that day** has landed on a **colored** square.

- the child chooses something from the goodie menu for that day.

Day Two

Parents determine that the child has successfully completed the predetermined criteria.

- parents put their initial in the box for day two. The child moves to the next square.

Parents determine that the child has **not** successfully completed the predetermined criteria.

- parents do **not** put their initials in the box for day two. The child remains in the same box in the grid, frozen on the game board until successful at task completion. The child chooses a punisher from the punishment list for that day.

The child is successful with task completion and for **that day** has landed on a **colored** square.

- the child chooses something from the goodie menu for that day.

Developing a Contract

- Good contracts need to provide a return on your children's investment.
- Have children talk about what they would find interesting and what their motivators would be for them to buy into the contract.
- Establish the goal you want to be attained, again be very specific.
- Decide who does what and how well. There has to be a renegotiation date and it has to be signed by parent, child and some other individual. It is this triad that provides greater authenticity to the contract.
- Answer the question of what to do if the contract does not work or children do not comply. A Screw-Up Plan needs to be developed that will kick in if the contract does not work.
- The longest period of time for a given contract is 30 days. One goal at a time is used and it must be specific. Examples for goals are clothing picked up off the floor five out of seven days, bathroom cleaned every other day and so on. Use observable, quantifiable behavior when setting goal for contract.

CONTRACT

WHO:
DOES WHAT:
HOW WELL:
REWARD UPON COMPLETION:
CLAUSE:

RE-NEGOTIATION DATE:

SIGNED_____
SIGNED_____
SIGNED_____

Organization of One's Room: Thoughts and Life in General

There needs to be a place for everything, a spot where things can be put away after children are done using them. Everything needs to be separated according to either use, need, or category. Eliminating the clutter that tends to surround ADD people allows them to think in a clearer manner. A schedule

should be established where once per week or once per month "stuff" is elim-
inated, papers and trash are thrown out and what is not needed is given or
thrown away. Once per year, closets need to be cleaned and those clothes not
worn during the year given away or sold at a local resale shop (you can make
money getting rid of stuff). Everything has a place and there is a place for
everything. Bins are set up, drawers and closets arranged to allow things to be
used and put back where they belong in a manner that is not taxing for the
ADD person.

Controversial Treatments that Are Still Being Researched

Biofeedback

Biofeedback is a technique that employs signals as "feedback" that allows
users to teach themselves to increase certain kinds of brain-wave activity and
decrease other kinds. The theory is to arouse certain areas of the brain and thus
decrease symptoms of ADD. However, lack of comprehensive research and
evidence of long-term results makes biofeedback a risky venture. Initial results
appear promising, however there is no support with follow-up studies. Studies
that have been conducted are few in number and flawed, providing questionable findings. While biofeedback remains proven highly effective for pain control, it has not shown substantial results with the ADD population.

Diets

There is failure to support the notion of a specific link between symptoms of
ADD and a particular diet. However, it has been found that ADD individuals
who suffer from allergies will benefit from a specific diet. This will improve
their physical state of being and thus allow them to function better from a physical perspective. However, any diet, any program, will offer more attention to
the ADD child, and ADD is a disorder of inattention. Therefore, attention that
provides increased structure, more one-on-one time and more monitoring will
automatically show improvement in the behavior and studies of the ADD child.

Chiropractic Adjustments

There is information to suggest that chiropractic adjustments of ADHD children who have misalignments in their spines that irritate the nervous system
have been helpful in alleviating their hyperactivity. It has been implied that
ADHD is related to these misalignments, which then contribute to their
hyperactivity. The idea proposed by the chiropractic community is that

adjustments to the spine calm the children by easing their irritation. Research again remains inconclusive regarding the effects of this treatment.

Massage

The use of massage therapy has been suggested as an adjunct to medication for treatment of ADHD with children. Massage has been found to decrease some of the side effects of medication, specifically headaches and sleep disturbances. Children are taught to massage themselves to address their symptoms of distractibility as a recentering process. There is a paucity of research available to document the above findings and this treatment remains in question as well. Barring any trauma incurred with regard to the massage process for children, outwardly, it would appear that teaching the child to soothe themselves with massage could be a useful endeavor.

Applied Kinesiology

This theory has emerged from the work with learning disabilities and purports that restoring the misalignment of two specific cranial bones to their proper position via specific bodily manipulations will correct the learning problem. This theory, however, has not been supported by research nor shown to have produced long-term effects.

Antimotion-Sickness Medication

There are advocates of an "inner ear" theory that assumes that ADD is the result of problems with the vestibular system. The theory also relates another area of the brain, the cerebellum, and the notion that problems with motion and balance may cause the symptoms of ADD. This theory is inconsistent with what we understand in terms of the chemical/electrical workings of the brain and has not been proven in clinical research.

Optometric Vision

This theory is based on the idea that visual disorders underlie reading problems and can be corrected by a series of vision-treatment programs using colored lenses. Very few studies have investigated the technique, thus it is highly criticized, viewed as unfounded, and not recommended for use.

Candida Yeast

This notion states that toxins produced by yeast overgrowth weaken the immune system and make the body susceptible to ADD. This theory is not supported. However, treatment programs to discourage yeast infections are helpful when warranted. ADD persons may have a tendency toward developing such infections as the result of poor eating habits and over-usage of fast foods.

Megavitamins and Mineral Supplements

Generally, research has not been able to prove that the use of vitamins will significantly alter the learning patterns of the ADD individual. Vitamins can be extremely helpful in treating the ADD adult, who usually suffers from an undue degree of stress and is therefore vulnerable to the effects of stress on their physical state.

There are some research studies currently being conducted on two specific products for the ADD population, both of which claim to be successful in treating the symptoms of ADD and improving the child's ability to function in the classroom situation. Pycnogenol, Super Green Algae, and Phyto Bears claim to have a generalized calming effect to significantly increase mental alertness and sustained attention, to increase organizational skills in the child or adult, to diminish impulsivity and aggressiveness and to develop control of overall behavior.

Clinically, we have not found such substances to be substantial in treating symptoms of ADD. We have evaluated children on these substances and found the symptoms of ADD still clearly exhibited. If anything, these nutritional supplements do provide some relief for distractibility because they appear to exert some calming effect on the individual, they *do* seem to be of benefit in the total functioning of the individual, improving the immune-system response and perhaps allowing for less medication to be taken (although this remains to be proven). These nutritional supplements and others provide the ability to flush the stored environmental and metabolic toxins out of the body, to intercept and neutralize free radicals within the blood stream, which becomes more necessary as we grow older.

Nutrition as an Added Ingredient to the Treatment of ADD

The antioxidants protect against many types of toxic substances that are now present in our environment. A type of choline has been found to be important in protecting brain cells and also operates as a preventive measure for the type of damage that strokes cause within the brain. Antioxidants protect against damage caused by what we call *free radicals*, which exist in the environment. These free radicals can react with other molecules and cause cell damage or DNA mutation. Higher levels of free radicals tend to cause increased damage to the cell and the effect is called oxidative stress. Oxidative stress can contribute to cardiovascular disease and cancer.

It has been noted that the supplements thiamine, riboflavin, niacin, pyridoxine, cholamine, folic acid, choline, pantothenic acid, inositol, iron, zinc, copper, chromium, taurine, carnitine, magnesium, tetrahydrobiopterin, tocopherol, tryptophan, and phenylalanine all impact such issues as carbohydrate sensitivity, neurotransmitter control, dementia, memory, fatigue, peripheral neuropathy, neurophysiologic problems, smell, taste, blood sugar, seizures, cognition and thinking, sleep disturbances, nervous exhaustion, and the catecholamine system in general (dopamine, norepinephrine and serotonin). Genetic and environmental factors all work together with nutritional factors in a well controlled system to keep brain function at its highest level of potential.

- It has been found that nutritional supplements can impact activities in all areas, e.g., the axons, synapses, the neurotransmitters, and for relief of the symptoms created by the lack of their availability.
- Nutritional supplements correct symptoms of the misuse and overuse of mood-altering substances found in coffee, tea, cocoa, and cola that impacts sleep, thinking, blood pressure and the peripheral (voluntary) nervous system.
- Excess alcohol use results in a depletion of several essential nutrients that can be replaced with nutritional supplements. The elderly as well as the head-injured population benefit from use of nutritional supplements.
- The immune system that has gone awry due to stress is much aided by nutritional supplements. When the system begins to overreact to everyday stimuli and fails to differentiate between hostile and friendly stimuli, there is a constant overreaction to all encounters that can be helped by nutritional supplements. Such overreaction results in a lowered immune-system response and greater susceptibility to colds and common viruses.
- Nutrition provides the help needed to allow the brain to operate at its fullest potential and to fight the impact of stress and daily living on the brain.
- We suggest using nutritional supplements primarily for the adolescent, adult and aged (unless addressing specific problem areas of the child).

Calcium is a Nutritional Supplement

We have found in our clinical practice that it is common for ADD individuals, particularly those without hyperactivity, to exhibit traits of anxiety. In fact, they tend to display symptoms of a generalized anxiety disorder that rests as a substrate, existing just below the surface. They really benefit from the effects of calcium, which seems to calm them. We find that calcium allows people to relax more and to be less fearful. At bedtime it also helps the child, adolescent, adult and aged population get to sleep and provides a more relaxed type of sleep.

Symptoms of anxiety can easily be tracked and documented in a person's family history. As a result, when these individuals begin with any form of stimulant medication, they quickly find themselves with increased anxiety that may range in degree from mild nervousness and agitation to full-scale panic reactions and feeling as if they could jump out of their skins at any moment.

A common complaint of stimulant medications is that they make people so nervous that all they can think about is the anxiety. They cannot even tell if their ADD symptoms are abated because they are so over-focused on the anxiety. In all probability, there is little impact on the ADD symptoms since their intolerance of the medication forces them to take very low doses. As a result, people will say the medication does not work when in fact it's simply that the low dosage they take is not enough to impact the ADD. One highly effective solution that we have found for these individuals (and usually this also impacts the adolescent and adult population) is to introduce calcium (a small amount such as 250 mg) with each and every dose of medication. This serves to calm the person down enough to tolerate the necessary dosage of medication and to correct the symptoms of the attentional disorder.

Calcium can operate as a key messenger system in the brain, helping with the opening and closing of cells and the transport system from neuron to neuron. It can also be a powerful mechanism to allow for more oxygen to reach the cells. Sometimes individuals who are lactose-intolerant and so avoid dairy products have a deficiency in calcium and display high levels of symptoms of anxiety that can be reversed with the use of calcium.

The problem for the young child is that we do not always know the absolute effects of these compounds. Botanicals (specifically measured vitamins that provide highly controlled targeting of symptoms), are suggested for usage with children to address sleeping, anxiety, and as a *first line of defense* against seizure activation. Thus, vitamins or nutritional supplements can be a wonderful adjunct to the ADD treatment process if used properly. Adolescents and adults benefit from the generalized use of these nutritional programs and with these age groups we would then recommend the Life Pak®. It is important to watch herbal remedies with children or any individual who is more fragile and sensitive physically due to reactions and interactions that can occur.

We are now learning that nutrition and diet can play a very important part in the life of the ADD child, adolescent, or adult. Specific nutritional interventions can improve not only physical health, but emotional health and the thinking abilities as well. It is very exciting to be able to look toward nutritional supplements as a means of addressing the issues that seem to plague the ADD individual.

It is clear from our clinical experience that ADD treatment primarily begins with the use of stimulants, however, there is a clear place for nutritional supplements to address the other issues that are present as well. We have found that nutritional supplements as an adjunctive therapeutic regime can benefit the young child as well as the aged population.

19

ADD versus Brain Damage: Does it Make a Difference?

19.1 There is Brain Impairment that Occurs Specific to ADD

There is a *particular pattern* that *occurs when there is a premorbid attentional disorder*, which does not necessarily occur in the absence of a premorbid ADD syndrome. Seizure activation becomes especially prominent in spatial areas of functioning, producing distortions in the copying of designs, in the ability to view the whole of things cognitively, and in part-whole relationships. Spatial functioning is pervasively impaired at levels of input as well as at the higher cognitive levels and is evidenced whenever operating as a variable in task performance. Spatial areas of brain functioning are targeted if the diagnosis is premorbid ADD without hyperactivity. It is weakened by the reorganization of brain functioning subsequent to the compensation of ADD symptoms. The right hemisphere tends to be impacted to a greater degree, given its ability to subserve both right- and left-hemisphere spatial functioning (whereas the left hemisphere subserves only left-hemisphere functioning).

When there is premorbid ADD and the individual suffers from head injury, the combination is particularly devastating. Typically, head injury, impacting memory and logical reasoning processes, results in diminishing the two compensatory mechanisms that the ADD individual (specifically ADD without hyperactivity) utilizes to compensate for deficits as a result of the premorbid attentional disorder. This often occurs as the consequence of seizure activity related to excitotoxicity processes occurring with head injury.

Mild trauma can result in the release of cytokines and excitatory amino acids impacting the cholinergic function of the region of the brain specific to memory functioning. This may result in the *consistent short-term memory deficits* that are observed following traumatic brain injury (TBI). Excitotoxicity processes that are elicited subsequent to brain injury set off a cascade of events leading to both biochemical and electrical changes within the brain, significantly altering the former status of brain functioning.

Seizure activity can often be difficult to observe, which is characteristic of absence seizures — nonmotoric seizures where the signs are more subtle and more difficult to diagnose. Research is beginning to document evidence that this type of seizure activity is more profound and more common than thought earlier. Seizure activity occurring prior to the age of 5 years poses the greatest risk to normal neural development and maturation. Regular seizures pose the greatest risk to normal cognitive development. Seizure activity tends to target the temporal area of brain functioning, which is the area responsible for memory abilities. It is a defined epileptogenic zone, meaning this area is more susceptible to seizure. Recent research has identified that seizures evidencing a minimal degree of motor activity and lack of consciousness were found to arise from temporal, temporoparietal or parieto-occipital areas as opposed to those seizures with accompanying motor phenomena and clear loss of consciousness, which arise generally from the frontal, frontocentral, central, or frontoparietal areas.

There is documented evidence through neuropsychological evaluation of the generalized impact to brain function, which is highly characteristic of seizure disorder that occurs with even mild head injury. Individuals appearing to have suffered only minimal impact to brain functioning — i.e., intact EEG recordings, nonsignificant CAT scans and MRIs — can still have sustained injury to the brain that is not observed through these measures. Their lifestyles have been altered: school performance has declined, and the family is aware of behavioral and emotional changes postinjury. Evidence on a neuropsychological evaluation will usually document impact to spatial and memory areas of brain functioning. At times, the motoric processes have been affected, varying in the impact on fine, gross, and coordinated movement. Ambidextrous movement may be reported as the dominant hand becomes weaker and receives increased assistance from the nondominant hand.

Memory is usually impaired and becomes more problematic with the interference of spatial stimuli or material. This will impact learning, especially when learning is based on pure memorization. Also notable in the learning pattern is much inconsistency. The individual is unable to recall previously learned information when in the process of learning new information. Therefore, the individual cannot accommodate and assimilate new information while retaining the old information. Learning becomes variable and dependent on the ability to cluster and retain the information by utilizing some type of structural framework.

The degree to which logical reasoning processes can intervene and code the information in some type of understandable manner determines the degree of impairment and whether the task will be performed within below-average or highly impaired limits vs. average or above-average limits. If able to somehow make sense of the material, functioning could increase to above average and superior levels dependent on the individual's intellectual potential. Evidence of *preserved frontal processes* is often seen in spite of considerable deficits to the spatial, motoric, and memory areas. Frontal processes, when not subject to interference, can reveal a substantially higher level of potential not seen elsewhere in an evaluation, thus documenting the capabilities of head-injured individuals when they are not having to continually compensate for deficits.

Attentional deficits are noted that compose characteristics of an attentional disorder. The question becomes whether such deficits represent an exacerbated premorbid attentional disorder or are the result of impact to brain functioning totally due to the head injury. While the capacity problem and distractibility could be the consequence of seizure activation impacting brain functioning subsequent to head injury, it becomes difficult to explain why the spatial functioning is targeted in the exact manner typically seen with the premorbid attentional disorders.

Learning skills may be essentially intact; these individuals are able to take in information and use it as feedback to modify their behavior. Learning, *but not the ability to learn*, is disturbed due to memory deficits and the deteriorated spatial functioning that has far-reaching consequences on academic functioning. This can result in the intellectual assessment representing globally repressed average to low or below-average overall functioning. Achievement evaluation also indicates diminished functioning subsequent to the impact of brain deterioration on both memory and spatial functioning, which has affected the ability to learn to the level of one's potential. Language skills and vocabulary development are hindered by the spatial deficits resulting from the premorbid ADD. There is an inability to visualize the whole word, in addition to an inability to purely memorize the nonsense syllables often used to develop word-attack skills. The mistake occurs when the professional uses the intellectual assessment and achievement evaluation as evidence of the individual's abilities without considering a more thorough evaluation that may pinpoint areas not affected by injury to the brain and be more representative of the individual's true level of potential.

There is clear documentation observed with the head-injured population that seizure activity might occur for only a brief duration of time (a matter of seconds). This seizure activity can occur continuously throughout the day or evening hours and what will be observed in the individual is clear ictal and interictal signs. Symptoms are varied and can range from intrusive thoughts or forced thinking, derealization, de-personalization, dreamy state, compulsive urges, hypergraphia, brief euphoria and sadness, and an altered time sense. Sleep walking, the blank stare, nonresponsive staring, complex automatic behavior, amnesic periods, drop-attacks, sudden intense emotion, the emotional outburst out of nowhere, the anger expressed that is clearly out of context for the situation or event, have all been documented as seizure related. Individuals experiencing seizure activity on a continual basis can experience polysensory phenomenona, such as confused behaviors, walking or looking around aimlessly, talking without engaging in conversation, hallucinations and delusions, inappropriate behaviors such as undressing or masturbating in public, a deepened emotionality, and the experience of false familiarity (the feeling of having seen objects before, heard sounds, voices or music before or having visited events or places before). Seizure activity can be associated with psychotic-like symptoms, creating a world of unreality and retreat for the head injured.

19.2 Seizure-Activity Symptoms

19.2.1   Tics or Seizures as Emotional Outbursts

- Panic attacks
- Blank staring
- Lack of memory
- Disorientation
- Periods of black or darkness
- Loss of moments of time
- Sleepwalking
- Thrashing in one's sleep
- Waking up tired like one did not sleep at all

The QEEG or quantitative analysis techniques utilize a method of mathematical processing of EEG, and provide a *finer* measure of the data obtained, often revealing abnormalities not seen otherwise. QEEG analysis, however, has been the subject of considerable review and debate. In our clinical practice, we find this method is quite helpful and adept in correlating with neuropsychological test findings to isolate seizure activation not seen otherwise. Additional techniques being utilized to measure seizure activation — e.g., fMRI, MRS, SPECT and FDG-PET — allow for further understanding of this elusive phenomenon.

19.3 Seizure Activity Is Often the Overlooked Phenomenon Occurring in Pediatric Head Injury

This silent activity is *slowly eroding brain functioning*, which has far-reaching consequences and is often evidenced post-accident as the academic environment becomes more demanding. Children who are injured at younger ages will appear intact until school becomes more demanding and complex. Attentional deficiencies are notable with the head-injured population, reflecting a diminished capacity to allocate resources. Children have a slower reaction time and the efficiency of neural operations is diminished subsequent to the injury. Poorly sustained attention is noticeable in their inability to complete tasks. Distractibility is highly evident. Children become easily distracted by any noise or sound occurring in their environment as well as by their own internal thoughts. Distractibility is evidenced in their speech patterns, inability to complete sentences or thoughts, inability to complete the tasks they begin, lack of organization, and failure to maintain eye contact. Often they will miss small details of instructions, directions, and conversation. In general, they are subject to being distracted by their own internal thoughts. Information processing is highly impacted by damage to the brain and is a main contributant to the loss of information. When logical processes remain relatively preserved, these individuals will use logical reasoning skills to put together the information available to them, but at the risk of developing erroneous conclusions of which they remain unaware. These traits are common characteristics of ADD without hyperactivity that are further exacerbated by injury to the brain.

Children can be easily misdiagnosed as ADHD subject to the impulsivity (often due to the distractibility or emotional lability of seizure activation), excessive distractibility (subsequent to the combination of both ADD and impact to brain functioning), and excessive movement that appears as overactivity (may be related more to anxiety). Children who have a family history of psychiatric disorder are at greater risk to develop psychiatric symptoms 3 to 6 months post injury. Children can appear demanding and persistent in the need for immediate gratification, however, this may be subject to tendencies of overfocused thinking, which permeates their thinking to the degree that one thing is all they think about, all they talk about, and all they want — until the next thing they decide to overfocus on. These children become demanding due to their own obsessive thinking and desire to complete the activity or event simply to relieve their own pervasive microscopic thought pattern.

The old theory that the younger the child the more benign the impact of head injury and the greater the ability of the child to recover is no longer substantiated. New research and evidence seen clinically clearly documents that this is not the case. The younger the age of injury the more children are at risk for future injury and academic problems. These children are placed in the position of playing catch up and trying to come back to where they were, while missing the new learning that should be occurring. During the building-block grades when new information becomes necessary for future learning and future learning is dependent on prior learning, this can be particularly devastating. The children injured in the first, second, or third grades are in process of attempting to recoup losses while missing the critical period of new learning. The result is that they often end up several grades behind despite the presence of intellectual potential or abilities that are above-average or even superior. Research confirms that rate of performance is the impairment that often impacts executive thinking, logical reasoning, and problem-solving abilities for those suffering from pediatric head injury. Therefore, injury occurring at earlier ages does not imply a more positive recovery, impacting both the efficiency of the brain and skill acquisition, especially if occurring prior to or during the building-block school years.

It is becoming well established that *TBI results in conversational impairment*, the ability to carry on some type of conversation, to express oneself suffi-ciently to ensure that one's needs are met. Research consistently identifies that those suffering from TBI are more susceptible to errors in their everyday conversation, which limits their ability to be social as well as to make requests. Information provided can be redundant, there are errors in the delivery system (tone and emotional prosody or effect), language lacks flu-ency, information is insufficient (often due to distractibility with result being dangling sentences), and not always appropriate to the situation. Messages are more inaccurate than accurate, and there is a lack of structure to the dis-course. Those who are more severe in their injury evidence errors associated with the more fundamental rules of conversational interaction. Excessive talkativeness, circular and tangential thinking, fixation on specific topics, diminished turn-taking skills, a difficulty contributing to and sustaining con-versation as well as the reduced ability to present their ideas in a logical man-ner, are common problems evidenced in the TBI population.

Competent communication requires the use of language in an everyday capacity to allow individuals to address the variety of possible interactions in their environment, ranging from the more superficial and social in nature to the more complex and educational in academic and work settings. Conversa-tion impacts these individuals' daily lives and results in the head-injured population (all ages) being unable to express themselves, address their needs verbally, or simply exchange feelings or information in a competent manner on a daily basis.

Socially, both *ADD children and children diagnosed with TBI were found to gen-erate fewer positive, assertive responses* and more indirect responses to their peer group. These children do not approach social situations confidently, their communication, both verbal and nonverbal, is not clear and often they do not follow group norms due to a lack of awareness of the appropriate social behavior for a given situation. Social abilities are diminished subsequent to information processing deficits and spatial dysfunctioning. The inability to perceive the total situation often results in the failure to anticipate conse-quences of their behavior, to know where to sit or place oneself physically in terms of proximity or distance, when or when not to talk. There is a tendency to interrupt conversations or speak inconsistently with the conversation that becomes socially disturbing. Distractibility may result in the interruption of speech for fear of forgetting what one wanted to say as well as the thinking of a prior topic unaware that the conversation has moved on to a new topic.

Minor head injury, which *can typically result in the presence of post-concussive symptoms* (PCS) occurs in approximately 50% of this population. The pres-ence of PCS tends to correlate with the presence of seizure activity. Those who have suffered a head injury are often subject to outbursts of anger and rage significant of seizure activation. Symptoms range over both degree and presence and include the following: constant headache, dizziness, fatigue, irritability, reduced concentration, insomnia, sleep disturbance, double vision, alcohol intolerance, short-term memory problems, emotional lability, anxiety, depression, and sensitivity to heat, noise, temperature, and light. Psychiatric syndromes lying dormant can be activated or reactivated. PCS was found to be an internally consistent syndrome. Despite the variance of complaints, they are related to a common etiological factor. Depression was not found to influence PCS as a premorbid variable. Anxiety was found to increase the subjective response of children who reported more symptoms despite the degree of neurological insult. Regardless of the fact that these symptoms are related to the head injury, parents report symptoms as attention deficits, hyperactivity, or conduct disorder, rather than PCS.

It is the symptoms of PCS that result in the mild head-injured population frequently being dismissed as not having a significant head injury or resolution of issues previously observed. In our practice, it is rare that symptoms observed post injury actually abate and unfortunately, because the individual outwardly appears intact, they are often dismissed as cured and it is only these individuals and their significant family members who are aware that the problems actually continue to exist and interfere with daily functioning. If children or adolescents are bright, they will perform within average ranges in the academic setting and it is mistakenly believed this means they are intact and no longer suffer from the consequences of head injury. It is the PCS symptoms that eventually, over a period of time, produce a personality that has formed around the continual (often undiagnosed) seizure activation, with the result of extensive emotional issues that often remain undiagnosed as well.

19.3.1 PCS Misdiagnosed as Conduct Disorder, Anxiety, ADHD, and Oppositional Defiant Disorder

- Easily fatigued
- Balance-coordination difficulties
- Noise sensitive
- Heat sensitive
- Touch sensitive
- Whines a lot
- Little noises
- Once upset cannot get them back
- Blank emotionless stare
- Emotional lability
- Emotional reaction or overreaction to situation
- Easily upset
- Stress increases all of the above

- Sleepwalking
- Incontinence
- Restless legs
- Tired when they wake up in the morning
- Aggression out of nowhere (swearing, inappropriate behavior)
- Panic out of nowhere (does not fit situation)
- Constant headaches
- Dizziness, nausea
- Short-term memory loss
- Irritability
- Distractibility
- OCD symptoms
- Automatisms, repetitive movements
- Slow thinking speed
- Appetite decreases

To truly understand the impact of head injury, these individuals' premorbid functioning needs to be comparatively analyzed with their postmorbid skills. Many evaluators are utilizing norms that are either not appropriate or have such a wide range (from one to two standard deviations either side of the mean) that comparisons are no longer appropriate or relevant. The difficulty of assessing the mild TBI population is that brain imaging does not support evidence of the injury, which does not necessarily mean there is no injury. Often survivors report persistent effects 6 to 12 months or longer of post-injury symptoms characteristic of PCS.

Professionals trained to examine for evidence of head injury may report no findings or significant findings often depending on which side of the litigation they support. The trained evaluator needs to address issues of malingering, premorbid status, environment, motivation, physical and emotional health, impact of medications, errors in scoring and misinterpretation. Research has noted that 98% of this population revealed mild effects that were transitory with the academic measures indicating no immediate or long-term effects. Variability of findings increased with the severity of the injury. Outcomes of individuals 5 years post-trauma indicate that the most frequent sign of residual impairment was headaches. Balance difficulties and fatigue or weakness were observed secondarily.

TBI and PCS clearly result from different factors and present a different etiologic pathway. PCS can occur in the absence of head injury for years subsequent to the head injury. PCS tends to show up after the changes that occur within the brain following a head injury and can indicate seizure activity. The presence of PCS can be used as an indicator to determine the individual's ability to cope with stress factors following the injury. Pre-injury factors such as age, education, occupation, personality, emotional adjustment, and post-injury factors such as pain, family support, compensation, stress, expectancy, interact with cognitive factors and directly impact PCS.

Trauma associated with either the accident or type of injury as well as events occurring subsequent to the injury can create symptoms of PTSD. Trauma occurs when events happen in individuals' lives with which they are unprepared to cope. Usually this involves either events that are unlikely to occur again or an ongoing situation such as a dysfunctional alcoholic family system where children are too young to cope with the events occurring on an everyday basis in their lives. Often the continual evaluation and events related to the litigation regarding more involved or significant TBI cases can create trauma and symptoms of PTSD. This was noticeable in the evaluation of a 7-year-old child who was far more comfortable meeting professionals and attending doctor appointments than a child should be at that chronological age. The child had adopted adult characteristics of handling himself in these situations, which is highly characteristic of PTSD. PTSD is not always a prerequisite in TBI patients and does not provide adequate explanation for amnesia about the events of the injury. Failure to recall events prior to or subsequent to injury are primarily due to neurological factors and the loss of memory. Those TBI patients meeting some qualifications of PTSD were found to be suffering from biochemical, genetic substrates of depression or anxiety, and the post-traumatic amnesia was their method of protecting themselves against disturbing memories. There is an overlap of PTSD and PCS and the need to separate out the symptoms belonging to each of these disorders.

19.4 A Sense of Self

The adolescent asks "Who am I and where do I belong?" Self-esteem that is already altered by the presence of ADD becomes even more diminished when head injury occurs.

Temperament traits, life experiences and additional issues of premorbid diagnoses such as ADD, depression, anxiety, all play a considerable role in the development of attachment and one's individual value system. These factors, singly and interactively, impact the developmental process of determining and implementing moral rules in life. The manner in which people proceed through life to construct, test and apply rules of behavior is highly affected in positive and negative directions by these factors. The process of attaining autonomy and self-individuation is often a rather convoluted course (people zig when they should have zagged) and is filled with ups and downs as they attempt to carve out a value system and mode of operation specifically tailored to their needs, goals, and desires.

The manner in which people emerge from adolescence impacts the way in which they continue to approach the world. This is only altered through an equally determined course of analysis, insight, and behavior changes. Research supports the notion that unresolved conflicts in adolescence remain unresolved. The daughter who feels worthless and unloved by her maternal figure remains unloved and unworthy, destined to spend the remainder of her life searching for both attention and outward signs of love and admiration that will never be fulfilling enough to fill the void or gap left by the loss of that maternal love. ADD symptoms prevent academic success and leave the daughter unresolved as to where to attain a sense of herself and where to receive positive feedback and establish prowess in something. As self-esteem continues to deteriorate, the female becomes increasingly attached to her outer appearance as the means to attain some measure of success. It is not unlikely that eating disorders develop from that point onward and suicide becomes more prevalent. The daughter who is already unable to seek approval due to the effect of ADD symptoms becomes even more disconsolate with the effects of head injury, and the occurrence of head injury may only confirm the downward spiral of events in her life.

ADD or head injury symptoms can prevent the son from receiving the necessary approval of his father. He then spends his life proving, again and again, how successful, important, and masterful he is. Each new acquisition is one step closer to being the most important and the most masterful. The unfulfilled son either becomes the dutiful son, attempting to please the father and competing with anyone or anything to accomplish this task, or the defiant son, rebelling against the perceived lack of tolerance and acceptance from the father figure. The rebellious son becomes the antithesis of the father's beliefs. Feeling and believing in the rejection of his father, the son feels unworthy, and anticipates and fears failure. Eventually, he enters into a downward self-fulfilling prophesy of failure that continues to plummet downward until there is nowhere to go. But, having hit bottom, the son may begin to value his own opinion in order to rebuild his life.

Children or adolescents who are head injured or ADD feel less than, not acceptable, and not equal to their peers. If head injured, they can often feel as if they are a burden to their families. They are the ones being trotted off to the doctor. They are the sick ones who are so important that the parent misses work because their doctor appointment cannot wait as it can for other members of the family. The head-injured child is the recognized child in the family, receiving all of the attention, especially immediately post-accident. Family members are so grateful to have the child alive and seeming to be intact, that they give endlessly to the child.

If the child or adolescent had an initial injury that was severe enough to require hospitalization, their initial presentation to the parent is one that evokes horror. Parents recoil from the tubes connected to their children, the black eyes, the sunken faces and so on. They are so grateful to have their children returned to them, to have them home and safe, that they overindulge them in their demands for attention and neediness. Once such children are recovered outwardly and appear intact, parents do not want to acknowledge or recall the accident.

This can result in parents being poor documenters of their children's symptoms and behavior post accident. They do not want to notice the symptoms of ongoing seizure activation, they want to ignore any little nuances that may make them face that their children are not fully recovered from the accident. When the professional points out certain behaviors as problematic or asks parents about their occurrence, the first tendency on the part of parents is to minimize or deny any difficulties or problems. *Everything is fine*, the message being *let's forget that all of this occurred*. Ignore it and it will go away. Head injury is traumatic. If parents feel responsible in any manner, the desire to forget is even stronger. If such parents feel guilty they will tend to skew the information regarding their children, usually minimizing the symptoms. The idea that they might have had a role in any event that resulted in injury to their child is impossible to even consider.

Given the additional diagnosis of ADD, and the fact that it emerged genetically through one or both of the parents, can further accentuate their guilt. The result may be a high degree of over-protectiveness (over-reaction to the injury) or ambivalence, fueled by the necessity of denial, toward their children, their accomplishments, or difficulties or deficits. When such deficits impact school performance this carries considerable weight and the parents will eventually be inundated by professionals with suggestions for change. The children's doctors, teachers, aunts, uncles, grandparents, etc. will observe things in the children that the parents may resent even being discussed. Also, head injury results in increased vulnerability should another similar injury recur, and ADD individuals can be more prone to accidents and injuries associated with sports activities.

19.5 Adult Head-Injured Patients, Strangers to Their Formerly Familiar World

Despite attempts to establish a routine, things simply are not the same. Short-term memory problems are very upsetting when attempting to function on an everyday basis. Each day is fraught with oversights, disappointments and problems. Distractibility and confusion as well as information-processing deficits result in poor work performance and miscommunication with family members. Often the person appears intact outwardly; they look fine although often they don't act fine. Family members desperately want the adult to resume his or her former activities and duties within the family system and household. They just want to forget what has occurred and negate the perceived guilt of parent or spouse. Unconsciously, pressure is placed on the head-injured to get well as soon as possible. Coerced by family members who want the adult to get better as quickly as possible, TBI patients return to work too quickly, go home from the hospital too soon, downplay the severity of their symptoms to appear more intact than they actually are or feel.

In response to repeated failures, self-esteem lowers, there is an increasing sense of worthlessness and depression sets in. Anxiety becomes ever present and doubt sets in as to what one will be able to accomplish on any given day. Functioning remains so variable subject to neurological factors and ongoing seizure activation, that the individual is left bewildered, frightened, unsure of any of their abilities, and unable to trust themselves. Psychological symptoms following the ongoing seizure activity create an increased emotionality and sensitivity that heightens this whole process. Emotional outbursts and out-of-control aggression become more commonplace as stress triggers seizures. People significant to the head injured become frightened, wary and distant in their inability to predict their behavior. The head injured also become distant because of their own inability to predict their behavior and the escalating fear of physically or emotionally harming the person they love.

ADD adults who suffer a head injury lose either one or both of the two methods of compensation they have used on a daily basis to cope with symptoms of the premorbid ADD and thus function. Methods of compensation using logical reasoning skills are compromised due to the inefficiency of the brain subsequent to injury or direct impact to that area of brain functioning. Memory deficits are the most common complaint, whereas prior to the injury the individual could memorize information and with their excellent memory manage to make up for other deficits. Language skills were developed using memorization via a whole-word approach. Post injury, the individual is no longer able to compensate in this way. Often, those suffering from head injury and never diagnosed with a premorbid ADD present increased attentional symptoms for which they were formerly able to compensate. They will self-report poor sustained attention, loss of information, distractibility, forgetting and losing things, shifting from one uncompleted activity to another, poor eye contact, inability to complete thoughts or sentences, missed appointments, misunderstood conversations and needing instructions and directions repeated. They will confirm that these problems have always been present in their lives, but after the injury have increased and are no longer controllable.

The head injury will increase or exacerbate any underlying emotional disorder that was present pre-injury. Depression, anxiety, bipolar disorder, psychosis, emotional disorders will reveal an increase in symptoms due to the impact of injury on the brain. The individual is no longer able to compensate and contain emotional issues due to the impairment of brain functioning. Frontal processes associated with psychological status and control of one's emotions are diminished, either generally due to changes occurring within the brain and decreased neural efficiency, or directly due to specific impact. When the impact is more general and not subject to specific factors, underlying emotions will rise to the surface no longer contained or controlled. If the impact is specific, however, emotionality then becomes subject to the area of the frontal processes, producing a range of symptoms from aggressiveness and irritability to apathy and a total lack of emotions.

ADD symptoms and head injury may overlap, but they are two different and distinct disorders. Head injury will exacerbate the premorbid condition of ADD. ADD as a premorbid disorder can be documented and ruled in or out subsequent to head injury. Both conditions create symptoms that need to be addressed via coping mechanisms and medical management. It is important to realize the far-reaching impact of head injury and not assume that these individuals are recovered simply because their outward appearance is intact.

20

Summary of Issues Critical to Understanding ADD

The model that is presented begins with addressing the originating problem of thinking, emotional, or physical issues. This is accomplished via a specific evaluation designed to determine the degree of severity and impact of symptoms of the attentional disorder on the individual's functioning. A good genetic, familial history is taken to eventually arrive at an integrated treatment program that combines the use of therapy, group support, exercise, diet, environmental counseling and, finally, nutritional pharmacology.

20.1 Facts About ADD (Attention Deficit Disorder)

20.1.1 A Recap of ADD

ADD is a disorder of the frontal-lobe supervisory system, and the parietal lobe and its connections. Symptoms of ADD resemble what has traditionally been termed a "frontal-lobe disorder," characterized by problems with planning and organization, sequencing, utilization of feedback, modification of behavior as a consequence of feedback, and maintaining and switching sets and information-processing skills. There is decreased arousal and vigilance resulting in inconsistent and variable behavior. Behavioral symptoms include a loss of enthusiasm, a craving for stimulation, forgetfulness, carelessness, lack of frustration tolerance, avoidance and procrastination, hypo- and hyperactivity, inappropriate behavior, miscommunication, distractibility, lack of insight and awareness, and both excessively slow and quick movement. Diagnosis based on behavioral symptoms is deceiving, resulting in misdiagnosis and confusion. Behavioral symptoms can be caused by many different factors, including a coexisting underlying disorder. ADD people are individual, unique, and very different from each other, yet have similar patterns that allow the two subtypes, ADD without hyper-activity and ADD with hyperactivity, to be distinguished from each other.

ADD is also represented as an attention and concentration disorder, theoretically involving subcortical connections to the frontal lobe that serve as a gating mechanism in the brain. Irrelevant information needs to be gated out to allow the individuals to focus on some information and not be overwhelmed by all of the incoming stimuli from their external environment.

ADD is a biochemical disorder involving neurotransmitters or brain messengers. The disorder is basically genetic and a consequence of a bio-chemical imbalance in the brain with which one is simply born. Those with the disorder usually present symptoms quite early in life and continue to present symptoms throughout their adult lives and into aging. This is not a disorder that can be outgrown, as formerly believed. By adulthood the entire fabric of the individual's life has been affected.

Deficiencies present in early childhood are chronic in nature. They do improve with maturation but deficits persist and can be observed when compared with same-age peers. Deficiencies can lead to social problems and increased necessity of controlling responses by those in the external environment. Lack of success to control this disorder leaves those signifi-cant in the individuals' lives frustrated and ADD individuals feeling rejected. Often, the fear of failure keeps individuals from seeing all of their abilities, assets, and capabilities.

To truly understand ADD, "attention" must be understood as a global process and not just an issue of being able to attend, focus, and sustain attention to task. This has been a primary mistake in truly understanding just what ADD means to children, adolescents, or adults and how it impacts their lives. Therefore, attention is a combination of events that are both cog-nitive (thinking) and behavioral processes. Attention is the ability to control and select stimuli and responses, take in some information, gate out other information, select and control how that information is utilized, and select and control the outcome or response. Attention is therefore not seen as a single process that can be specified to any one area of the brain. This con-clusion is confirmed by a vast amount of research, experimental and clinical findings. Those areas of the brain that are involved vary and change, depending on the demands of the task involved. Different processes are used for different functions and, depending on what is needed, determine what area of brain functioning is involved. Only the parietal and frontal areas of the brain are involved in ADD, because that is where the neu-rotransmitters, or brain messengers dopamine and norepinephrine, pre-dominantly operate.

ADD affects everyone differently. There is a wide range across specific areas and the disorder occurs in varying degrees. Thus, two individuals may share the diagnosis of an attentional disorder without hyperactivity yet exhibit distinctly different problems, patterns, and coping skills in the way they handle certain tasks. It is important to remember that there is a great amount of diversity in examining the attention disordered or ADD population as a whole.

20.1.2 Common Conditions Associated with ADD

1. Conduct problems
   - 60% and more experience conduct or behavior problems
   - Oppositional defiant behavior
   - Temper tantrums
   - Anger outbursts
   - Destructiveness
   - Verbal and physical aggression
2. Academic performance problems
   - 90% and more experience academic problems
   - Underachievement
   - Variability of performance
   - Learning disability
3. Emotional immaturity
   - 50% and more experience emotional immaturity
   - Overreaction to situations
   - Low frustration tolerance
   - Low self-esteem
4. Social skills problems
   - 50% and more problems with social skills
   - Selfish, self-centered
   - Rejected by peers due to intrusive, aggressive behavior
   - Little regard for social consequences
   - Immature play and social interests
   - Poor self-awareness
5. Immature motor coordination
   - 30 to 60% have immature motor coordination
   - Bed-wetting (20%)
   - Involuntary defecation (10%)
   - Allergies, colds, ear infections

- Increased minor physical anomalies (including seizure activity, nonmotor type)
- Increased sleep disturbance (30%)

20.2 ADD — More Definition

ADD is a developmental disorder characterized by

- Poor sustained attention
- Ability to maintain vigilance is problematic
- Impulsivity
- Difficulty with delay of gratification
- Increased variability of task performance

The syndrome develops in early childhood and is not accounted for by other gross disturbances or impairments within the brain.

I. **ADD without hyperactivity** — These children appear to have the most predominant general trait of inattentiveness. The following behaviors can be observed

- Excessive daydreaming, "spacey" appearance
- Cognitive sluggishness (processing disorder is possible)
- Hypoactive, lethargic
- Excessive confusion or mental "fogginess"
- Information-processing deficits resulting in missed details of instructions, directions, and communication in general
- Inconsistent memory retrieval (based on missing information)
- Increased anxiety and depression
- Socially reticent or diminished social involvement
- Rarely aggressive or oppositional (unless attempting to avoid failure)
- Rarely impulsive (unless reactive to over-control, increased tension, and need to escape)
- Fear of failure followed by avoidance and procrastination

These children will be classified in the DSM-IV as Attention Deficit Hyperactivity Disorder, Predominantly Inattentive Type. Children must have at least six items from the following list and there is a disturbance of 6 months' duration. The items must be to the degree of being developmentally inappropriate and there is no evidence of impulsivity or hyperactivity for the past 6 months.

1. Often fails to give close attention to details or makes careless mistakes in schoolwork, work, or other activities.
2. Often has difficulty sustaining attention in tasks or play activities.
3. Often seems not to listen when spoken to directly.
4. Often does not follow through on instructions and fails to finish schoolwork, chores, or duties in the workplace (not due to oppositional behavior or failure to understand instructions).
5. Often has difficulty organizing tasks and activities.
6. Often avoids, dislikes, or is reluctant to engage in tasks that require sustained mental effort (such as schoolwork or housework).
7. Often loses things necessary for tasks or activities (e.g., toys, school assignments, pencils, books, or tools).
8. Often is easily distracted by extraneous stimuli.
9. Often is forgetful in daily activities.

II. ADD with hyperactivity — The disorder is to be classified predominately as a disturbance of hyperactive-impulsive behavior that can be associated with inattention. According to the DSM-IV, the age of onset is around 7 years, there is a disturbance of 6 months' duration, and it is classified as Attention Deficit Disorder, Predominantly Hyperactive-Impulsive Type. There is no evidence of inattention for the past 6 months.

Hyperactivity
1. Often leaves seat in classroom or in other situations in which remaining seated is expected.
2. Often fidgets with hands or feet and squirms in seat.
3. Often runs about or climbs excessively in situations in which it is inappropriate (in adolescents or adults, may be limited to subjective feelings of restlessness).
4. Often has difficulty playing or engaging in leisure activities quietly.
5. Often is "on the go" or often acts as if "driven by a motor."
6. Often talks excessively.
Impulsivity
7. Often interrupts or intrudes on others (i.e., butts into other children's games).

8. Often blurts out answers to questions before they have been completed.

9. Often has difficulty waiting for his or her turn in games or group situations.

The Basic Characteristics are

- Inattention
- Impulsivity
- Hyperactivity
- Diminished rule-governed behavior
- Variability of task performance

There is a combined-type disorder if both criteria of inattention and hyperactive-impulsivity have been met for a duration of 6 months.

There must be clear evidence of significant impairment in social, academic, or occupational functioning. The above is in accordance with the DSM-IV. However, clinically, this does not appear to be the case. What would qualify as the combined type of disorder may well be the overfocused subtype.

20.3 Overfocused Subtype of Attention Deficit Disorder without Hyperactivity

The *Overfocused subtype* tends to describe a category of individuals who are generally more physically and emotionally vulnerable, sensitive and, to varying degrees, fragile. They are more prone to immune-system disorders and are more physically at risk.

Hallmark symptoms are as follows

- Emotionally reactive and sensitive
- Overfocuses on a situation, idea, thing, or event and thinks about it so much that it must happen — can think or talk of nothing else until this occurs
- Makes small thing into big things — mountains out of molehills
- Everything is a major deal — things are blown out of proportion
- Do not like transition — they don't want to go, but once they get there, they don't want to leave
- Mood changes frequently — emotional lability
- Sensitive to certain types of clothing — don't like anything tight at collars or cuffs
- Chews pills — cannot swallow them

- Colic in infancy — don't sleep
- Prone to asthma and allergies
- Anxious — prone to worry, become mired in "what if this" and "what if that"
- Tendency to ruminate — over-think, over-analyze, over-predict, over-anticipate
- Self-critical — self-derogatory thinking, judgmental of self, and then others
- Fear of failure — avoidance and procrastination, especially after over-analysis
- Fear of change — more comfortable with routine and structure
- Extreme emotions — work hard, play hard, Type A personality, intense
- Can develop seizure activation — nonmotor type

Other Diagnoses — *Oppositional Defiant Disorder* is viewed as a disorder of hostile and defiant behavior toward others, arising in childhood and frequently culminating in *Conduct Disorder.*

To be defined as Oppositional Defiant Disorder, children must display four characteristics from the following list

1. Often loses temper
2. Argues with adults
3. Actively defies or refuses adults' requests or rules
4. Deliberately does things that annoy other people
5. Blames others for his or her own mistakes or misbehavior
6. Often touchy or easily annoyed by others
7. Angry and resentful
8. Often spiteful or vindictive

To be defined as Conduct Disorder, the individual must have at least three of the following 15 items in the past 12 months with at least one criterion present in the past 6 months.

Aggression to people and animals

1. Bullies, threatens, or intimidates others.
2. Often initiates physical fights with others.
3. Has used a weapon that can cause serious physical harm to others (such as a bat, broken bottle, knife, gun).
4. Has been physically cruel to people.
5. Has been physically cruel to animals.

6. Has stolen while confronting a victim (such as mugging, purse snatching, extortion or armed robbery).

7. Has forced someone into sexual activity.

Destruction of property

8. Has deliberately engaged in fire setting with the intention of causing serious damage.

9. Has deliberately destroyed others' property (other than by fire setting).

Deceitfulness or theft

10. Has broken into someone else's home, building or car.

11. Often lies to obtain goods or favors or obligations (i.e., "cons" others).

12. Has stolen items of nontrivial value without confronting a victim (such as shoplifting but without breaking and entering, forgery).

Serious violations of rules

13. Often stays out at night despite parental prohibitions, beginning before the age of 13 years.

14. Has run away from home overnight at least twice while living in parental or parental surrogate home (or once for a lengthy period of time).

15. Often is truant from school beginning before 13 years of age.

Behaviors or symptoms noted above can be seen as a result of other issues. Fear of failure can be so overwhelming that someone would rather appear oppositional and defiant than risk failing at something. Traits of oppositionality and defiance can also be seen with such disorders as Post Traumatic Stress Disorder as a protective mechanism as well as with certain personality types, Borderline Personality Disorder, Depressive, Aggressive, and Negativistic personality traits.

20.4 Follow Up Data: Attention Deficit Disorder — Adults (Residual Form)

Of those diagnosed as having ADD, 70% continue to be affected into adulthood. The following characteristics (some but not all) are observed in adults

- Inability to complete tasks
- Impulsivity and non-reflectiveness (which leads to poor judgment in both personal and work decisions)

- Highly distractible (cannot maintain eye contact, interrupts conversations, does not finish thoughts before moving to a new thought)
- Shifting from one unfinished task to another without completing anything
- Unable to operate at level of true potential
- Low self-esteem, need for approval from others, does not like conflict
- Fear of failure, avoid and procrastinate, fearful of taking risks when performance is involved
- Problematic interpersonal relationships
- Lack of insight
- Hot or explosive temper
- Lack of organization
- Lack of reward system, lack of feedback system (which leads to a chronic unhappiness and dissatisfaction with frequent job changes and relationship changes)
- Low stress tolerance
- Vulnerable to stress
- Flies off the handle quickly
- Planning disorder
- Low frustration tolerance
- Carelessness
- Lack of foresight
- Absentmindedness
- Difficulty keeping promises
- Problem with day-to-day organization of family life
- Mental and physical restlessness
- Note-taking and paperwork problems
- Financial problems
- Missed appointments: missing times, dates, and events
- Mild to severe communication problems
- Not able to express feelings and describe thoughts
- Miscommunication due to missing small details of date, times, places, and communication in general
- Difficulty with instructions and directions, often needs oral direction repeated
- Cannot think from a whole perspective

- Right-left confusion; directions of north, south, east, and west confused
- Does not like to dance (due to spatial issues and right-left confusion)

It has been shown through research that adults suffering from residual ADD exhibit the following

- More auto accidents (due to spatial problems)
- More geographically mobile (location change more often)
- More antisocial behavior in general
- More involvement with the legal authorities
- Poor performance in later schooling
- Less job success
- Self-esteem problems (low self-esteem)
- Relationship problems
- Problems increase with the complexity of life, job, marriage, and family as well as the aging process
- Cannot keep agreements

According to the DSM-IV, adult ADD can be characterized by symptoms of both Inattention and Hyperactive–Impulsive behavior.

Inattention
1. Trouble directing and sustaining attention
2. Difficulty completing projects; follow-up and following through in general
3. Easily overwhelmed by tasks of daily living
4. Inability to maintain an organized living or work place; things become chaotic
5. Inconsistent work performance, yet self-critical and judgmental
6. Lacks attention to detail, yet compulsive and perfectionistic

Hyperactivity–Impulsivity
1. Makes decisions impulsively, fails to anticipate consequences of behavior.
2. Difficulty delaying gratification, involved in stimulation-seeking actions.
3. Restless and fidgety, constantly on the move.
4. Makes statements and comments without considering their impact.

5. Impatient and easily frustrated.

6. Frequent traffic violations.

Overlap between the two categories occurs due either to the presence of an underlying coexisting disorder or presence of the symptom due to another reason. Frequently anxious individuals are over-diagnosed as hyperactive. Over-focused individuals who think too much and finally just act on it, are over-diagnosed as impulsive.

Positive Attributes

- Life is exciting and interesting
- Movers and shakers
- Builders of businesses
- Great in sales
- Passionate individuals
- Risk takers
- Self-employed individuals
- Good in any situation where a great deal of emotionality is helpful

20.4.1 Adult ADD List of Cognitive Mistakes

1. Do you find that you read something and need to read it again because you have no idea of what you just read?

2. Do you walk into a room and forget what you came to get, only to leave and return again still forgetting what you left another part of the house for?

3. Do you fail to hear people speaking to you because you are thinking about something else? Do you miscommunicate on the date, time, place of an appointment, swearing that you never received that information?

4. Do you have important letters that have gone unanswered for days? They got lost in a pile that you forgot about.

5. Do you fail to see what you want in the supermarket even though it is there? Do you feel overwhelmed by too many items clustered together?

6. Do you find that you forget what you wanted when you walked into the store to buy it, after being so overwhelmed by all of the sights and sounds?

7. Do you find that you forget what you wanted to say even though it is on the *tip of your tongue*?

8. Do you find that there are times that you can't think of anything to say because your mind is full of too many thoughts at one time?

9. Do you find yourself throwing away things that you did not mean to throw away because you were thinking of something else at the time and not paying attention?

10. Does your mind wander while watching TV? Do you use the clicker to change in the middle of a program and never watch the entire program?

11. Do you have difficulty sustaining conversation when there are other voices or noises occurring in the house?

12. Do you find yourself not listening to someone with whom you are in a conversation and your mind just wandered off without your realizing it?

13. Do you find yourself suddenly losing track of what it was that you were saying while you are still in the middle of speaking?

14. Do find yourself starting to do something, becoming distracted and then find yourself doing something else?

15. Do you find it difficult to do more than one thing at a time?

16. Do you find yourself not finishing your sentences or starting a new sentence before you have finished the last one?

17. Do you speak in half-thoughts and the rest of the thought remains in your head, unspoken?

18. Do you think that you said something when everyone around clearly states that you did not?

20.4.2 ADHD is Over-Diagnosed. ADD Without Hyperactivity is Under-Diagnosed

In our clinical practice we have found it extremely critical to be able to separate out the two disorders. These two disorders represent very different issues for treatment and very different relationships with family members and other significant individuals in these people's lives. There are different expectations related to each disorder based on different abilities and different ways the disorder has an impact on their thinking and performance. Diagnosis and separation of ADD with hyperactivity from ADD without hyperactivity allows for treatment that is designed specifically to address the problems related to each individual disorder.

The ADHD individual may lie, display manipulative and secretive behaviors and resembles more of the behavioral profile characteristic of

delinquency, addictive personal, and Oppositional Defiant Disorder. These behaviors arise not from an attempt to defend and protect oneself as in the case with the ADD without hyperactivity individual, but as part of the manifestations of the disorder itself. Aggressive individuals may be seen with this disorder, especially when it is severe in nature. The impulsivity may be truly there and also involve another neurotransmitter, serotonin, in addition to the dopamine imbalance. ADHD tends to involve the RAS, the frontal areas of the brain, and primarily the neurotransmitter dopamine. This disorder is more associated with learning disabilities for reading, writing, and spelling due to the inability to learn related to problems of the frontal processes as well as structural changes within the brain.

ADD without hyperactivity involves a capacity problem, slow cognitive thinking, thalamus as the relay system, and parietal areas of the brain. Difficulty in school with reading, writing, and spelling problems tend to be related to spatial problems characterized by visual neglect, an inattention to the whole, problems at the phonemic level, and not seeing the word in a whole manner to develop a sight vocabulary. The spatial area or the parietal area is more impacted. Other spatial problems can appear, such as gauging distances while driving, anticipation of consequences in terms of visualizing the whole, and the impact of a specific action on the whole situation. Norepinephrine tends to be the neurotransmitter most involved with ADD without hyperactivity and these individuals will benefit from medications targeting that system.

The task is to try to distinguish one disorder from the other as much as possible. There is controversy as the two disorders overlap each other. It is believed that they do not. It is proposed that the behavioral symptoms of the Overfocused Subtype of the attentional disorder without hyperactivity and the clinical symptoms of ADD without hyperactivity actually compose the diagnostic criteria for the combination subtype. Children can appear oppositional and defiant, which may not be a behavior related to ADHD, but instead a means of defending against feeling insecure due to incompetence subject to symptoms of the attentional disorder. There are different correlated or comorbid symptoms associated with each disorder that result from the different combinations of neurotransmitter imbalances. Both the ADD without hyperactivity and the ADHD individual are very sensitive and vulnerable, however, the disorder will appear in different ways and is exemplified by different behaviors.

ADD without hyperactivity is often misdiagnosed as ADHD due to the extreme degree of anxiety these individuals have in both their family history and throughout their lifetime. These individuals are fear based and the disorder of ADD without hyperactivity is highly correlated with anxiety and depression. There is a clear genetic familial history of anxiety and anxiety-related somatic symptoms. These individuals appear overactive due to being so anxious and it is not uncommon to see both children and adults exhibit anxiety in their continuous leg, knee, or foot movements. Sleep problems are prevalent, as these individuals shift and move throughout the night contributing to what may be called a "Restless Leg Syndrome."

20.5 ADD Without Hyperactivity Is More Common

ADD without hyperactivity is the more common disorder. Generally ADD will be correlated with

- Reading disorders
- Problems with the parietal and temporal areas of the brain
- Spatial problems
- Hypoglycemia/hypothyroid
- Asthma

Physical symptoms seen with this disorder are as follows

- Hypoglycemia and eating problems
- Fatigue
- Stress
- Headaches
- Sleeping problems
- Irritability and nervousness
- Stomach upset
- Aches and pains
- Rapid heartbeat
- Dizziness-lightheadedness
- Vomiting and nausea
- Diarrhea
- Constipation
- Weakness
- Confusion
- Dry mouth
- Mental and physical restlessness

ADHD is seen less often and tends to be correlated to

- Hyperthyroid
- Learning disability
- Tourette's Syndrome

The Overfocused Subtype of ADD without hyperactivity is a subgroup more vulnerable to physical symptoms such as the following.

- They chew and can't swallow pills
- Upset stomach
- Colicky as infant
- Cannot stand tightness at cuff or collar
- Easily stressed and frightened
- Sleep problems, sleep deprivation
- Fatigue, can't sleep
- Low blood sugar, hypoglycemia

20.6 How To Get a Good Diagnosis

20.6.1   Why Is This Important?

It is very important to obtain a good diagnosis that will tell you exactly what the problem areas are. Just to define whether someone has an attention disorder means nothing. What they do about it is the question. This is where it becomes so critical to be able to exactly define the specific problem areas. Once these areas are identified they become easier to remedy or fix.

Often the problem occurs when people are unable to exactly define all the different problem areas. If all problem areas are not identified, fixing one problem only allows another to surface. This can become very frustrating, leaving people to think that the situation cannot ever be fixed.

Therefore you want a testing battery that is going to define, *in very clear terms,* the exact problems or specific issues that block these individuals' ability to work to the level of their potential. We suggest neuropsychological evaluation: the use of brain behavior measures to identify exactly what is occurring.

20.6.2   What to Ask for to Make Sure You are Getting a Thorough Evaluation

These issues need to be measured

- Distractibility
- Missing information
- Information processing
- Capacity
- Sustained attention and focus
- Slow thinking speed (this would mean that time measures do not provide an accurate measure of someone's abilities or skills)
- Frontal process and the use of logic. The ability to
  - Sequence
  - Switch sets
  - Think in a flexible manner and generate solutions to problems

20.6.2   Questions to Be Addressed by Evaluation

1. Is there a learning disability or are the reading, spelling, writing, and math problems due to something else?
2. Are there other issues such as damage to the brain, low blood sugar or some other condition operating?
3. Test scores must be compared with the person's potential. What can we expect of them? What are they really able to do?
4. After answering these questions, self-report measures can be used to support the testing data. What are the additional coexisting diagnoses to consider? (Tourette's Syndrome, emotional disorders, issues that may be increased by the use of stimulant medication.)

20.6.2.1   Points to Consider

- We suggest that you do not rely on the self-report measures alone to determine a diagnosis of ADD.
- We suggest that the IQ assessment be understood in relation to the ADD disorder if it exists.
- There is benefit to identifying the problem areas to develop specific coping skills and treat ADD symptoms.
- It is very important to determine exactly what the problem areas are before attempting to resolve them.

- The brain is not differentiated until the age of 13 years or beyond; changes can occur and areas of the brain can be retrained or enhanced.
- ADD without hyperactivity needs to be treated differently from ADHD. These two disorders are very different from each other. The person needs to be understood from a whole perspective by understanding what is wrong and what other factors are involved. The issues and concerns are very different for each of these two subtypes.

Finally, a good diagnosis also helps with choice of medication as well as providing some prediction of what to expect from its use. It is important to pay attention to any other factors besides ADD that may arise, especially when using stimulant medication.

Looking at ADD from a whole perspective and treating it with

- Coping skills for each problem area
- Ways to retrain the brain
- Ways to increase skill level and develop problem areas such as reading and poor vocabulary
- Address health issues and good diet and nutrition
- Identify coexisting conditions and other issues that add to problems created by ADD symptoms
- Medicate to directly treat biochemical problem

Bibliography

Adler, C. H. (1997) Treatment of restless legs syndrome with gabapentin, *Clinical Neuropharmacology,* 20(2), 148–151.

Alexrod, B. N., Goldman, R. S., Heaton, R. K., Curtiss, G., Thompson, L. L., Chelune, G., and Kay, G. G. (1996) Discriminability of the Wisconsin card sorting test using the standardization sample, *Journal of Clinical and Experimental Neuropsychology,* 18, 338–342.

Ammerman, R. T. and Patz, R. J. (1996) Determinants of child abuse potential: Contribution of parent and child factors, *Journal of Clinical Child Psychology,* 25(3), 300–307.

Arnold, E. Harvey, O'Leary, S. G., and Edwards, G. H. (1997) Father involvement and self-reported parenting of children with attention deficit hyperactivity disorder, *Journal of Consulting and Clinical Psychology,* 65(2), 337–342.

Barber, B. L. and Eccles, J. S. (1992) Long term influence of divorce and single parenting on adolescent family- and work-related values, behaviors, and aspirations, *Psychological Bulletin,* 111(1), 108–126.

Barkley, R. A. (1997) Behavioral inhibition, sustained attention and executive functions: Constructing a unifying theory of ADHD, *Psychological Bulletin,* 1, 65–94.

Barkley, R. A. (1997) Parents as shepherds, not engineers, *ADHD Report,* 5(6), 1–4.

Barkley, R. A. (1998) Age-dependent decline in ADHD: a final rejoiner, *ADHD Report,* 6(1), 7–10.

Barkley, R. A., Grodzinsky, G., and DuPaul, G. (1992) Frontal lobe functions in attention deficit disorder with and without hyperactivity: A review and research report, *Journal of Abnormal Child Psychology,* 20, 163–188.

Barkley, R., Koplowitz, S., Anderson, T., and McMurray, M. B. (1997) Sense of time in children with ADHD: Effects of duration, distraction, and stimulant medication, *Journal of the International Neuropsychological Society,* 3, 359–369.

Barnhill, J. L. and Horrigan, J. P. (1997) Tourette's syndrome in patients with developmental disorders, ANPA Abstracts *Journal of Neuropsychiatry and Clinical Neurosciences,* 9(1), 139, P30.

Baron-Cohen, S. and Hammer, J. (1997) Parents of children with asperger syndrome: what is the cognitive phenotype?, *Journal of Cognitive Neuroscience,* 9(4), 548–554.

Bear, D. M. (1995) Psychiatric presentations of epilepsy, In *Neurology of Behavior and Cognition,* Seminar held at the Knickerbocker Hotel, Chicago, Illinois, December 12–16, 1995.

Berkowitz, E. (1998) Psychosocial issues and treatment approaches with children and adolescents, *The ADHD Challenge,* 12(1), 5–9.

Berti, A., Ládavas, E., and Corte, M. D. (1996) Anosognosia for hemiplegia, neglect dyslexia, and drawing neglect: Clinical findings and theoretical considerations, *Journal of the International Neuropsychological Society,* (2), 426–440.

Beydoun, A., Sackellares, J. C., Shu, V., and The Depakote Monotherapy for Partial Seizures Study Group (1997) Safety and efficacy of divalproex sodium monotherapy in partial epilepsy: A double blind, concentration-response design clinical trial, *Neurology,* 48, 182–188.

Bidman, C. L., Sherling, M., and Bruun, R. D. (1995) Combined pharmacotherapy risk, *Journal of American Academy of Child and Adolescent Psychiatry* 34(3), 263–264.

Borcherding, B., Thompson, K., Krusei, M., Bartko, J., Rapoport, J. L., and Weingartner, H. (1988) Automatic and effortful processing in attention deficit/hyperactivity disorder, *Journal of Abnormal Child Psychology,* 16, 333–345.

Bouma, P., Bovenkerk, A. C., Westendorp, G. J., and Brouwer, O. F. (1997) The course of benign partial epilepsy of childhood with centrotemporal spikes: A meta-analysis, *Neurology,* 48, 430–437.

Bourgeois, B. F. D. (1995) Valproic acid, clinical use, In *Antiepileptic Drugs,* 4th ed., Levy, R. H., Mattson, R. H., and Meldrum, B. S., Eds., Raven Press, Ltd., New York, 633–640.

Braaten, E. B. and Rosén, L. A. (1997) Emotional reactions in adults with symptoms of attention deficit hyperactivity disorder, *Personality and Individual Differences,* 22(3), 355–361.

Brady, K. D. and Gerring, J. P. (1997) Cognitive recovery following pediatric closed head injury: role of age at injury and lesion location, ANPA Abstracts, *Journal of Neuropsychiatry and Clinical Neurosciences,* 9(1), 135.

Braswell, L. (1998) Self-Regulation training for children with ADHD: Response to Harris and Schmidt, *ADHD Report,* 6(1), 1–3.

Bray, G. A. (1988) Sympathetic nervous system and a nutrient balance model of food intake, In *Nutritional Modulation of Neural Function,* Morley, John E., Sterman, M. Barry, and Walsh, John H., Eds., San Diego, Academic Press Inc., 87–94.

Bremer, D. A. and Stern, J. A. (1976) Attention and distractibility during reading in hyperactive boys, *Journal of Abnormal Child Psychology,* 4, 381–387.

Brown, R.T. and Wynne, M. E. (1982) Correlates of teacher ratings, sustained attention, and impulsivity in hyperactive and normal boys, *Journal of Clinical Child Psychology,* 11, 262–267.

Burrows, G. D. and Kremer, C. (1997) Mirtazapine: Clinical advantages in the treatment of depression, *Journal of Clinical Psychopharmacology,* 17(2) (Suppl. 1), 34S–39S.

Casey, B. J., Castellanos, F. X., Giedd, J., and Marsh, W. L. (1997) Implication of right frontostriatal circuitry in response inhibition and attention-deficit hyperactivity disorder, *Journal of the American Academy of Child and Adolescent Psychiatry* 36(3), 374–383.

Castellanos, F. X. et al. (1997) Controlled stimulant treatment of ADHD and comorbid Tourette's syndrome: Effects of stimulant and dose, *Journal of American Academy Child and Adolescent Psychiatry,* 36, 589–96. Referenced in *Journal Watch for Psychiatry,* 3(7), 54.

Castellanos, F. X., Giedd, J. N., Eckburg, P., Marsh, W. L. et al. (1994) Quantitative morphology of the caudate nucleus in attention deficit hyperactivity disorder, *American Journal of Psychiatry,* 151(12), 1791–1796.

Chadwick, David (1995) Gabapentin, clinical use, In *Antiepileptic Drugs,* 4th ed., Levy, R. H., Mattson, R. H., and Meldrum, B. S., Eds., Raven Press, New York, 851–856.

Chang, K., Neeper, R. , Jenkins, M., Penn, J., Bollivar, L., Israeli, L., Malloy, P., and Salloway, S. (1995) Clinical profile of patients referred for evaluation of adult attention-deficit hyperactivity disorder, ANPA Abstracts, *The Journal of Neuropsychiatry and Clinical Neurosciences,* 7(3), 401.

Chappelle, P. B., et al. (1995) Guanfacine treatment of comorbid attention deficit hyperactivity disorder and Tourette's syndrome: Preliminary clinical experience, *Journal of the American Academy of Child and Adolescent Psychiatry* 34, 1140–1146.

Chaskelson, M., (1991) Identification of "hidden" cognitive deficits associated with attention deficit disorders, *CHADDer Box*, January, 1991, reprinted.

Cicerone, K. D. and Kalmar, K. (1997) Does premorbid depression influence postconcussive symptoms and neuropsychological functioning? *Brain Injury,* 11(9), 643–648.

Clark, D. B., Lesnick, L., and Hegedus, A. M. (1997) Traumas and other adverse life events in adolescents with alcohol abuse and dependence, *Journal of American Academy of Child and Adolescent Psychiatry* 36, 1744–1751.

Cohen, D.J. and Leckman, J. F. (1994) Developmental psychopathology and neurobiology of Tourette's Syndrome, *Journal of American Academy of Child and Adolescent Psychiatry,* 33(1), 2–15.

Coltheart, M. and Coltheart, V. (1997) Reading comprehension is not exclusively reliant upon phonological representation, *Cognitive Neuropsychology,* 14(1), 167–175.

Corbetta, M., Shulman, G. L., Conturo, T. E., Snyder, A. Z., Akbudak, E., Peterson, S., Marcus E., Raichle, E. (1997) A functional magnetic resonance imaging (fMRI) study of visuospatial attention, *Neurology,* 48 (Suppl.), S62.006.

Cunningham, C. E. (1997) Readiness for change: applications to the management of ADHD, *ADHD Report*, 5(5), 6–9.

de Groot, C. M., Yeates, K. O., Baker, G. B., and Bornstein, R. A. (1997) Impaired neuropsychological functioning in Tourette's syndrome subjects with co-occurring- compulsive and attention deficit symptoms, *The Journal of Neuropsychiatry and Clinical Neurosciences,* 9(2), 267–272.

DeLuca, J. W., Moore, G. J., Mueller, R. A. Slovis, T. L. And Chugani, H. T. (1997) Right hemisphere learning disability syndrome: differential findings from PET and MRS, ANPA Abstracts *Journal of Neuropsychiatry and Clinical Neurosciences,* 9(1), 131, P3.

Devor, E. J. (1994) A developmental-genetic model of alcoholism for genetic research, *Journal of Consulting and Clinical Psychology,* 62(6), 1108–1115.

Doran, S. (1997) Fragile X syndrome and attention deficit hyperactive disorder,*ADHD Report*, 5(1), 8–11.

Drake, D. D., Johnson, C., and Clark, M. (1997) Acute improvement in alertness and cognition following methylphenidate in attention-deficit hyperactivity disorder (ADHD) predicts chronic cognitive improvement, ANPA Abstracts *Journal of Neuropsychiatry and Clinical Neurosciences,* 9(1), 141, P37.

Drake, D. D., Johnson, C., and Clark, M. (1997) Pupillometry-predicted alerting methylphenidate dosage also predicts cognitive improvement in nonvigilant, inattentive attention deficit hyperactivity disorder (ADHD) ANPA Abstracts *Journal of Neuropsychiatry and Clinical Neurosciences,* 9(1), 141, P38.

Eiraldi, R. B., Power, T. J., and Nezu, C. M. (1997) Patterns of comorbidity associated with subtypes of attention-deficit hyperactivity disorder among 6- to 12-year-old children, *Journal of the American Academy of Child and Adolescent Psychiatry* 36(4), 503–514.

Elterman, R., Glauser, T., Ritter, F. J., Reife, R., Wu, S.-C., and Raritan, N. J. (1997) Efficacy and safety of topiramate in partial seizures in children, *Neurology,* 48, 1729.

Faraone, S. V. et.al. (1996) A prospective four-year follow-up study of children at risk for ADHD: Psychiatric, neuropsychological, and psychosocial outcome, *Journal of the American Academy of Child and Adolescent Psychiatry* 35(11), 1449–1459.

Faraone, Stephen V. (1996) Discussion of "Genetic influence on parent-reported attention-related problems in a Norwegian general population twin sample", *Journal of the American Academy of Child and Adolescent Psychiatry* 35(5), 596–598.

Ferguson, H. B. and Rapoport, J. L. (1983) Nosological issues and biological validation, In *Developmental Neuropsychiatry,* Rutter, M., Ed., New York: The Guilford Press, 369–384.

Ferraro, L. et al. (1997) Modafinil: A new kind of stimulant, *Biological Psychiatry,* 42, 1181–1183.

Filipek, P. A., Semrud-Clikeman, M., Steingard, R. J., Renshaw, P. F., Kennedy, D. N., and Biederman, J. (1997) Volumeric MRI analysis comparing subject having attention-deficit hyperactivity disorder with normal controls, *Neurology,* 48, 589–601.

Fischer, M., Barkley, R. A., Fletcher, K. E., and Smallish, L. (1993) The adolescent outcome of hyperactive children: Predictors of psychiatric, academic, social and emotional adjustment, *Journal of the American Academy of Child and Adolescent Psychiatry,* 32, 324–332.

Fisher, N. J. and DeLuca, J. W. (1997) Verbal learning strategies of right hemisphere learning-disabled adolescents and adults, ANPA Abstracts *Journal of Neuropsychiatry and Clinical Neurosciences,* 9(1), 169, P135.

Foodman, A. (1996) ADD and soft signs, *Journal of the American Academy of Child and Adolescent Psychiatry,* 35(7), 841–842.

Frazer, A. (1997) Pharmacology of antidepressants, *Journal of Clinical Psychopharmacology,* 17(2), (Suppl. 1) 2S–18S.

Fristoe, N. M., Salthouse, T. A., Woodard, J. L. (1997) Examination of age-related deficits on the Wisconsin card sorting test, *Neuropsychology,* 11(3), 428–436.

Fuster, J. M. (1997) *The Prefrontal Cortex, Anatomy, Physiology, and Neuropsychology of the Frontal Lobe,* 3rd ed., Lippincott-Raven, Philadelphia, New York.

Gardner, D. M. (1997) Olanzapine, *Child and Adolescent Psychopharmacology News,* 2(6), 1–5.

Garth, J., Anderson, V., and Wrennall, J. (1997) Executive functions following moderate to severe frontal lobe injury: Impact of injury and age at injury, *Pediatric Rehabilitation,* 1(2), 99–108.

Gaub, M. and Carlson, C. L. (1997) Behavioral characteristics of DSM-IV ADHD subtypes in a school-based population, *Journal of Abnormal Child Psychology,* 25(2), 103–111.

Gerring, J. P., Brady, K., D., Miller, G., Christiansen, J., Bryan, R. N., and Denckla, M. B. (1997) Psychiatric disorders and MRI pathology after closed head injury in children, ANPA Abstracts, *Journal of Neuropsychiatry and Clinical Neurosciences,* 9(1), 135.

Goldstein, P. C., Rosenbaum, G., and Taylor, M. J. (1997) Assessment of differential attention mechanisms in seizure disorders and schizophrenia, *Neuropsychology,* 11(2), 309–317.

Goldstein, S. (1997) What I've learned from 25 years in the field of hyperactivity/ ADHD, *ADHD Report,* 5(6), 4–6.

Goldstein, S., (1991) Young children at risk: The early signs of attention-deficit hyperactivity disorder, *CHADDer Box,* January, 1991, reprinted.

Gorenstein, E. E., Mammato, C. A., and Sandy, J. M. (1989) Performance of inattentive-overactive children on selected measures of prefrontal-type function, *Journal of Clinical Psychology,* 45(4), 619–631.

Grados, M. A., Gerring, J. P., Bryan, R. N., and Denckla, M. B. (1997) Obsessive-compulsive disorder (OCD) in children and adolescents with moderate to severe injury, ANPA Abstracts, *Journal of Neuropsychiatry and Clinical Neurosciences,* 9(1), 135.

Greene, R. W. et al. (1996) Toward a new psychometric definition of social disability in children with attention-deficit hyperactivity disorder, *Journal of the American Academy of Child and Adolescent Psychiatry,* 35(5), 571–578.

Griffiths, T. D., Rees, A., Witton, C., Cross, P. M., Shakir, R. A., and Green, G. G. R. (1997) Spatial and temporal auditory processing deficits following right hemisphere infarction: A psychophysical study, *Brain,* 120, 785–794.

Grinspoon, L. and Bakalar, J. B. (1995) Marijuana as medicine: A plea for reconsideration, *JAMA,* 273(23), 1875–1876.

Halligan, P. W. and Marshall, J. C. (1994) Toward a principled explanation of unilateral neglect, *Cognitive Neuropsychology,* 11(2), 167–206.

Hallowell, E. M. and Ratey, J. J. (1993) Suggested diagnostic criteria for ADD in adults, *ADDult News,* Winter.

Hallowell, N. (1993) Living and loving with attention deficit disorder: Couples where one partner has ADD, *Chadder: A Publication by C.H.A.D.D.,* Spring/Summer, 13–19.

Hauser, P., Zametkin, A. J., Martinez, P., Vitiello, B. (1993) Attention deficit–hyperactivity disorder in people with generalized resistance to thyroid hormone, *New England Journal of Medicine,* 32B(14), 997–1001.

Hécan, H. and Albert, M. L. (1978) *Human Neuropsychology,* New York, Wiley.

Hechtman, L. (1996) Families of children with attention deficit hyperactivity disorder: A review, *Canadian Journal of Psychiatry,* 41(6), 350–360.

Heilman, K. (1997) The neurobiology of emotional experience, *The Journal of Neuropsychiatry and Clinical Neurosciences,* 9(3), 439–448.

Heilman, K. M. (1994) Emotion and the brain: A distributed modular network mediating emotional experience, In *Neuropsychology,* Zaidel, D. W., Ed., San Diego, Academic Press, 139–158.

Heilman, K. M. (1997) The neurobiology of emotional experience, *Journal of Neuropsychiatry,* 9(3), 439–438.

Heilman, K. M. and Valenstein, E., Eds. (1979) *Clinical Neuropsychology,* New York, Oxford University Press.

Heilman, K. M., and Valenstein, E., Eds. (1993) *Clinical Neuropsychology,* 3rd ed., New York, Oxford University Press.

Heilman, K. M., Chatterjee, A., and Doty, L. C. (1995) Hemispheric asymmetries of near-far spatial attention, *Neuropsychology,* 9(1), 58–61.

Heilman, K. M., Voeller, K. K. S., and Nadeau, S. E. (1991) A possible pathophysiological substrate of attention deficit hyperactivity disorder, *Journal Child Neurology,* 6 (Suppl.), S76–S81.

Heilman, K. M., Voeller, K. K. S., and Nadeau, S. E. (1991) A possible pathophysiological substrate of attention deficit hyperactivity disorder, *Journal of Child Neurology,* 6, 76–81.

Hendriks, A. W. and Kolk, H. H. J. (1997) Strategic control in developmental dyslexia, *Cognitive Neuropsychology,* 14(3), 321–366.

Henik, A. (1996) Paying attention to the Stroop effect, *Journal of the International Neurological Society,* 2(5), 467–470.

Henik, A. (1996) Paying attention to the Stroop effect? *Journal of the International Neuropsychological Society,* (2), 467–470.

Hermann, D. and Parenté (1994) The multimodal approach to cognitive rehabilitation, *NeuroRehabilitation,* 4(3), 133–142.

Hermans, H. J. M. (1996) Voicing the self: From information processing to dialogical interchange, *Psychological Bulletin,* 119(1), 31–50.

Hern, K. L. (1997) Plasticity in functional recovery: is it a question of all or none? ANPA Abstracts *Journal of Neuropsychiatry and Clinical Neurosciences,* 9(1), 139, P32.

Hernandez, T. D. and Naritoku, D. K. (1997) Seizures, epilepsy, and functional reovery after traumatic brain injury: A reappraisal, *Neurology,* 48, 803–806.

Hill, J. C. and Schoener, E. P. (1998) The age-dependent decline of ADHD, *ADHD Report,* 6(1), 4–6.

Hilton, C. (1997) Changes to the Individuals with Disabilities Education Act (IDEA) *The ADHD Challenge,* 11(6), 9.

Hilton, D. K. Martin, C. A., Heffron, W. M., Hall, B. D., and Johnson, G. L. (1991) Imipramine treatment of ADHD in a fragile X child, *Journal of American Academy of Child and Adolescent Psychiatry,* 30(5), 831–834.

Holmes, V. M. and Standish, J. M. (1996) Skilled reading with impaired phonology: A case study, *Cognitive Neuropsychology,* 13(8), 1207–1222.

Horner, B. R. and Scheibe, K. E. (1997) Prevalence and implications of attention-deficit hyperactivity disorder among adolescents in treatment for substance abuse, *Journal of the American Academy of Child and Adolescent Psychiatry,* 36, 30–36.

Hublin, C., Kaprio, J., Partinen, M., Heikkilä, K., and Koskenvuo, M. (1997) Prevalence and genetics of sleepwalking: A population-based twin study, *Neurology,* 48, 177–181.

Hughes, J. R. (1997) Substance abuse and ADHD, American Journal of Psychiatry, 154(1), 132.

Hynd, G. W., Hern, K. L., Novey, E. S., Eliopulos, D. et al. (1993) Attention deficit disorder and asymmetry of the caudate nucleus, *Journal of Child Neurology,* 8, 339–347.

Janzen, T., Graap, K., Stephanson, S., Marshall, W., and Fitzsimmons, G. (1995) Differences in baseline EEG measures for ADD and normal achieving preadolescent males, *Biofeedback and Self Regulation,* 20(1), 65–82.

Javorsky, J. (1996) An examination of youth with ADHD and attention-deficit/hyperactivity disorder and language learning disabilities: A clinical study, *Journal of Learning Disabilities,* 29(3), 247–258.

Jeste, D. V., Heaton, S. C., Paulsen, J. S., Ercoli, L. et al. (1996) Clinical and neuropsychological comparison of psychotic depression with nonpsychotic depression and schizophrenia, *American Journal of Psychiatry,* 153(4), 490–496.

Jibson, M. D. and Tandon, R. (1996) Special report: A summary of research findings on the new antipsychotic drugs, *The Psychiatry Forum*, 16, 1–6.

Johnston, C. and Freeman, W. (1997) Attributions for child behavior in parents of children without behavior disorders and children with attention deficit-hyperactivity disorder, *Journal of Consulting and Clinical Psychology*, 65(4), 636–645.

Kant, R., Smith-Seemiller, L., Issac, G., and Duffy, J. (1997) Tc-HMPAO SPECT in persistent post-concussion syndrome after mild head injury: Comparison with MRI/CT, *Brain Injury*, 11(2), 115–124.

Kasper, S. (1997) Efficacy of antidepressants in the treatment of severe depression: The place of mirtazapine, *Journal of Clinical Psychopharmacology*, 17(2), (Suppl. 1), 19S–28S.

Keck, P. E., Jr. and McElroy, S. L. (1996) Outcome in the pharmacologic treatment of bipolar disorder, *Journal of Clinical Psychopharmacology*, 16(2), (Suppl. 1), 15S–23S.

Keck, P. E., Jr., McElroy, S. I., Vuckovic, A., and Friedman, L. M. (1992) Combined valproate and carbamazepine treatment of bipolar disorder, *The Journal of Neuropsychiatry and Clinical Neurosciences*, 4, 319–322.

Keenan, K. and Shaw, D. (1997) Developmental and social influences on young girls' early problem behavior, *Psychological Bulletin*, 1, 95–113.

Kelly, K. and Ramundo, P. (1993) *You mean I'm not lazy, stupid, or crazy?! A self-help book for adults with attention deficit disorder*, Tyrell and Jerem Press, Cincinnati.

Kelly, M. D. (1995) Neuropsychological assessment of children with hearing impairment on trail making tactual performance and category test, *Assessment*, 2(4), 305–312.

King, B. and Lynn, D. (1997) Psychopharmacology of self-injurious behavior in children and adolescents, *Child and Adolescent Psychopharmacology News*, 2(5), 1–4.

Kinsbourne, M. (1974) Lateral interactions in the brain. In *Hemispheric Disconnection and Cerebral Function*, Kinsbourne, M. and Smith, W. L., Eds., Springfield, MA, Thomas, 239–259.

Kinsbourne, M. (1994) Neuropsychology of attention, In *Neuropsychology*, Zaidel, D. W., Ed., Academic Press, San Diego, 105–123.

Kirby, M. Y. and Long, C. J. (1996) Minor head injury: Attempts at clarifying the confusion, *Brain Injury*, 10(3), 159–186.

Klove, H., Troland, K., and Ellertsen, B. (1995) Children at risk: Diagnostic and treatment consideration, *Journal of the International Neuropsychological Society* 1(4), 321.

Knivsberg, A.-M. (1997) Urine patterns, peptide levels and IgA/IgG antibodies to food proteins in children with dyslexia, *Pediatric Rehabilitation*, 1(1), 25–33.

Kolata, G. (1990) Advance in hyperactivity research, Thursday, November 15, *The New York Times*, reprinted.

Koob, G. F., and Nestler, E. J. (1997) The neurobiology of drug addiction, *Journal of Neuropsychiatry*, 9(3), 482–497,

Kranzler, H. R. and Anton, R. F., (1994) Implications of recent neuropsychopharmacologic research for understanding the etiology and development of alcoholism, *Journal of Consulting and Clinical Psychology*, 62(6), 1116–1126.

Kraus, M. F. and Maki, P. (1977) The combined use of amantadine and L-dopa/carbidopa in the treatment of chronic brain injury, *Brain Injury*, 11(6), 455–460.

Kulynych, J. J., Vladar, K., Jones, D. W., and Weinberger, D. R. (1994) Gender differences in the normal lateralization of the supratemporal cortex: MRI surface-rendering morphometry of Heschl's gyrus and the planum temporale, *Cortex*, 4(2), 107–118.

Kuperman, S., Johnson, B., Arndt, S., Lindgreen, S. et al., Quantitative EEG differences in a nonclinical sample of children with ADHD and undifferentiated ADD, *Journal of the American Academy of Child and Adolescent Psychiatry,* 35(8), 1009–1017.

Kutja, K. S., Voeller, R., Bogoian, G., Geffken, C., Wilson, P., Edge, M., Garofalakis, P., and Mutch, J. (1997) Comorbidity of ADHD and dyslexia in adults, ANPA Abstracts *Journal of Neuropsychiatry and Clinical Neurosciences,* 9(1), 149, P64.

Langdon, D. W. and Warrington, E. K. (1997) The abstraction of numerical relations: A role for the right hemisphere in arithmetic?, *Journal of the International Neuropsychological Society,* 3, 260–268.

Latham, P. H. (1997) ADD and test accommodation under the ADA, Several court cases shed light on who qualifies, *Attention,* Fall, 41–42.

Latham, P. S. and Latham, P. H. (1997) Equal Employment Opportunity Commission issues new guidance on psychiatric disabilities and the ADA, *Attention,* Fall, 38–40.

Lavenstein, B. L. (1997) Modification of the "on off" effect induced by stimulants in patients with ADHD utilizing propranolol, *Neurology,* 48(Suppl), P05.004.

Leach, J. P. and Brodie, M. J. (1995) Lamotrigine, Clinical Use, In *Antiepileptic Drugs,* 4th ed., Levy, R. H., Mattson, R. H., and Meldrum, B. S., Eds., Raven Press, Ltd., New York , 889–896.

Leach, M. J., Lees, G., and Riddall, D. R. (1995) Lamotrigine, Mechanisms of Action, In *Antiepileptic Drugs,* 4th ed., Levy, R. H., Mattson, R. H., and Meldrum, B. S., Eds., Raven Press, Ltd., New York , 861–870.

Leone, M. et al. (1997) Alcohol use is a risk factor for a first generalized tonic-clonic seizure, *Neurology,* 48, 614–620.

Loiseau, P. and Duché (1995) Carbamazepine, clinical use, In *Antiepileptic Drugs,* 4th ed., Levy, R. H., Mattson, R. H., and Meldrum, B. S., Eds., Raven Press, Ltd., New York , 555–566.

Lubar, J. F., Swartwood, M. O., Swartwood, J. N., and O'Donnell, P. H. (1995) Evaluation of the effectiveness of EEG neurofeedback training for ADHD in a clinical setting as measured by changes in TOVA scores, behavioral ratings and WISC-R performance, *Biofeedback and Self-Regulation,* 20, 83–99.

Lubow, R. E. and Josman, Z. E. (1993) Latent inhibition deficits in hyperactive children, *Journal of Child Psychology and Psychiatry,* 34(6), 959–973.

Lynch, W. J. (1995) Achievement testing in traumatic brain injury: Two new approaches, *Journal Head Trauma Rehabilitation,* 10(5), 95–98.

MacLeod, D. and Prior, M. (1996) Attention deficits in adolescents with ADHD and other clinical groups, *Child Neuropsychology,* 2, 1–10.

Masamitsu, S., Yamanaka, T., and Furuya, T. (1993) Attention state in electrodermal activity during auditory stimulation of children with attention-deficit hyperactivity disorder, *Perceptual and Motor Skills,* 77, 331–338.

Matte, R. and Bolaski, J. A. (1998) ADHD, the brain and neuroimaging: a review of literature, *The ADHD Challenge,* 12(1), 3–8.

Max, J. E., Lindgren, S. D., Robin, D. A., Smith, W., L. Jr., Sato, Y., Mattheis, P. J., Castillo, C. S., and Stierwalt, J. A. G. (1997) Traumatic brain injury in children and adolescents: Psychiatric disorders in the second three months, ANPA Abstracts, *Journal of Neuropsychiatry and Clinical Neurosciences,* 9(1), 137, P25.

Mayes, S. D. et al. (1994) Methylphenidate and ADHD: Influence of age, IQ, and neurodevelopmental status, *Developmental Medicine and Child Neurology,* 36(12), 1099–1107.

McDonald, R. M. (1997) Students with LD/ADD win landmark court decision over Boston University, *Attention*, Fall, 36–37.

McGlinchey-Berroth, R., Bullis, D. P., Milberg, W. P., Verfaellie, M., Alexander, M., and D'Esposito, M. (1996) Assessment of neglect reveals dissociable behavior but not neuroanatomical subtypes, *Journal of the International Neuropsychological Society*, (2), 441–451.

McGrath, J. (1997) Cognitive impairment associated with post-traumatic stress disorder and minor head injury: A case report, *Neuropsychological Rehabilitation*, 7(3), 231–239.

McHugh, P. R. (1993) Multiple Personality disorder, *The Harvard Mental Health Letter*, 10(3), 4–6.

Mega, M. S., Cummings, J. L., Salloway, S., and Malloy, P. (1997) The limbic system: An anatomic, phylogenetic, and clinical perspective, *The Journal of Neuropsychiatry and Clinical Neurosciences*, 9(3), 315–330.

Mendez, M. F., Engebrit, B., Doss, R., Miller, B. L., and Cummings, J. L. (1997) Clinical characteristics of epileptic aura with cognitive manifestations, ANPA Abstracts *Journal of Neuropsychiatry and Clinical Neurosciences*, 9(1), 145, P51.

Mesulam, M.-M. (1995) Association Cortex and Networks; Frontal lobes, In Neurology of Behavior and Cognition, Seminar held at the Knickerbocker Hotel, Chicago, IL, December 12–16, 1995.

Mesulam, M.-M. (1995) Limbic system and neurology of memory, In Neurology of Behavior and Cognition, Seminar held at the Knickerbocker Hotel, Chicago, IL, December 12–16, 1995.

Mesulam, M.-M. (1995) Right hemisphere specialization and spatial neglect, In Neurology of Behavior and Cognition, Seminar held at the Knickerbocker Hotel, Chicago, IL, December 12–16, 1995.

Michael and Hall (1994) 'Blunts' are more potent, more dangerous, *Psychopharmacology Update*, 5(12), 6.

Milberger, S., Biederman, J., Faraone, S. V., and Chen, L. (1997) ADHD is associated with early initiation of cigarette smoking children and adolescents, *Journal of the American Academy of Child and Adolescent Psychiatry* 36(1), 37–44.

Milberger, S., Biederman, J., Faraone, S. V., Chen, L. et al. (1996) Is maternal smoking during pregnancy a risk factor for attention deficit disorder in children? *American Journal of Psychiatry*, 153(9), 1138–1142.

Millichap, G. J. (1997) Use of CNS stimulants for attention-deficit disorders, ANPA Abstracts *Journal of Neuropsychiatry and Clinical Neurosciences*, 9(1), 150, P69.

Minshew, N. J., Goldstein, G., and Siegel, D. J. (1997) Neuropsychologic functioning in autism: Profile of a complex information processing disorder, *Journal of the International Neuropsychological Society* 3, 303–316.

Miozzo, M. and Caramazza, A. (1997) On knowing the auxillary of a verb that cannot be named: Evidence for the independence of grammatical and phonological aspects of lexical knowledge, *Journal of Cognitive Neuroscience*, 9(1), 160–166.

Mittenberg, W., Wittner, M. S., and Miller, L. J. (1997) Postconcussion Syndrome Occurs in Children, *Neuropsychology*, 11(3), 447–452.

Mooney, G. and Speed, J. (1997) Differential diagnosis in mild brain injury: understanding the role of non-organic conditions, *NeuroRehabilitation*, 8, 223–233.

Moriarty, M. B., Varma, A. R., Stevens, J., Fish, M., Trimble, M. R., and Robertson, M. M. (1997) A volumetric MRI study of Gilles de la Tourette's syndrome, *Neurology*, 49, 410–415.

Murphy, K. and Barkley, R. A. (1996) Attention deficit hyperactivity disorder adults: Comorbidities and adaptive impairments, *Comprehensive Psychiatry*, 37(6), 393–401.

Nada-Raja, S., Langley, J. D., McGee, R., Williams, S. M. et al. (1997) Inattentive and hyperactive behaviors and driving offenses in adolescence, *Journal of the American Academy of Child and Adolescent Psychiatry* 36(4), 515–522.

Nigg, J. T., Hindshaw, S. P., and Halperin, J. M. (1996) Continuous performance test in boys with attention deficit hyperactivity disorder: Methylphenidate dose response and relations with observed behaviors, *Journal of Clinical Child Psychology*, 25(3), 330–340.

Nigg, J. T., Swanson, J. M., and Hinshaw, S. P. (1977) Covert visual spatial attention in boys with attention deficit hyperactivity disorder: Lateral effects, methylphenidate response and results for parents, *Neuropsychologia*, 35(2), 165–176.

Nobre, A. C., Sebestyen, G. N., Gitelman, D. R., Mesuam, M. M., Frackowiak, R. S. J., and Frith, C. D. (1997) Functional localization of the system for visuospatial attention using positron emission tomography, *Brain*, 120, 515–533.

Nuwer, M. (1997) Assessment of digital EEG, quantitative EEG, and EEG brain mapping: Report of the American Academy of Neurology and the American Clinical Neurophysiology Society, *Neurology*, 49, 277–292.

Paradiso, S., Andreasen, N. C., O'Leary, D. S., Arndt, S. et al. (1996) Cerebellar size and cognition: Correlations with IQ, verbal memory and motor dexterity, *Neuropsychiatry, Neuropsychology and Behavioral Neurology*, 10(1), 1–8.

Pelham, W. E., Hoza, B., Kipp, H. L., Gnagy, E. M., and Trane, S. T. (1997) Effects of methylphenidate and expectancy on ADHD children's performance, self-evaluations, persistence, and attributions on a cognitive task, *Experimental and Clinical Psychopharmacology*, 5(1), 3–13.

Phelan, T. W. (1998) Who's in charge at your house?, *The ADHD Challenge*, 12(1), 1–7.

Phône-Poulenc Rorer Pharmaceuticals Inc. (1995) DDAVP Nasal Spray, Collegeville, PA.

Pickworth, W. B., Rohrer, M. S., and Fant, R. V.(1997) Effects of abused drugs on psychomotor performance, *Experimental and Clinical Psychopharmacology* 5(3), 233–241.

Pineda, D., Rosselli, M., Cadavid, C., and Ardila, A. (1997) Neurobehavioral characteristics of 7- to 9-year-old children with attention deficit hyperactivity disorder (ADHD) ANPA Abstracts *Journal of Neuropsychiatry and Clinical Neurosciences*, 9(1), 137, P26.

Pineda, D., Rosselli, M., Cadavid, C., and Ardila, A. (1997) Neurobehavioral characteristics of 10- to 12-year-old children with attention deficit hyperactivity disorder (ADHD) ANPA Abstracts *Journal of Neuropsychiatry and Clinical Neurosciences*, 9(1), 138, P27.

Piven, J., Palmer, P., Jacobi, D., Childress, D., and Arndt, S. (1997) Broader autism phenotype: Evidence from a family history study of multiple-incidence autism families, *American Journal of Psychiatry* 154(2), 185–190.

Pliszka, S. R. (1992) Comorbidity of attention-deficit hyperactivity disorder and overanxious disorder, *Journal of American Academy of Child and Adolescent Psychiatry* 31(2), 197–203.

Pliszka, S. R., McCracken, J. T., and Maas, J. W. (1996) Catecholamines in attention deficit hyperactivity disorder: Current perspectives, *Journal of the American Academy of Child and Adolescent Psychiatry* 35(3), 264–272.

Plizka, S. R., McCracken, J. T., and Maas, J. W. (1996) Catecholamines in attention-deficit hyperactivity disorder: Current perspectives, *Journal of the American Academy of Child and Adolescent Psychiatry,* 35(3), 264–272.

Post, R. B. et al. (1997) Carbmazepine in bipolar disorder, *Child and Adolescent Psychopharmacology News,* 2(3), 6.

Post, R. B., Chaderjian, M. R., Lott, L. A., and Maddock, R. J. (1997) Effects of lorazepam on the distribution of spatial attention, *Experimental and Clinical Psychopharmacology,* 5(2), 143–149.

Powell, A. L., Yudd, A., Zee, P., and Mandelbaum, D. E., (1997) Attention deficit hyperactivity disorder associated with orbitofrontal epilepsy in a father and a son, *Neuropsychiatry, Neuropsychology, and Behavioral Neurology,* 10(2), 151–154.

Powell, J. H., Al-Adawi, S., Morgan, J., and Greenwood, R. J. (1996) Motivational Deficits after brain injury: Effects of bromocriptine in 11 patients, *Journal of Neurology, Neurosurgery and Psychiatry,* 60, 416–421.

Rafal, R. And Robertson, L. (1995) The neurology of visual attention, In *The Cognitive Neurosciences,* Michael S. Gazzaniga, Ed., Cambridge, MA: MIT Press, 625–648.

Ramsey, J. M., Horwitz, B., Donohue, B. C., Nace, K., Maisog, J. M., and Andreason, P. (1997) Phonological and orthographic components of word recognition: A PET-rCBF study, *Brain,* 120, 739–759.

Raskin, S. A. (1997) The relationship between sexual abuse and mild traumatic brain injury, *Brain Injury,* 11(8), 587–603.

Ratey, J. J. (1991) Paying attention to attention in adults, *Chadder: A Publication by C.H.A.D.D.,* Fall/Winter, 13–14.

Ratey, J. J. and Hallowell, E. M. (1993) 50 Tips on the management of adult attention deficit disorder, *The CH.A.D.D.ER Box,* 6(1), 1–8.

Ratey, J. J., Hallowell, E. M., and Miller, A. C. (1995) Relationship dilemmas for adults with ADD: The biology of intimacy, In *A Comprehensive Guide to Attention Deficit Disorder in Adults, Research, Diagnosis and Treatment,* Nadeau, K. G., Ed., New York: Brunner/Mazel Publishers, 218–235.

Reitan, R. M. and Davidson, L. A., Eds. (1974) Clinical neuropsychology: Current status and applications, Washington, DC: Hemisphere Publishing Corp.

Reitan, R. M. and Wolfson, D. (1986) Traumatic brain injury. Vol. I Pathophysiology and neuropsychological evaluation, Tucson, AZ: Neuropsychology Press.

Reitan, R. M. and Wolfson, D. (1988) Traumatic brain injury. Vol. II Recovery and rehabilitation, Tucson, AZ: Neuropsychology Press.

Reitan, R. M. and Wolfson, D. (1992) Neuroanatomy and neuropathology: A clinical guide for neuropsychogists, 2nd ed., Tucson, AZ: Neuropsychology Press.

Reitan, R. M. and Wolfson, D. (1992) Neuropsychological evaluation of older children, Tucson, AZ: Neuropsychology Press.

Reitan, R. M. and Wolfson, D. (1993a) The Halstead-Reitan neuropsychological test battery and clinical interpretation, 2nd ed., Tucson, AZ: Neuropsychology Press.

Reitan, R. M. and Wolfson, D. (1994) A selective and critical review of neuropsychological deficits and the frontal lobes, *Neuropsychology Review,* 4, 161–198.

Reitan, R. M. and Wolfson, D. (1994b) Aphasia and sensory-perceptual deficits in children, 2nd ed., Tucson, AZ: Neuropsychology Press.

Reitan, R. M. and Wolfson, D. (1994c) Aphasia and sensory-perceptual deficits in adults, 2nd ed., Tucson, AZ: Neuropsychology Press.

Reitan, R. M. and Wolfson, D. (1994d) A selective and critical review of neuropsychological deficits and the frontal lobes, *Neuropsychology Review,* 4, 161–198.

Reitan, R. M. and Wolfson, D. (1995a) The category test and the trail making test as measures of frontal lobe functions, *The Clinical Neuropsychologist,* 9, 50–56.

Reitan, R. M. and Wolfson, D. (1996a) Can WISC-R IQ values be computed validly for learning disabled children? *Applied Neuropsychology,* 3, 15–20.

Reitan, R. M. and Wolfson, D.(1996b) Differential relationships of age and education to WAIS subtest scores among brain-damaged and control groups, *Archives of Clinical Neuropsychology,* 11, 303–311.

Reitan, R. M. and Wolfson, D.(1996c) The diminished effect of age and education on neuropsychological performances of learning-disabled children,*Child Neuro-psychology,* 2, 11–16.

Reitan, R. M. and Wolfson, D.(1996d) Relationships between specific and general tests of cerebral functioning, *The Clinical Neuropsychologist,* 10, 37–42.

Reitan, R. M. and Wolfson, D.(1996e) Relationships of age and education to Wechsler Adult Intelligence Scale IQ values in brain-damaged and non-brain-damaged groups, *The Clinical Neuropsychologist,* 10, 293–304.

Remington, G. (1997) Selecting a neuroleptic and the role of side effects, *Child and Adolescent Psychopharmacology News,* 2(2), 1–9.

Robin, A. L. et al. (1997) The empirical study of personality in ADHD adults: A new beginning, *ADHD Report,* 5(6), 11–15.

Roitman, S. E. Lees, B. S., Cornblatt, B. A., Bergman, A., Obuchowski, M., Mitropoulou, V., Keefe, R., Silverman, J. M., and Siever, L. J. (1997) Attentional functioning in schizotypal personality disorder, *American Journal of Psychiatry,* 154 (5), 655–660.

Rose, F. D., Johnson, D. A., and Attree, E. A. (1997) Rehabilitation of the head-injured child: Basic research and new technology, *Pediatric Rehabilitation,* 1(1), 3–7.

Ross, E. (1995) Neurological perspectives on human aggression, In Neurology of Behavior and Cognition, Seminar held at the Knickerbocker Hotel, Chicago, IL, December 12–16, 1995.

Ross, E. D. (1995) Aprosodias, Director, Mesulam M., M.D., Presented at December 12–16, 1995 Conference, Neurology of Behavior and Cognition, 131–135.

Ross, R. G., Hommer, D., Breiger, D., Varley, C., and Radant, A. (1994) Eye movement task related to frontal lobe functioning in children with attention deficit disorder, *Journal of the American Academy of Child and Adolescent Psychiatry* 33, 869–874.

Ryan, N. D. (1990) Heterocyclic antidepressants in children and adolescents. The safe and effective use of psychotropic medications in adolescents and children,*Journal of Child and Adolescent Psychopharmacology,* 1(1), 21–31.

Salanova, V., Andermann, F., Rasmussen, T., Olivier, A., and Quesney, L. F. (1995) Parietal lobe epilepsy, clinical manifestations and outcome in 82 patients treated surgically between 1929 and 1988, *Brain,* 118, 607–627.

Satz, P., Zaucha, K., McCleary, C., Light, R., and Becker, D. (1997) Mild head injury in children and adolescents: A review of studies (1970–1995) *Psychological Bulletin,* 122(2), 107–131.

Scheffer, I. E. and Berkovic, S. F. (1997) Generalized epilepsy with febrile seizures plus a genetic disorder with heterogeneous clinical phenotypes, *Brain,* 120, 479–490.

Schlaepfer, T. E., Pearlson, G. D., Wong, D. F., Marenco, S., and Dannals, R. F. (1997) PET study of competition between intravenous cocaine and [^{11}C] raclopride at dopamine receptors in human subjects, *American Journal of Psychiatry,* 154(9), 1209–1213.

Schmitter-Edgecombe, M. (1996) The effects of divided attention on implicit and explicit memory performance, *Journal of the International Neurological Society,* 2 (2), 111–125,

Schmitter-Edgecombe, M. (1996) The effects of divided attention on implicit and explicit memory performance, *Journal of the International Neuropsychological Society,* (2), 111–125.

Schwartz, R. L., Adair, J. C., D. Na, Williamson, D. J. G., and Heilman, K. M. (1997) Spatial bias: Attentional and intentional influence in normal subjects, *Neurology,* 48, 234–242.

Segalowitz, S. J., Dywan, J., and Unsal, A. (1997) Attentional factors in response time variability after traumatic brain injury: An ERP study, *Journal of the International Neuropsychological Society,* 3, 95–107.

Seidman, L. J., Biederman, J., Faraone, S. V., and Weber, W. (1997) A pilot study of neuropsychological function in girls with ADHD, *Journal of the American Academy of Child and Adolescent Psychiatry,* 36(3), 366–373.

Seidman, L. J., Faraone, S. V., Biederman, J., Weber, W., and Ouellette, C. (1997) Toward defining a neuropsychology of attention deficit-hyperactivity disorder: Performance of children and adolescents from a large clinically referred sample, *Journal of Consulting and Clinical Psychology,* 65(1), 150–160.

Shallice, T. (1994) Multiple levels of control processes, In *Attention and Performance XV,* Umiltà, Carlo and Moscovitch, Morris, Eds., Cambridge, MA, MIT Press, 395–420.

Shapiro, S. K. and Hynd, G. W. (1993) Psychobiological basis of conduct disorder, *School Psychology Review,* 22(3), 386–402.

Shekim, W.O. (1990) Adult attention deficit hyperactivity disorder, residual state (ADHD,RS) *Chadder: A Publication by C.H.A.D.D.,* Spring/Summer, 16–18.

Sher, K. J., Martin, E. D., Wood, P. K., and Rutledge, P. C. (1997) Alcohol use disorders and neuropsychological functioning in first-year undergraduates, *Experimental and Clinical Psychopharmacology,* 5(3), 304–315.

Sherman, D. K., McGue, M. K., and Iacono, W. G., (1997) Twin concordance for attention deficit hyperactivity disorder: A comparison of teachers' and mothers' reports, *American Journal of Psychiatry,* 154(4), 532–535.

Simeon, D., Gross, S., Guralnik, O., Stein, D. J., Schmeidler, J., and Hollander, E., (1997) Feeling unreal: 30 cases of DSM-III-R Depersonalization Disorder, *American Journal of Psychiatry,* 154(8), 1107–1113.

Simeon, J. G. (1997) Propranolol in aggressive children and adolescents, *Child and Adolescent Psychopharmacology News,* 2(3), 11–12.

Sirven, J. I., Liporace, J. D., French, J. A., O'Connor, M. J., and Sperling, M. R. (1997) Seizures in temporal lobe epilepsy: I. Reliability of scalp/sphenoidal ictal recording, *Neurology* (48), 1041–1046.

Sisodiya, S. M., Free, S. L., Stevens, J. M., Fish, D. R., and Shorvon, S. D. (1995) Widespread cerebral structural changes in patients with cortical dysgenesis and epilepsy, *Brain,* 118, 1039–1050.

Smid, H. G. O. M. et al. (1997) Differentiation of hypoglycemia induced cognitive impairments: An electrophysiological approach, *Brain,* 120, 1041–1056.

Smith, G. P. (1976) The arousal function of central catecholamine neurons, *Annual New York Academy of Science,* 270, 45–55.

Snow, P., Douglas, J., and Ponsford, J. (1997) Conversational assessment following traumatic brain injury: a comparison across two control groups, *Brain Injury,* 11(6), 409–429.

Spencer, T. J. et al. (1996) Growth deficits in ADHD children revisited: Evidence for disorder-associated growth delays?, *Journal of the American Academy of Child and Adolescent Psychiatry,* 35(11), 1460–1469.

Starbuck, V., Bleiberg, J., and Kay, G. C. (1995) d-Amphetamine-mediated enhancement of the P300 ERP: A placebo-crossover double-blind case study, *Neuropsychiatry, Neuropsychology, and Behavioral Neurology,* 8(3), 189–192.

Stein, M. B., Walker, J. R., Hazen, A. L., and Forde, D, R. (1997) Full and partial posttraumatic stress disorder: findings from a community survey, *American Journal of Psychiatry,* 154(8), 1114–1119.

Stothard, S. E., Snowling, M. J., and Hulme, C. (1996) Deficits in phonology but not dyslexic?, *Cognitive Neuropsychology,* 13(3), 641–672.

Sturm, W., Willmes, K., Orgass, B., and Hartje, W. (1997) Do specific attention deficits need specific training?, *Neuropsychological Rehabilitation,* 7(2), 81–103.

Sutker, P. B., Uddo, M., Brailey, K., Vasterling, J. J., and Errara, P. (1994) Psychopathology in war-zone deployed and nondeployed operation desert storm troops assigned graves registration duties, *Journal of Abnormal Psychology,* 103(2), 383–390.

Tannock, R. (1997) Television, videogames, and ADHD: Challenging a popular belief, *ADHD Report,* 5(3) 3–7.

Thapar, A., Hervas, A., and McGuffin, P. (1985) Childhood hyperactivity scores are highly heritable and show sibling competition effects: Twin study evidence, *Behavior Genetics,* 25, 537–544.

Thomasson, M. (1998) Organizational skills for adults with attention deficit disorder, *The ADHD Challenge,* 12(1), 9–10.

Tran, P., Hamilton, S. H., Kuntz, A., Potvin, J. H. (1997) Double-blind comparison of olanzapine versus risperidone in the treatment of schizophrenia and other psychotic disorders, *Journal of Clinical Psychopharmacology,* 17(5), 407–418.

Trzepacz, P., Mahlab, R., Butters, M., and Soety, E. (1997) Weintraub-Mesulam cancellation tests (WMCT), ANPA Abstracts *Journal of Neuropsychiatry and Clinical Neurosciences,* 9(1), 168, P131.

Van Reekum, R., Bayey, M., Gardner, S. et al. (1995) N of 1 study: Amantadine for the amotivational syndrome in a patient with traumatic brain injury, *Brain Injury,* 9, 49–53.

Vargha-Khadem, F., Carr, L. J., Isaacs, E., Brett, E., Adams, C., and Mishkin, M. (1997) Onset of speech after left hemispherectomy in a nine-year-old boy, *Brain,* 120, 159–182.

Warschausky, S., Cohen, E. H., Parker, J. G., Levendosky, A. A., and Okun, A. (1997) Social problem-solving skills of children with traumatic brain injury, *Pediatric Rehabilitation,* 1(2), 77–81.

Weiss, G. (1983) Long-term outcome: Findings, concepts, and practical implications, In *Developmental Neuropsychiatry,* Rutter, M., Ed., New York: The Guilford Press, 422–436.

Weiss, G. and Hechtman, L. T. (1993) Hyperactive children grown up, 2nd ed., ADHD in children, adolescents, and adults, New York: Guilford Press.

Weiss, G., Hechtman, L., Perlman, T., Hopkins, J., and Wener, A. (1979) Hyperactives as young adults. A controlled prospective ten-year follow-up of 75 children, *Archives of General Psychiatry,* 36, 675–681.

Weiss, M. and Walkup, J. T. (1997) Clinically appied pharmacokinetics of the SSRI's and SNRI's, *Child and Adolescent Psychopharmacology News,* 2(3), 1–9.

Whalen, J., McCloskey, M., Lesser, R., P., and Gordon, B. (1997) Localizing arithmetic processes in the brain: evidence from a transient deficit during cortical stimulation, *Journal of Cognitive Neuroscience*, 9(3), 409–417.

Whyte, J., Polansky, M., Cavallucci, C., Fleming, M., Lhulier, J., and Coslett, B. H. (1996) Inattentive behavior after traumatic brain injury, *Journal of the International Neuropsychological Society*, (2), 274–281.

Wilder, B. J. (1995) Phenytoin, clinical use, In *Antiepileptic Drugs*, 4th ed., Levy, R. H., Mattson, R. H., and Meldrum, B. S., Eds., New York: Raven Press, Ltd., 339–344.

Wirrell, E. C., Camfield, C. S., Camfield, P. R., Gordon, K. E., and Dooley, J. M., (1997) Long-term prognosis of typical childhood absence epilepsy: Remission or progression to juvenile myoclonic epilepsy, *Neurology*, 47, 912–918.

Worthington, A. D. (1996) Cueing strategies in neglect dyslexia, *Neuropsychological Rehabilitation*, 6(1), 1–17.

Young, I. T. et al. (1997) Acute treatment of bipolar depression with gabapentin, *Biological Psychiatry*, 42, 851–853.

Zald, D. H. and Kim, S. W. (1996) Anatomy and function of the orbital frontal cortex, I. Anatomy, neurocircuitry, and obsessive-compulsive disorder, *The Journal of Neuropsychiatry and Clinical Neurosciences*, 8(2), 125–138.

Zald, D. H. and Kim, S. W. (1996) Anatomy and function of the orbital frontal cortex, II. Function and relevance to obsessive-compulsive disorder, *The Journal of Neuropsychiatry and Clinical Neurosciences*, 3, 249–26.

Zohar, A. H., Pauls, D. L., Ratzoni, G., Apter, A., Dycian, A., Binder, M., King, R., Leckman, J. F., Kron, S., and Cohen, D. J., (1997) Obsessive-compulsive disorder with and without tics in an epidemiological sample of adolescents, *American Journal of Psychiatry*, 154(2), 274–276.

Index

A